Computational Vision in Neural and Machine Systems

Computational vision deals with the underlying mathematical and computational models for how visual information is processed. Whether the processing is biological or machine, there are fundamental questions related to how the information is processed. How should information be represented? How should information be transduced in order to highlight features of interest while suppressing noise and other artifacts of the image capture process? *Computational Vision in Neural and Machine Systems* addresses these and other questions in 15 chapters, the book being divided into three sections, which overlap between biological and computational systems: dynamical systems; attention, motion and eye-movements; and stereovision. The editors have brought together the best and brightest minds in the field of computational vision, combining research from both biology and computing and enhancing the developing synergy between computational and biological visual modeling communities. Aimed at researchers and graduate students in computational or biological vision, neuroscience, and psychology.

LAURENCE HARRIS is Professor of Psychology at York University, Ontario, Canada. An expert in the brain's processing of information from multiple senses, especially regarding self-motion and orientation in normal and unusual environments, particularly space, his research involves work on the International Space Station and in environments simulated using virtual reality.

MICHAEL JENKIN is Professor of Computer Science and Engineering at York University, Ontario, Canada. His research interests include perception and guidance for autonomous robotic systems, and the development and analysis of virtual reality systems. In 2005 he was the recipient of the CIPPRS/ACTIRF award for research excellence and service to the Canadian Computer and Robot Vision research community.

COMPUTATIONAL VISION IN NEURAL AND MACHINE SYSTEMS

Edited by

LAURENCE R. HARRIS
York University,
Toronto, Ontario, Canada

MICHAEL R. M. JENKIN
York University,
Toronto, Ontario, Canada

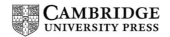
CAMBRIDGE
UNIVERSITY PRESS

CAMBRIDGE UNIVERSITY PRESS
Cambridge, New York, Melbourne, Madrid, Cape Town, Singapore, São Paulo

Cambridge University Press
The Edinburgh Building, Cambridge CB2 2RU, UK

Published in the United States of America by Cambridge University Press, New York

www.cambridge.org
Information on this title: www.cambridge.org/9780521862608

© Cambridge University Press 2007

First published 2007

Printed in the United Kingdom at the University Press, Cambridge

A catalog record for this publication is available from the British Library

ISBN-13 978-0-521-86260-8 hardback
ISBN-10 0-521-86260-4 hardback

For Carolee and Heather

The CD-ROM that accompanies this book contains colour imagery and video clips associated with various chapters and the York Vision Conference itself. The CD-ROM is presented in HTML format, and is viewable with any standard browser (e.g., Netscape Navigator or Microsoft Internet Explorer). To view the videos on the CD-ROM you will need Quicktime, which is available free from Apple. To view the CD-ROM, point your browser at the file **index.htm** on the CD-ROM.

Laurence Harris
Michael Jenkin

Contents

Contributors

Pierre Baldi
School of Information and Computer Science, Office 424C
Bioinformatics
University of California, Irvine
Irvine, CA 92697-3425, USA

Patrick Bouthemy
IRISA/INRIA
Campus universitaire de Beaulieu
35042 Rennes Cedex, France

Frédéric Cao
IRISA/INRIA
Campus universitaire de Beaulieu
35042 Rennes Cedex, France

Yang Cheng
Jet Propulsion Laboratory
California Institute of Technology
4800 Oak Grove Drive
Pasadena, CA 91109, USA

James J. Clark
Centre for Intelligent Machines
McConnell Engineering Building
McGill University
3480 University St.
Montreal, Quebec, Canada, H3A 2A7

Charles E. Connor
Zanvyl Krieger Mind/Brain Institute and Department of Neuroscience
Johns Hopkins University
Baltimore, MD 21218, USA

J. Douglas Crawford
Centre for Vision Research and Department of Psychology
York University
4700 Keele Street
Toronto, Ontario, Canada, M3J 1P3

Jian Ding
Department of Cognitive Sciences
Institute for Mathematical Behavioral Sciences
Department of Neurobiology and Behavior
University of California
Irvine, CA 92697-5100, USA

Norma Graham
Department of Psychology
Columbia University, New York, NY 10027, USA

Ziad M. Hafed
Systems Neurobiology Laboratory
Salk Institute for Biological Studies
10010 North Torrey Pines Rd.
La Jolla, CA 92037, USA

Laurence R. Harris
Centre for Vision Research and Departments of Psychology and Biology
York University
4700 Keele Street
Toronto, Ontario, Canada, M3J 1P3

Laurent Itti
Computer Science Department
University of Southern California
Hedco Neuroscience Building
3641 Watt Way, HNB-30A
Los Angeles, CA 90089, USA

Piotr Jasiobedzki
MDA Space Missions
9445 Airport Rd.
Brampton, Ontario, Canada, L6S 4J3

Michael Jenkin
Centre for Vision Research and Department of Computer Science and Engineering
York University
4700 Keele Street
Toronto, Ontario, Canada, M3J 1P3

Li Jiek
Centre for Intelligent Machines
McGill University
3480 University St.
Montreal, Quebec, Canada, H3A 2A7

Andrew Johnson
Jet Propulsion Laboratory
California Institute of Technology
4800 Oak Grove Drive
Pasadena, CA 91109, USA

Mark Maimone
Jet Propulsion Laboratory
California Institute of Technology
4800 Oak Grove Drive
Pasadena, CA 91109, USA

Larry Matthies
Jet Propulsion Laboratory
California Institute of Technology
4800 Oak Grove Drive
Pasadena, CA 91109, USA

Jane Mulligan
University of Colorado at Boulder
Boulder, CO 80309-0430, USA

Matthias Niemeier
Centre for Vision Research and Department of Life Sciences
University of Toronto
1265 Military Trail
Toronto, Ontario, Canada, M1C 1A4

Marc Pollefeys
Department of Computer Science
University of North Carolina at Chapel Hill
Chapel Hill, NC 27599-3175, USA

Steven L. Prime
Centre for Vision Research and Department of Psychology
York University
4700 Keele Street
Toronto, Ontario, Canada, M3J 1P3

Arlene Ripsman
Centre for Vision Research and Department of Computer Science and Engineering
York University
4700 Keele Street
Toronto, Ontario, Canada, M3J 1P3

Sudipta Sinha
Department of Computer Science
Campus Box 3175, Sitterson Hall
University of North Carolina at Chapel Hill
Chapel Hill, NC 27599-3175, USA

Mikhail Sizintsev
Centre for Vision Research and Department of Computer Science and Engineering
York University
4700 Keele Street
Toronto, Ontario, Canada, M3J 1P3

George Sperling
Department of Cognitive Sciences
Institute for Mathematical Behavioral Sciences
Department of Neurobiology and Behavior
University of California
Irvine, CA 92697-5100, USA.

Carlo Tomasi
Department of Computer Science
Duke University
Box 90129, Durham, NC 27708-0129, USA

Thomas Veit
IRISA/INRIA
Campus universitaire de Beaulieu
35042 Rennes Cedex, France

Preeti Verghese
The Smith-Kettlewell Eye Research Institute
2318 Filmore St.
San Francisco, CA 94115, USA

Richard P. Wildes
Centre for Vision Research and Department of Computer Science and Engineering
York University
4700 Keele Street
Toronto, Ontario, Canada, M3J 1P3

Reg Willson
Jet Propulsion Laboratory
California Institute of Technology
4800 Oak Grove Drive
Pasadena, CA 91109, USA

S. Sabina Wolfson
Department of Psychology
Columbia University, New York, NY 10027, USA

Jingyu Yan
Department of Computer Science
University of North Carolina at Chapel Hill
Chapel Hill, NC 27599-3175, USA

1 Computational vision in neural and machine systems

Michael Jenkin and Laurence Harris

1.1 Introduction

The ability to process visual information streams is a critical requirement for both biological systems as well as for a wide variety of robotic devices. The fundamental need for effective visual information processing in biological systems is illustrated in Figure 1.2. These three snapshots show a cheetah emerging from the long grass in Tanzania. Being able to discern the shape emerging from the tall grass *early* is a critical survival skill. Biological systems that are unable to process the visual information in a timely fashion are unlikely to succeed in the wild. Similarly, in the machine vision domain, timely effective processing of visual information is often key. Figure 1.3 shows the AQUA robot, a visually guided amphibious robot that is capable of unsupervised operation (Dudek *et al.*, 2005). This vehicle relies primarily on visual information obtained from forward facing cameras to reason about its external environment. Without the ability to process its multiple video camera inputs in a timely fashion, the robot would be unable to operate.

In 1991 (over 15 years ago), the Centre for Vision Research at York University held the first in what has become a bi-annual conference on vision. The 1991 conference – which resulted in the book *Spatial Vision in Humans and Robots* – examined how biological and machine systems address the task of processing the rich visual field in order to recover information about the spatial surround. Fifteen years later, the York Vision Conference has re-visited this fundamental issue: the relationship between computational models of visual information processing and research into biological visual information processing.

The past fifteen years have seen astounding advances in both artificial and biological vision. Driven (at least in part) by advances in the technology available to explore how biological systems process visual information, and the orders of magnitude performance improvements in the computational power that can be brought to the task of

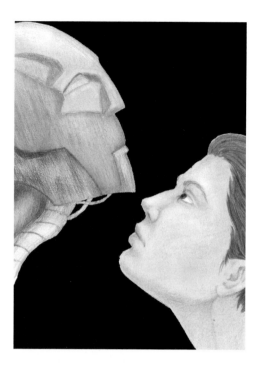

Figure 1.1. Computational vision in neural and machine systems. Appears with the kind permission of Emma Jenkin.

processing visual imagery, visual models have advanced from processing a single image viewed in isolation to a stream of embedded visual information processing within an ongoing spatio-temporal relationship. In the computational field, this has lead to the consideration of visual information processing not as the evaluation of an isolated static image, but rather as the task of processing an image stream within the context of some wider task. In the biological fields, this has lead to a wide range of advances including the emergence of models of multi-modal fusion of information from different perceptual systems.

As visual information processing is considered within a temporal context, many of the problems that occur "naturally" in the biological community become apparent in the computational one. This includes tasks such as integrating information from multiple views, searching for specific objects within a wide visual display, and attending to salient features within the environment.

David Marr (1982) distinguished three levels of visual processing: computational, algorithmic, and implementational. His computational level consisted of a description of what computation needs to be performed and what information is available to perform the computations on. His algorithmic level specified how the computational level might be performed. Algorithms performed biologically are likely to be very different from those performed on a computer. For example there are many levels of parallel

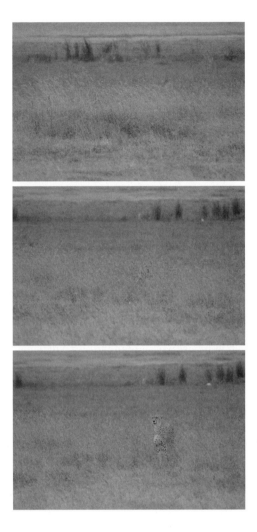

Figure 1.2. Vision is a critical perceptual ability for many biological systems. Early detection of visual events – such as that depicted above – can be essential for an individual's survival.

processing in the brain, which is unusual in a digital computer. The implementation level is the act of performing the selected algorithm, either in the brain or in a digital computer. This book places more emphasis on the first of Marr's three stages, outlining the principles of the computational processes to be performed with less emphasis on the actual algorithms that might be employed to run them.

This volume is divided into three parts, centred around the topics of dynamical systems; attention, motion and eye movements; and stereo vision. Dynamical systems deals with adaptation, motion detection, robotic vision systems, shape recovery from image sequences, and the reconstruction of objects from parts and attributes processed separately. The section on attention deals with attention and action, visual search in clutter, the memory of visual features accross saccades, and modelling gaze in natural images. Finally, the section on stereo describes a number of algorithms and approaches that reflect the current state of the art in stereo vision algoirthms and models of stereo information processing.

In each of these sections we find papers that examine spatial information processing and how it interacts with the temporal domain. In Part I, for example, Norma Graham and Sabina Wolfson examine specific adaptation processes in human visual information processing. They question how various levels of visual information processing adapt to the absolute levels of illumination that are available and the time course of this adaptation. In Part II, Steven Prime, Matthias Niemeier, and Douglas Crawford examine how visual information is maintained across visual saccades, a problem that is critical to biological systems that utilize eye movements to integrate larger portions of the visual field than are available in a single gaze, and which is also critical in machine systems which must use camera and vehicle motion to deal with the limited field of view of existing camera technologies. Finally in Part III, Jane Mulligan examines how stereo image processing can be made sufficiently "computationally efficient" that it can be embedded within machine vision systems and used as a building block for telepresence systems.

Beyond these three examples we find a collection of chapters that seek to address spatial vision information processing in both the computational and biological fields. These chapters illustrate just how detailed our understanding of basic visual information processing has come, and how much remains to be discovered. They also demonstrate how similar the problems are that are encountered by biological and computational systems and how similar are the underlying information processing models (algorithms). Much has been accomplished in the fifteen years since the first York Vision Conference on Spatial Vision in Humans and Robots. As we observed in the introduction to the book that arose from that conference, the two communities can learn a great deal from each other. That observation seems just as true today.

1.2   The CD-ROM

Enclosed with this volume is a CD-ROM that contains video, colour imagery, and other digital media associated with the text. A complete copy of this volume in PDF format can also be found on the CD-ROM. The material on the CD-ROM can be accessed using a standard browser (such as Internet Explorer or Firefox). Videos on the CD-ROM are viewable with Quicktime, while viewing of the presentations on the CD-ROM will require a PowerPoint viewer.

References

Dudek, G., Jenkin, M., Prahacs, C. *et al.*, (2005). A visually guided swimming robot. *Proc. IROS 2005*. Edmonton, Alberta.

Harris, L. and Jenkin, M. (1993). *Spatial Vision in Humans and Robots*. New York:

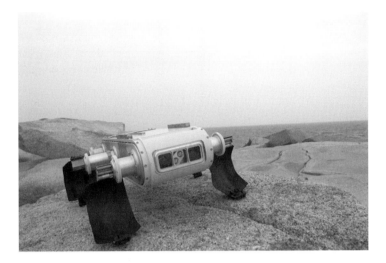

Figure 1.3. The AQUA Robot. A visually guided amphibious robot (Dudek *et al.*, 2005).

Cambridge University Press.

Marr, D. (1982) *Vision: a Computational Investigation into the Human Representation and Processing of Visual Information.* San Francisco: W. H. Freeman.

Part I

Dynamical systems

2 Exploring contrast-controlled adaptation processes in human vision (with help from *Buffy the Vampire Slayer*)

Norma Graham and
S. Sabina Wolfson

We have been interested for many years in intermediate levels of visual processing: levels which are lower than the perception of "objects" and "scenes" but higher than the pointwise processing of the retina and LGN.[1] Many of these intermediate processes are concerned with the initial analyses of pattern and form. Much of their action can be well modeled by what are technically linear operations – in particular, multiple analyzers sensitive to different ranges of spatial frequency and orientation.[2] However, some of their action cannot be modeled this way as it is fundamentally nonlinear. We have recently become interested in the dynamics of these intermediate nonlinear processes, and more particularly in questions about how the visual system sets its sensitivity based on the recent history of stimulation.

This chapter affords us an opportunity to be informal and to relate past work to present work in ways that are uncommon in journal papers. We are happy to take advantage of this opportunity. We will use informal speech and explanations and also personal anecdotes. And we will give many fewer references to published literature than is our wont, but instead will try to guide the reader to places where such references can be found.

Computational Vision in Neural and Machine Systems, ed. L. Harris and M. Jenkin. Published by Cambridge University Press. © Cambridge University Press 2007.

[1] The terms "lower" and "higher" are only approximate, of course, since information travels "downstream" as well as "upstream." Lennie (1998) presents interesting hypotheses – and an overall view – about the function and nature of the processes that have physiological substrates from V1 up to V4 and MT.

[2] The psychophysical research on these multiple analyzers, and a small amount of the physiological research, is described in Graham (1989) and summarized in Graham (1992).

Two sets of psychophysical experiments – and the models that were tested by their results – are described in this chapter. The first is described briefly and the second at length.

The first set was designed to investigate behaviorally the dynamics of luminance-controlled processes like light adaptation in the retina or LGN. Strictly speaking, these processes are lower than the level that we have been most interested in and were done with a third major collaborator, Don Hood, who is very interested in that level. Further, this set is already published for the most part. Thus we will describe it quite briefly. However, we do describe it because it both inspired the second set and also gave us distinct expectations about how the second set would turn out.

The second set of experiments was designed to investigate the dynamics of contrast-controlled processes. We started out to study one such process that had proved necessary to explain our previous results with textured patterns (done in collaboration with other investigators, in particular Jacob Beck and Anne Sutter). But the results of this second set of experiments ended up suggesting the existence of an entirely different contrast-controlled process, and one that we had not previously even imagined. This second set of experiments and the new process they suggested will be the focus of most of this chapter.

2.1   Dynamics of luminance-controlled adaptation processes (light adaptation)

2.1.1   Flickering the luminance of spatially homogeneous backgrounds and measuring thresholds for superimposed luminance probes

The first set of experiments, that we will only discuss briefly here, was intended to investigate the dynamics of luminance-controlled adaptation processes (e.g. light adaptation in the retina). Figure 2.1 shows the spatial and temporal characteristics of this paradigm, which is often called the probed-sinewave paradigm.

In probed-sinewave experiments, the luminance of a spatially homogeneous background is flickered sinusoidally in time during each trial. At some point during the trial a luminance-defined probe is introduced (of intensity ΔI, an increment in the figure, but decrements have been used as well). It is typically a smaller disk in the middle of the flickering background.

You can see movies of these stimuli on the CD-ROM accompanying this book. Video 1 shows the flickering background disk by itself. Video 2 shows the flickering background disk with a probe increment introduced.

Results from one typical observer from one study are shown in Figure 2.2 (with separate frequencies of flickering background in separate panels) and then again in Figure 2.3 (with the results at different frequencies superimposed in one panel). Probe threshold is plotted as a function of phase, and, to help show trends in results, the phases are plotted through two cycles on the horizontal axis. The results in Figures 2.2 and 2.3 show typical features of experimental results from this paradigm. Of particular

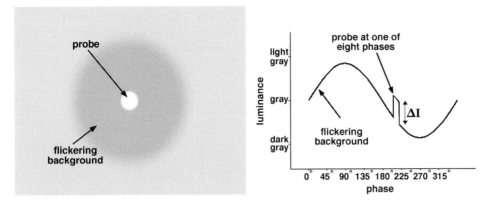

Figure 2.1. The probed-sinewave paradigm used to study luminance-controlled adaptation (light adaptation) processes. Spatial paradigm on left, and temporal paradigm on right. The luminance in the probe ΔI is adjusted until the observer can just discriminate between the background-alone and the background-plus-probe.

importance to the story here, note the large general increase in probe threshold magnitude (the upward displacement of the curves) as the background's flicker frequency is raised from lower (lighter and thinner lines and symbols) to higher (darker and bigger lines and symbols). The probe thresholds decrease at still higher frequencies – not shown here – until they are back down on average to the same level as at very low frequencies.

Many other studies – using different conditions and different observers – have been done by various groups of investigators. While the studies differed among themselves in a number of ways, they all showed a big general increase in probe threshold magnitude as the frequency of the flickering background increased from low to middling. (Many were compared in Graham, Wolfson, and Chowdhury, 2001.)

2.1.2 What do the results imply for models of light adaptation?

This empirical result – the general increase in probe threshold with increase in background flicker frequency – has turned out to be very powerful in discriminating among different models, or, more generally, in discriminating among different ideas of how light adaptation might work. Indeed Hood *et al.* (1997) showed that this empirical result completely rules out a large class of previously successful models containing the best features of the two earlier modeling traditions (the merged models of Graham and Hood, 1992). This empirical result could not, however, immediately rule out in the same dramatic way a new model suggested by Wilson (1997). The Wilson model, based on explicit physiological pieces, could be trivially modified to do a satisfactory job to at least a good first approximation (Hood and Graham, 1998, as was subsequently shown also with a fuller set of results by Wolfson and Graham 2000, 2001a). But the Wilson model has some drawbacks (see discussion in Wolfson and Graham, 2001a,b). The best current candidate in our opinion is the more abstract

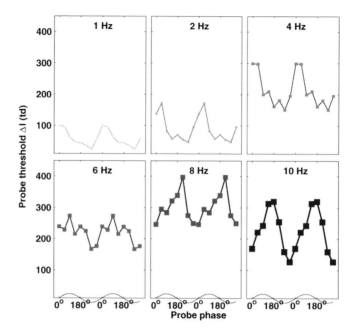

Figure 2.2. Experimental results from the probed-sinewave paradigm, plotted as probe threshold ΔI versus phase. Two cycles of the background are shown for help in displaying the patterns in the results but the points in the second cycle are identical to those in the first cycle. Experimental data from observer JG in Figure 4 of Hood *et al.* (1997).

model of Snippe, Poot, and van Hateren (2000, 2004) shown in Figure 2.4. The Snippe *et al.* model with its three general kinds of processes easily handles the empirical result we have been talking about, that is, the general elevation of probe threshold as background flicker frequency increases from low to middling. The model does so by adding a contrast-gain-control process to the previously suggested subtractive and divisive stages of luminance-controlled processes (light adaptation). See the figure legend for some more details. (The actual processes themselves are described precisely in Snippe *et al.*, 2000.)

The contrast-gain-control process in the model of Figure 2.4 presumably acts before any stage at which there is substantial binocular combination, and therefore its physiological substrate is likely to be the in the retina or LGN. This presumption comes from a further empirical result: In the probed-sinewave paradigm, most of the general elevation with increasing flicker frequency does not show interocular transfer (Wolfson and Graham, 2001b).

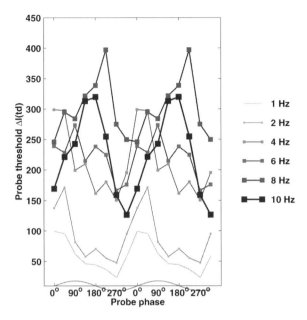

Figure 2.3. The experimental results for different frequencies in Figure 2.2 superimposed in one panel. In general, the probe thresholds tend to increase as frequency of the flickering background is varied from low (lighter-colored and thinner symbols and lines) to middling (darker and thicker symbols and lines).

2.1.3 About some terms: additive or subtractive, multiplicative or divisive, and gain control

The Snippe *et al.* model (Figure 2.4) has distinct processes labeled "divisive" and "subtractive." This labeling distinction is quite suggestive and often useful. It sometimes causes difficulty, however. Consider the following: If a process simply multiplies two values (its inputs) to produce its output, what happens if you now redefine the inputs and outputs to be the logarithms of the originals? The process now adds the two newly defined inputs to be its newly defined output. Any difference between the old and new case is simply a matter of exactly what you say "input" and "output" mean. In the situations where the distinction is useful, the process is more complicated and/or the outputs and inputs do not lend themselves naturally to being redefined as logs (or antilogs). In general, it pays to be cautious about these terms and take them merely as suggestive.

The contrast-controlled process in the Snippe *et al.* model (Figure 2.4) is called a "contrast-gain control", and is more of a multiplicative (or divisive) than a subtractive (or additive) process. Most of the processes for which people use the words "gain control" seem to have such a multiplicative nature, and the word "gain" often refers to

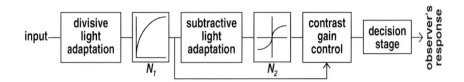

Figure 2.4. A diagram of the model of Snippe *et al.* (2000, 2004). This is the model for light adaptation that we currently find the most promising. They used three main processes because (in their words, p. 451, Snippe *et al.*, 2000): "From psychophysical experiments on light adaptation (mainly using background steps), it has been concluded that light adaptation contains both divisive (also referred to as multiplicative) and subtractive components (see Hayhoe *et al.*, 1992; Graham and Hood, 1992). Our model follows this tradition. It has been suggested previously that the elevation of test thresholds on modulated backgrounds above the test detection level for a steady background could arise from a contrast gain control process (Hood *et al.*, 1997; Wu *et al.*, 1997). This gain control would be activated by the temporal contrast of the background modulation, which would decrease the transmission gain for the test pulse, and hence its detectability. The third module in our model, contrast gain control, is a quantitative implementation of this suggestion." Precise description and equations for the separate processes are given in their articles. This diagram here is modified slightly from theirs (Snippe *et al.*, 2000, Figure 2) by some changes in notation and making further explicit the decision stage that leads to an observer's response. We added the decision-stage box to emphasize the fact that the assumptions relating the outputs of processes relatively early in visual processing to an observer's response are critical in the testing of any such model. Often quite straightforward assumptions prove reasonable and useful, however, and such is the case here.

a multiplicative constant relating the ratio of output to input.

We will use the words "luminance-controlled" and "contrast-controlled" adaptation processes to mean that either the luminance or contrast, respectively, of preceding visual stimulation is changing the responsiveness to new stimulation. By using these more general terms, we want to imply that the control at issue is not necessarily of the multiplicative sort that would be implied by "luminance-gain control" or "contrast-gain control."

2.2 Dynamics of contrast-controlled adaptation processes

2.2.1 Flickering the contrast of patterned backgrounds and measuring the thresholds of superimposed patterned probes

In the second set of experiments – intended to investigate the dynamics of contrast-controlled adaptation processes – the contrast of a spatially patterned background is

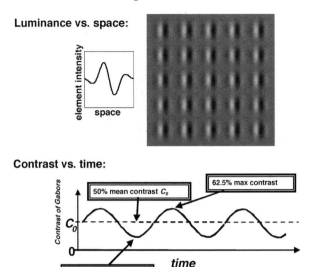

Background Pattern

Figure 2.5. Diagram of the spatially patterned flickering background stimulus used in our contrast adaptation experiments. The upper panel shows a piece of the background pattern with only 5×5 of the 15×15 Gabor-patch elements used in the experiment. The small inset on the left shows the Gabor function that describes the spatial profile of an individual element. The functions at the bottom show the temporal profile – contrast as a function of time – of each Gabor-patch element.

flickered sinusoidally in time during each trial. At some point during the trial a spatially patterned probe is introduced.

You can see movies of these stimuli on the CD-ROM accompanying this book. Video 3 shows the flickering patterned background by itself. Video 4 shows the background with a probe introduced. The next few paragraphs and figures describe these stimuli further.

Figure 2.5 shows the general spatial and temporal characteristics of the flickering background in this kind of experiment. The upper part of Figure 2.5 shows a piece of pattern. (This piece contains an array of 5×5 Gabor patches, whereas we used 15×15 in the experiments and in the movies.) The lower part of Figure 2.5 shows the contrast in any one of these Gabor patches as a function of time. The values of the flickering background's contrast at the mean, peak, and trough that were used in the experiments reported here are labeled on the figure.

Figure 2.6 illustrates the presentation of a short-duration probe stimulus. The right-hand panel of Figure 2.6 shows a piece of the background with probe at the moment the probe is presented, in other words, a test stimulus. To prevent confusion, it is impor-

Background + Probe = Test Pattern

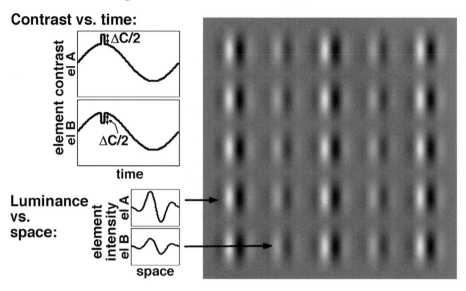

Figure 2.6. Example of the background-plus-probe or test pattern. The right panel shows a piece of the test pattern. The two types of Gabor patches that define alternating columns are called *element A* and *element B*, which are abbreviated *el A* and *el B*. The spatial profiles of these two element types are in the panels at the lower left showing luminance as a function of spatial position. The temporal profiles of the two element types are plotted in the panels at the upper left showing contrast as a function of time. The probe is an increase in contrast for *el A* and a decrease for *el B*. The increase and decrease are of equal magnitude $\Delta C/2$, so the total contrast difference between the two element types in the probe is ΔC. Note that the word "test" here explicitly means the combination of background and probe. The word "probe" refers to the change that is made in the background pattern in order to produce the test pattern. In some contexts, either word can be used to the same effect, but in others (particularly later in this chapter) it will be useful to keep the meanings distinct.

tant to note that we will use the word "test" here to explicitly mean the *combination of background and probe*. The word "probe" refers to the change that is made to the background pattern. Thus, the test stimulus is the sum of the background stimulus and the probe stimulus. In Figure 2.6 the illustrated test stimulus (the probe plus background) looks like alternating columns (vertical stripes) of different-contrast Gabor elements. Test stimuli can also be alternating rows (horizontal stripes) of Gabor patches (as in Figure 2.7 left panel). We will call the two types of Gabor patches that define alternating rows or columns by the names *element A* and *element B*, abbreviated as *el A* and *el B* in Figure 2.6. The luminance of element A and element B as a function of spatial

Observer's task:
Horizontal vs. Vertical

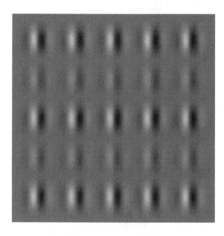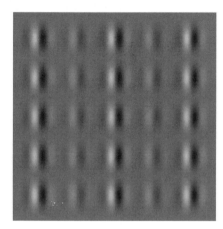

Figure 2.7. The observer's task is to identify the orientation of the contrast-defined stripes as being either horizontal (left panel) or vertical (right panel). ΔC is varied to find the value at which the observer can just discriminate at criterion level between the two orientations. That value of ΔC is called the probe threshold.

position is plotted in the lower left drawings of Figure 2.6.

The temporal characteristics of the probe presentation are shown in the upper left of Figure 2.6. Contrast is plotted as a function of time for the two element types. The probe illustrated in Figure 2.6 is composed of an increase in contrast for one type of element (*el A* in this case) and an equal-sized decrease in contrast for the other element. The total contrast in the probe will be called ΔC, and so the contrast increase (*el A*) and decrease (*el B*) are each equal to half that quantity ($\Delta C/2$) as indicated in the figure. (A forewarning: This symmetry between increase and decrease in contrast was true for all probes used in the experiments we are about to describe. However, later in the chapter, this will not be true, as we will explicitly point out at the appropriate point.)

The observer's task in our experiments reported here was always to identify the orientation of the contrast-defined stripes as being either vertical or horizontal (see Figure 2.7) and, of course, these possibilities were randomly presented from trial to trial.

Further details of the experiments reported here (for the interested reader) On half the trials, the orientation of all the individual Gabor patches in a pattern was vertical as in the examples here. On the other half of the trials (randomly intermixed) the Gabor patches were all horizontal. Note that there is undoubtedly nonlinear distortion in all the illustrations here (the movies and the figures) but in the actual experiments, the stimuli were very carefully calibrated. For the experiments reported below, the spatial frequency of the Gabor patches was 2 c/deg, and the other spatial attributes of the pattern were as pictured here. The background pattern flickered for a total of several seconds. The probe was presented approximately in the middle of the flickering period as dictated by the following constraints: There was always at least one second of flicker before and after the probe, and the flicker always started and stopped at positive zero-crossings. The probe could occur at 1 of 8 equally spaced phases (randomly chosen on each trial) ranging from $0°$ to $315°$. Between the periods of flicker the screen was a homogeneous field at the mean luminance of 58 cd/m^2. The probe duration was 82 ms (7 frames at the CRT's refresh rate of 85 Hz) for observers JW and EG, and 35 ms (3 frames) for observers KF and SH. The observer responded to indicate whether the contrast-defined stripes were perceived as horizontal or vertical (see Figure 2.7). The probe's contrast levels were determined on each trial using simple 1-up-3-down staircases. The probe threshold was calculated as the value of ΔC such that the observer can just discriminate (at a criterion of 81% correct) between the two orientations. Observers were instructed not to fixate rigidly in order to avoid after-images. They were given feedback about correctness of their responses.

2.2.2   Why we used these patterns and what we expected to find

We used this type of pattern in these experiments because we already knew a great deal about their perception by human observers. What we knew made it sensible to believe the following, which we will briefly state and then elaborate upon.

The flickering background pattern (e.g. Figure 2.5) should drive a particular contrast-gain-control process.

But it should NOT stimulate the pathway detecting the probe stimulus.

Thus, when we varied the temporal frequency of the flickering background and the phase of the probe with respect to this background and we then measured the observer's sensitivity to the probe, we hoped for the following outcome. We hoped that we would be measuring the dynamic properties of the contrast-gain-control process and that we would NOT be measuring (to any substantial extent) the dynamic properties of the pathway detecting the probe.

The following text, and the illustrations in Figures 2.8 and 2.9, give a little more substance to the general idea just sketched.

The test pattern formed by the background-and-probe (see image in Figure 2.6) is an example of the *element-arrangement textures* introduced by Jacob Beck and his colleagues in the early 1980s (e.g. Beck, Prazdny and Rosenfeld, 1983) and studied by many people, including us, since then. These textures are defined by the difference between two types of elements, in our experiments here the different levels of contrast in otherwise identical Gabor-patch elements. The particular arrangement of the two types of elements is striped in the example here, although other arrangements – in particular checked – have been used.

Note also that Gabor-patch element-arrangement textures like those used here (where contrast is the only difference between element types, e.g., Figure 2.6) are very very similar to stimuli usually called *contrast-modulated noise* or *contrast-modulated sinusoidal gratings*. The spatial frequency and orientation of the Gabor patches in the

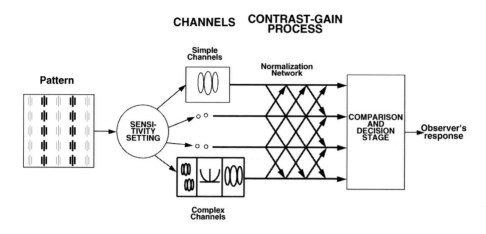

Figure 2.8. Our general model as it existed before the experiments described in this chapter. This framework includes complex channels and a contrast-gain control of the normalization type. See text for more details about these nonlinear processes. The "sensitivity setting" stage shown in this figure preceding the simple and complex channels would, in general, contain early local nonlinearities like retinal and LGN light adaptation. But we have shown that for experiments using texture element-arrangement patterns within the range of contrasts and luminances used here, this stage is effectively linear.

element-arrangement textures play the role of the carrier spatial frequency and orientation in the contrast-modulated noise or sinusoidal gratings. The spatial frequency and orientation of the stripes defined by the contrast differences in the element-arrangement textures play the role of the modulation signal in the contrast-modulated noise or sinusoidal gratings. Thus many results using contrast-modulated noise and sinusoidal gratings can be used also to support the statements we are about to make.

Thus one can say the following. A wide variety of experimental results using element-arrangement textures and other similar patterns can be explained on the basis of *spatial-frequency and orientation-selective channels* (which are linear filters), but – and it is a big caveat – only if at least two, dramatically different, nonlinear processes are also included in the model. We will describe these nonlinear processes in the next several paragraphs. We will not list all the many references for the statements we are going to make, but the interested reader can find the omitted references in the following publications: Graham and Sutter (1998, 2000), Graham and Wolfson (2001), Landy and Graham (2003), and Wolfson and Graham (2005a). These list many references to the studies that provide evidence for the existence of these nonlinear processes, their possible functions, and their general properties, as investigated by us and by many others.

As well as *spatial-frequency and orientation-selective channels* that are linear fil-

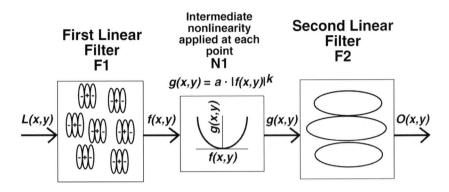

Figure 2.9. More details of the structure of a complex channel. Later in the chapter we will refer to this as the "original" kind of complex channel. $L(x, y)$ is luminance at position (x, y); $O(x, y)$ is the output of the complex channel; f and g represent functions specifying the outputs at intermediate stages within the channel; and a and k are parameters specifying the exact form of the intermediate nonlinearity $N1$.

ters (which we call *simple channels* in Figure 2.8 and which are sometimes called *first-order channels*), it is necessary to postulate a nonlinear kind of channel. We call these nonlinear channels *complex channels*, and they are also sometimes called *second-order channels* or *non-Fourier channels*. As sketched in the bottom middle of Figure 2.8 and drawn with details in Figure 2.9, these complex channels contain two layers of linear filtering $F1$ and $F2$ separated by a nonlinearity $N1$. This kind of structure is often called, for short, an FNF structure. The nonlinearity sandwiched between the two linear filters is something like a full-wave or half-wave rectification applied to the output of the first filter at each spatial position and at each moment in time. (In particular, the output of $N1$ is never less than zero.) The first linear filter $F1$ is characterized by a relatively small receptive field (spatial weighting function) and the second linear filter $F2$ is characterized by a substantially larger one.

In the case of element-arrangement textures made with Gabor patches, a simple linear channel would not be able to detect the striped element arrangement at all, but a complex channel would. We do not have the space here to go through this argument, but an interested reader can find a demonstration of this argument with an element-arrangement texture in Figure 11 of Graham, Beck, and Sutter (1992) and with another kind of pattern in Figure 4 of Landy and Graham (2003).

In addition to the rectification-type nonlinear process in the complex channels, we had discovered there was another and very dramatic nonlinearity. It depended upon the contrast of the patterns, and it was already very compressive for very low contrasts. We showed eventually that this compressive effect can definitely NOT be explained by any relatively early local process occurring before the level of the channels. In particular, therefore, it cannot be explained by a luminance-controlled process like light adaptation. We also showed that a contrast-gain-control process of the type frequently called *normalization* could explain this dramatic compressive effect. This normalization process involves inhibition among channels. Any given channel is inhibited by other channels in its *normalization pool*, where this inhibition acts in such a way (divisively) that it "normalizes" the response of the inhibited channel with respect to the total response from a rather large set of channels.

A normalization process of this sort can be shown to have a number of attractive functional properties that might explain why evolution produced such a process in the visual system. For example, it prevents overload on higher levels while it allows the channels to preserve their sensitivity and also their selectivity (e.g. for orientation) over a wide range of contrasts by changing the effective operating range on the contrast dimension. More recently it has also been suggested that such a process has the appropriate characteristics to help encode natural images efficiently.

For our element-arrangement patterns, with appropriate simplifying assumptions, we have previously derived a simple equation giving the predictions from the general model shown in Figure 2.8. This equation – incorporating the normalization process as well as simple and complex channels with very few parameters – produces quantitative predictions that can account for a large body of results (see Graham and Sutter, 2000).

Now let us use the general framework of Figure 2.8 to translate the general expectations given at the beginning of this section into more specific statements about what we expected to find from the experiments using flickering patterned backgrounds.

First note that the observer's ability to identify the orientation of the element-arrangement test stimulus (see Figures 2.6 and 2.7) is mediated by the appropriately tuned complex channels. By "appropriately tuned" we mean the complex channels that have first-stage receptive fields matched in spatial frequency and orientation to the Gabor-patch elements, and second-stage receptive fields matched in spatial frequency to the striped arrangement (and sensitive to either vertical or horizontal orientation).

The flickering background (Figure 2.5) produces NO response in these appropriately tuned complex channels that can identify the test stimulus orientation because there is no striped arrangement in the background stimulus, and thus nothing for the second filter of these complex channels to respond to.

But the flickering background does drive the signal from the normalization pool up and down because it stimulates many simple channels and may also stimulate other complex channels that respond to the Gabor patches although they cannot identify the orientation of the striped arrangement.

Hence any effect of the flickering background on the response to the probe would be via its effect on the contrast-gain normalization process and not contaminated (to any large extent) by dynamic characteristics of the direct response to the probe.

On the assumption that the measured effects would be reflecting the characteristics of a contrast-gain control pathway of something like the normalization type, we planned to compare quantitatively the results of these experiments to predictions from a number of proposed models in the literature or constructed by us. The models included: the Carandini, Heeger, and Movshon (1997) model of normalization in V1 cells; the Wilson and Humanski (1993) model of a contrast-gain control based on some psychophysical results; a model consisting of a general purpose contrast-gain control stage something like that in the Snippe *et al.* (2000) model of light adaptation (Figure 2.4 here).

Although we had not done extensive quantitative predictions at the time we started collecting results from the experiments on flickering patterned backgrounds reported below, we knew quite a good deal about the general form of the predictions based on the above expectations.

In general there would be phase-specific effects and the precise form of them would change with temporal frequency of the background, reflecting the general dynamics of the normalization pool's inhibiting effect on the channel detecting the probe.

Some of the models would predict that, in spite of these phase-specific effects that depend on temporal frequency, the probe thresholds averaged across phase would not change very much with temporal frequency.

Other models, however, would predict a general elevation effect like that found in the earlier light adaptation results (Figures 2.2 and 2.3) where the thresholds would generally elevate as temporal frequency increased from low to middling. Indeed it was exactly that effect that the Snippe *et al.* (2000) contrast-gain-control process (see Figure 2.4) was designed to predict. And thus if we took their process as a model of the contrast-gain, the general probe-threshold elevation with background frequency would also be predicted for the contrast adaptation experiments.

2.2.3   The results on flickering patterned backgrounds

Of course it took us much longer than we planned to finally get usable results from these contrast adaptation experiments when we did start trying to run them. The usual sorts of delays intervened including equipment breakdowns, software mistakes, and trouble getting the stimulus parameters in a range to produce measurable performance from typical observers (performance greater than chance and less than perfect). But this time we had another delay with nobody to blame but ourselves: when we finally collected usable results, we did not believe them. This delay cost us weeks. How could this happen? To explain our blindness, lets look at the experimental results and compare them to our expectations.

The results from one typical observer are shown in Figure 2.10 (different panels for different frequencies of background) and again in Figure 2.11 (results for different frequencies juxtaposed) following the same conventions as Figures 2.2 and 2.3 for the light-adaptation experiments. Probe threshold (this time ΔC rather than ΔI, however) is plotted versus the phase of the probe and, to help show trends in results, the phases are plotted through two cycles on the horizontal axis.

At low temporal frequencies of flicker, the results were in line with our expectations. In particular, the probe thresholds generally followed the contrast of the background as one might expect from some process that was fast compared to the frequency of the background. This is like the earlier light-adaptation results.

However, look what happened across the range of frequencies. The curves in Figures 2.10 and 2.11 are on average moving dramatically downward as background frequency increases. They are moving downward rather than staying at roughly the same level (which we had thought they might) or going upward (which we had also thought they might as in the light adaptation results of Figures 2.2 and 2.3). To put it in other

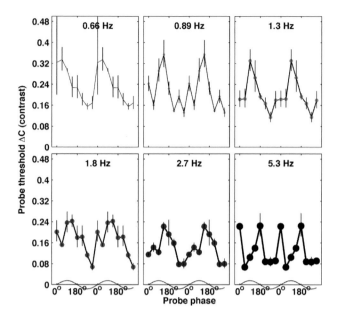

Figure 2.10. Results of the contrast-adaptation experiments for a typical observer (JW). Patterned probe thresholds (vertical axis) are plotted as a function of phase (horizontal axis) for various flicker frequencies of the patterned background (different panels). The data points show the mean ±1 SE bars from three estimates of each threshold (done in three different sessions). In each session trials of all eight phases were randomly intermixed.

words, as the frequency of the flickering patterned background increases, the observer is generally becoming dramatically more sensitive to the patterned probe. This was completely outside the range of effects we had led ourselves to expect.

2.2.4 Functional fixity, the effects of expectancy, and the Buffy idea

So what did we do? What humans often do. Namely we refused to believe our eyes (refused to believe the new evidence) and believed our preconceptions instead. Psychologists have various names for effects of this sort: mental set, functional fixedness, confirmation bias. In the long course of evolution, one presumes these effects have been useful heuristics. But they clearly can be overdone.

We spent weeks proving once more that there were no artifacts in the experimental procedure, no mistakes in the experimental set-up and no errors in the computer program. We collected results from four observers to make sure that the first was not fooling us (or herself) somehow. We kept getting the same results and kept having trouble believing them. And we certainly could not understand them. And we were

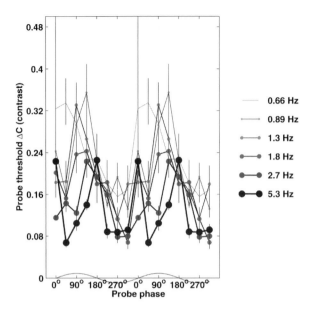

Figure 2.11. The contrast-adaptation results shown in Figure 2.10 but with the re-sults from all background flicker frequencies superimposed in one panel. In general, the probe thresholds tend to decrease as the frequency of the flickering background is varied from the lowest (lighter-colored and thinner symbols and lines) to the highest (darker and thicker symbols and lines). The light-adaptation results in Figure 2.3 show the opposite trend with background frequency.

sorely tempted to stop this line of experimentation altogether.

On the other hands, the experimental results were striking, repeatable, and contin-ued nagging at us. And eventually we broke the effects of expectancy. The college-age daughter of one of us (NG) came home for a bad wisdom-teeth extraction operation, and then wanted to spend the rest of Thanksgiving weekend watching *Buffy the Vampire Slayer*. Her mother gave in to daughter's pleas for company. So mother and daughter watched two full seasons of Buffy in four days. Mother sat at the dining-room table occasionally looking at the experimental results of Figures 2.10 and 2.11 and occa-sionally sketching diagrams of predictions from the kinds of models outlined above. Daughter lay on the couch occasionally examining the homework she was supposed to be doing. The predictions from mother's preconceived ideas continued to disagree with the experimental results. Buffy continued to slay vampires. But some place during those four days, Buffy turned mother's mind to sufficient mush that the preconceived ideas vanished from it. And a glimmer of an alternative idea took their place. (What happened to daughter's homework is lost to history, but she passed the semester.)

Although this glimmer of an alternative idea took months to become a full-fledged model, it did turn out to account quantitatively for the major features of the experimental results that were so unexpected to us originally. It now makes the results perfectly believable to us although still somewhat surprising on other grounds. The idea – and its various accompaniments – will be labeled here "Buffy" in honor of its inspiration and for lack of better labels (although in the future we will try to find more traditionally respectable and descriptive names).

It is now hard to believe we were so surprised by these results. Indeed, in retrospect it is hard even for us to understand why. This in our experience is typical also. Once a fixity or expectational set has been broken, people are amazed they were so blind. And forget for the next occasion that they might again be blind.

For the reader to understand the Buffy idea more easily, we think it best to postpone the direct presentation of the idea until later and instead present first some further experimental results we collected to test the idea when it was still a glimmer.

2.3 Using Buffy and Regular Steady-State backgrounds

2.3.1 Limits as background frequency gets very low or very high

We constructed two new experimental conditions – called *Regular Steady-State* and *Buffy Steady-State* here – to study what happens at very low and very high frequencies of the flickering spatially patterned background. To understand these conditions, let us first look at what happens as the flicker frequency gets very low (Figure 2.12) or very high (Figure 2.13) while keeping the phase of the probe constant with respect to the flickering background. The contrast of the stimulus seen by the observer is plotted vertically and time is plotted horizontally. Consider an interval of arbitrary length just before the moment at which the probe is added to the background. This interval is shown as a shaded area in these two figures.

Consider Figure 2.12. As the background flicker frequency gets lower, the function relating the flickering background's contrast to time, which starts out showing several cycles of sinusoidal fluctuation (top of Figure 2.12), flattens and becomes closer and closer to a horizontal line during the interval just before the probe (bottom of Figure 2.12). Or, to say it another way, as the flicker frequency gets lower, the background stimulus during the before-probe interval becomes more and more like a stimulus of constant contrast. Or, to say it still a third way, the function that relates the flickering background's contrast to time during the interval before the probe reaches a conventional limit: its limit is the function where contrast equals a constant during that interval.

If you look more closely at Figure 2.12, you can also see that (as background frequency gets lower and lower) the contrast level of the limiting function depends on the phase that the probe was in with respect to the background before the limit was reached. In the example of Figure 2.12, this phase is approximately midway between the trough (phase $270°$) and the next zero-crossing. We will call the limiting contrast level C_{BP} (where the B and P stand for background and phase); it is shown as a solid horizontal line in the bottom drawing of Figure 2.12. The dashed horizontal line in each drawing shows C_0, the mean contrast level of the background.

As background flicker frequency gets lower:

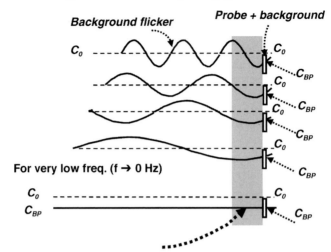

For very low frequencies, the background contrast in time
window before the probe is constant at C_{BP}

Figure 2.12. A sketch showing the interval before the probe pattern as the frequency of background flicker gets lower and lower while keeping the phase of the probe with respect to the background constant. The little vertical open rectangles represent the probe patterns; the top of the little rectangle is the contrast level of the higher-contrast Gabor patches, and the bottom of the rectangle is that of the lower-contrast Gabor patches. The wavy sinusoidal curve shows the contrast of the flickering background. The dashed horizontal line in each panel shows the mean contrast of the flickering background (C_0). The solid horizontal line in the bottom panel shows the contrast (C_{BP}) of the flickering background at the phase of the probe. The large shaded rectangular area in this figure simply marks the interval before the probe is presented.

What happens as the background flicker frequency gets higher (Figure 2.13), again keeping the probe phase constant? Now the function relating the flickering background's contrast to time does not approach a conventional limit at all. It just oscillates faster and faster (bottom of Figure 2.13).

But what if there is a process that integrates over recent contrast within a temporal window (e.g. the shaded area in Figure 2.13)? For such a process, the average contrast in the temporal window determines the state of the process at the time the probe is presented. And, to foreshadow later explanations, the existence of such a process forms one important part of the Buffy idea.

In Figure 2.13, at each frequency of background flicker, the average contrast during the temporal window before the probe is sketched as the thick black horizontal bar extending throughout the shaded area representing the temporal window. As you can

As background flicker frequency gets higher:

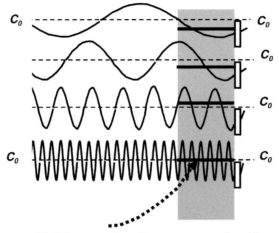

For very high frequencies, the average contrast in
time window before probe settles down at overall
mean contrast C_0.

Figure 2.13. Sketch showing what happens in the interval before the probe as the frequency of the background flicker gets higher and higher while keeping the phase of the probe with respect to the background constant. Symbols and conventions as in Figure 2.12 with the following additions. The large shaded vertical rectangle now more specifically indicates the temporal-integration window of a hypothetical process. And the thick horizontal bar in that shaded area indicates the average contrast of the flickering background during that temporal-integration window; thus the thick horizontal bar also indicates the state of the hypothetical process at the moment the probe is presented.

see in the figure, as background flicker frequency gets higher and higher (curves from top to bottom), the average contrast in that temporal window goes up and down, but the amplitude of the ups and downs gets smaller and smaller. Thus the average contrast in the window does reach a conventional limit. That limit equals the mean background contrast of the sinusoidal flicker C_0 (shown by the dashed horizontal line). And notice that this average contrast settles down at that same contrast *no matter what the phase of the probe relative to the background*.

2.3.2 The Regular Steady-State condition – to study very low frequencies

How can we study very low frequencies? The limiting situation shown in Figure 2.12 motivates our *Regular Steady-State* condition shown in Figure 2.14. The general Regular Steady-State paradigm is shown in the upper panel of this figure and examples at

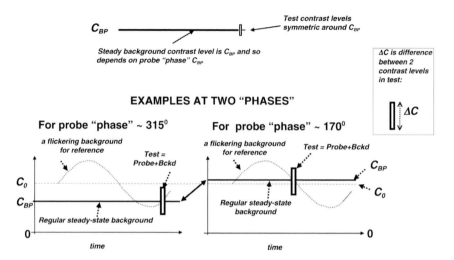

Figure 2.14. Sketch of time course of stimuli in the Regular Steady-State condition. The top panel shows a general case, and the bottom two panels indicate some of the details for two examples "phases". "Phase" here refers to the phase of the probe with respect to the flickering background (which was kept constant) as the frequency got lower and lower in the limiting process that motivated this steady-state condition (Figure 2.12).

two particular probe "phases" are shown in the lower panels.[3] As you can see in the figure, the Regular Steady-State condition is constructed by using a steady background – at the appropriate contrast C_{BP} for the "phase" one is considering – instead of using very-low-frequency flicker. The test stimulus remains the same as it was on the flickering background.

    To summarize: the Regular Steady-State condition has the following two properties.

(1) The steady background contrast (C_{BP}) changes depending on the "phase" of the probe.

(2) For all "phases" the contrasts of the two element types in the test stimulus are symmetric around the steady background contrast.

---

[3]*A terminological aside:* The use of the word "phase" in this steady-state condition (and below in another steady-state condition) is a bit odd. Thus we put it in quotation marks for this initial discussion although we will drop the quotation marks in what follows. Note that the "phase" in a steady-state condition is equal to the phase of the probe with respect to the flickering background (which was kept constant) as the frequency changed in the limiting process that motivated the steady-state condition (Figure 2.12 and, for the next steady-state condition, Figure 2.13).

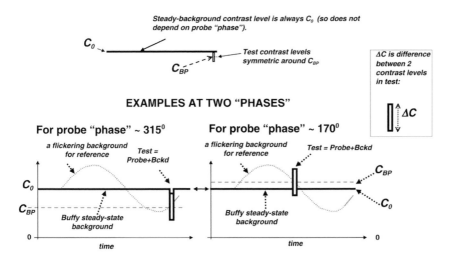

Figure 2.15. Sketch of time course of stimuli in the *Buffy Steady-State* condition. Same format as Figure 2.14. "Phase" here refers to the phase of the probe with respect to the flickering background (which was kept constant) as the frequency got higher and higher in the limiting process that motivated this steady-state condition (Figure 2.13).

Details of the Regular Steady-State condition   The methods for the steady-state experiments were identical to those for the flickering-background experiments (see above) with the following specifications: The steady-state background was on for about 2.6 s and the probe was approximately in the middle. There was always at least 1 s of steady background before and after the probe.

2.3.3   The Buffy Steady-State condition – to study very high frequencies assuming a temporal-integration process

How can we study very high frequencies given that it is impossible to generate very high frequency flickering backgrounds? The limiting situation shown in Figure 2.13 motivates the *Buffy Steady-State condition* shown in Figure 2.15. A general sketch is at the top and two example phases below.

   As you can see in the figure, the Buffy Steady-State condition is constructed by using a steady background instead of the desired very-high-frequency flicker. The steady background will be at the same contrast C_0 independent of phase. The test (background-plus-probe) stimulus remains the same as it was on the flickering background.

   To summarize, the Buffy Steady-State condition has the following two properties.

(1) The steady background contrast is C_0 for all "phases" of probe.

(2) The two contrasts in the test are NOT usually symmetric around the steady background contrast (which is always C_0). The two contrasts are symmetric around C_{BP} which changes depending on the phase of the probe.

Note that this condition is only a way to study very high temporal frequencies if there is a process that integrates over a temporal window. And even then it really is only studying certain aspects of behavior at very high frequencies. But, as mentioned above, the temporal-integration process is an important part of the idea we were trying to study.

Details of the Buffy Steady-State condition.   Other than the differences between the two steady-state conditions portrayed in Figures 2.14 and 2.15, all methods for the Buffy Steady-State were like those for the Regular Steady-State condition.

2.3.4   Experimental results from the two steady-state conditions

The results from the Regular and Buffy Steady-State conditions are shown in the left and right panels, respectively, of Figure 2.16 for the same observer JW whose results on flickering backgrounds were shown earlier (in Figures 2.10 and 2.11). Figure 2.17 shows the results from Figure 2.16 again; now they are superimposed on this observer's results for the flickering backgrounds shown earlier.

As can be seen in the figures, the results are rather as you would expect by extrapolation from the results on the flickering backgrounds to even lower and even higher frequencies. In particular, the Regular Steady-State thresholds are quite high like those on the lowest-frequency flickering backgrounds; the Buffy Steady-State thresholds are very low, somewhat lower even than the highest flicker frequency studied for this observer JW (5.3 Hz).

Another aspect of the Buffy Steady-State results is worth pointing out. They, like those on flickering backgrounds at the highest flicker frequencies, show almost complete frequency doubling. (The probe-threshold curves show two almost-identical maxima and two almost-identical minima per cycle of the background flicker.) Such complete frequency doubling (visible in every individual session from every observer) was much more dramatic than any frequency-doubling seen in the light-adaptation results and had initially surprised us when we had only collected the flickering-background results and had not yet had the glimmer of the Buffy idea.

2.3.5   Examining Buffy Steady-State results further: the extreme phases

Consider the phases that produce the extreme thresholds in the experimental results from the Buffy Steady-State condition. Phases at or near the zero-crossings ($0°$ and $180°$) lead to the maximal thresholds, and phases at or near the peak ($90°$) and trough ($270°$) lead to minimal probe thresholds (Figure 2.16). (Remember that "phase" here

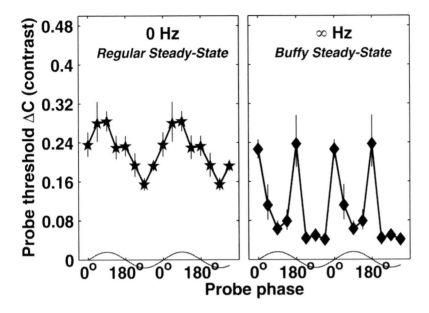

Figure 2.16. Results from the Regular (left panel) and Buffy (right panel) Steady-State conditions for the observer JW whose results on flickering backgrounds are shown in Figures 2.10 and 2.11. The results shown are the mean ±1 SE bars from 6 estimates of each threshold (done in 6 different sessions). In each session all eight phases were studied in randomly intermixed trials.

refers to the phase of the probe with respect to the background flicker in the limiting process shown in Figure 2.13.)

The stimuli corresponding to these extreme phases are illustrated further in Figure 2.18. The background stimulus (a steady field of contrast C_0) is presented to the observer for some period of time. This stimulus could also be called an "adapting stimulus" and is so called in Figure 2.18. In the experiments here, the duration of the adapting stimulus happened to be a bit more than 1 s, but anything that long or longer probably produces much the same result (and things somewhat shorter might also). Then the test stimulus (the combination of background-plus-probe) is presented briefly.

For the peak phase (90°), the average of the two contrast levels in the test stimulus is ABOVE the background contrast. Indeed usually it turns out that not only the average but both of the individual contrast levels in the test stimulus at threshold are above the background contrast.

For the zero-crossing phases (0° and 180°), the average contrast of the test stimulus is equal to that of the background stimulus, and the two levels at threshold therefore STRADDLE the background contrast.

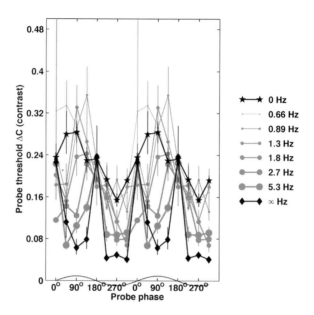

Figure 2.17. The steady-state and flickering-background contrast-adaptation results replotted from Figures 2.11 and 2.16.

For the trough phase $(270°)$, the average of the two contrast levels in the test stimulus is BELOW the background contrast. Usually it turns out that not only the average but both of the individual contrast levels in the test stimulus at threshold are below the background contrast.

Figure 2.19 displays numerically some results from the Buffy Steady-State for these three extreme phases for two observers (JW, the observer whose results have been shown in earlier figures, and another observer SH). The contrast levels in the test stimuli at threshold are given in one column and then the difference between those contrasts is given in the adjacent column.

As one would expect from the curves in Figure 2.16, right panel, the contrast difference at threshold is much larger for the test stimulus which STRADDLES the background (zero-crossing phase) than for either of the other test stimuli ABOVE or BELOW the background contrast. And the threshold contrasts for those other two are very similar to one another but on opposite sides of the background contrast. The observers cannot see that straddling stimulus well enough to identify the orientation of its stripes until the two contrast levels defining the stripes are very far apart, e.g. about 23% for observer JW and 41% for observer SH. For the test stimuli where both contrast levels are on one side of the steady background contrast, the threshold contrast differences range from 5% to 8%.

The results are particularly dramatic for observer SH. For this observer, the two

Three Phases in the Buffy Steady-State condition

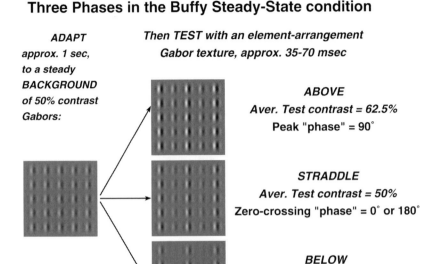

ADAPT
approx. 1 sec,
to a steady
BACKGROUND
of 50% contrast
Gabors:

Then TEST with an element-arrangement
Gabor texture, approx. 35-70 msec

ABOVE
Aver. Test contrast = 62.5%
Peak "phase" = 90°

STRADDLE
Aver. Test contrast = 50%
Zero-crossing "phase" = 0° or 180°

BELOW
Aver. Test contrast = 37.5%
Trough "phase" = 270°

Figure 2.18. Illustrations of three kinds of trials (the three extreme phases) in the Buffy Steady-State condition. The observer sees ("adapts") to a steady background of equal-contrast Gabor patches for a little more than 1 s and then sees a briefly presented test stimulus which has either vertical contrast-defined stripes (as in the figure) or horizontal. The observer is to say which orientation the stripes are. Notice that the test stimuli have patches of two contrast levels. Depending on the phase, these contrast levels can (1) average ABOVE, or (2) STRADDLE, or (3) average BELOW the contrast C_0 of the Gabor patches in the steady background.

contrast levels (70% and 30%) in the threshold for the STRADDLING test stimulus are literally further out from the background contrast level than are any of the contrast levels in threshold test stimuli ABOVE (66%, 59%) or BELOW (41%, 34%) the steady background.

To look at the results in a slightly different way: Which test stimulus is hardest for the observer? It is the middle one – the test stimulus in which the contrasts are STRADDLING the background contrast. Thus, when looked at in this way, the contrasts NEAREST to the adapting contrast are actually hardest for the observer to process (in whatever way is necessary for the observer to do this identification task). This seemed a surprising effect of adaptation to us, and we will return to this topic again in the last section. But first we will present a model that can explain the mechanism of this adaptation effect.

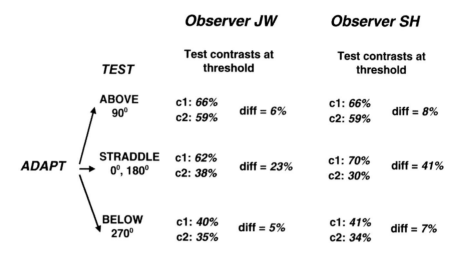

		Observer JW Test contrasts at threshold		**Observer SH** Test contrasts at threshold	
	TEST				
ADAPT	**ABOVE** 90⁰	c1: *66%* c2: *59%*	diff = *6%*	c1: *66%* c2: *59%*	diff = *8%*
	STRADDLE 0⁰, 180⁰	c1: *62%* c2: *38%*	diff = *23%*	c1: *70%* c2: *30%*	diff = *41%*
	BELOW 270⁰	c1: *40%* c2: *35%*	diff = *5%*	c1: *41%* c2: *34%*	diff = *7%*

Figure 2.19. Results from two observers for the three extreme phases of the Buffy Steady-State condition illustrated in Figure 2.18. For each observer, the contrast levels in the test stimuli at threshold are given in one column and then the difference between those contrasts in the adjacent column. (All contrasts were rounds to the nearest 1%. Since the thresholds plotted at 0° and 180° in Figure 2.16 are actually from the same straddling test stimulus, these were averaged together for the numbers displayed for the straddling test stimulus here.) Notice that the threshold for the stimulus that STRADDLES the adapting level is much higher than that for stimuli either ABOVE or BELOW the adapting level.

2.4   A new kind of complex channel with embedded contrast adaptation (the Buffy channel)

Let's return now to the glimmer of an idea that appeared during the days of watching *Buffy the Vampire Slayer*, the idea that helped us begin to understand the flickering-background results that we had found so surprising (see Figures 2.10 and 2.11). Figure 2.20 attempts to portray the idea as it first appeared. It was a vague idea that some adaptable "contrast comparison process" might be operating in these perceptions, a comparison process with the following characteristics:

The input to the possible comparison process is some kind of response that measures the local contrast at different positions in the visual field. For the texture patterns used here, measuring the local contrast is like measuring the contrast in each Gabor-patch element.

There is a "comparison level" (at each position in the visual field) and the process compares the current local contrast to that comparison level. The comparison level is shown by the arrow in the figure.

A possible comparison process

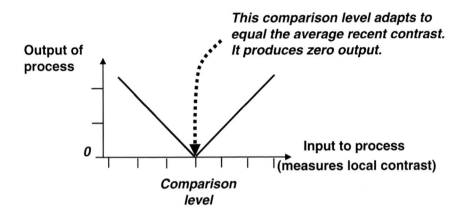

Figure 2.20. Diagram of a comparison process – an idea leading to a possible explanation for results like those in Figure 2.19.

And, most importantly, the comparison level is adaptable: It adapts to equal the average of its recent input (the input in some temporal interval before the current moment). Or, in other words, the comparison level equals the average recent local contrast.

The output of this possible comparison process (at any particular position) is then a measure of the difference between the current contrast and the average recent contrast (at that position). The output is zero when the current contrast and average recent contrast are equal, and it is positive when they are different, where the magnitude depends on just how different they are, but the direction of the difference is ignored. To get from this notion sketched in Figure 2.20 to something rigorous required some further steps.

2.4.1 How to measure local contrast for the input to this process

First, where could the input to this comparison process come from? That is, how can we measure local contrast to use as the input to this process? Figure 2.21 shows a structure that has been used by a number of people for this purpose. This particular filter–nonlinearity–filter (FNF) structure computes a measurement of the contrast in a particular spatial-frequency and orientation range (that corresponding to the first filter's receptive fields) at each position in the visual field.

The second filter in this structure is simply an excitatory-center-only receptive field. Thus it blurs the rectified output from the first filter. The second filter's excitatory-only center is about the size of a receptive field at the first filter, and thus it blurs over an area about the size of one such receptive field – which is approximately the size of the Gabor patches in our stimuli.

TO MEASURE LOCAL CONTRAST
(e.g. contrast in Gabor patch)

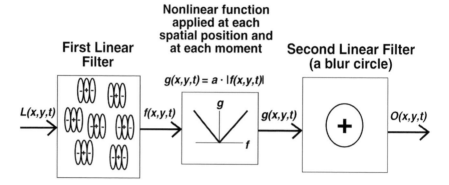

Figure 2.21. Diagram of a structure that can measure local contrast at the spatial frequency and orientation range corresponding to the receptive fields of the first-stage
filter. For the patterns used in the contrast adaptation experiments here (represented by
the function $L(x, y, t)$ in the figure), the output $O(x, y, t)$ of this structure (at any particular spatial position) will be a good measure of the contrast of a Gabor patch at that
position (assuming the Gabor patch has spatial frequency and orientation appropriate
for the first-stage filter). Functions specifying the outputs at intermediate stages within
the channel are represented by the symbols f and g, and a is an arbitrary constant. See
text for further description.

You would need multiple FNF structures like the one in Figure 2.21 to measure
the local contrast at all ranges of spatial frequency and orientation.

2.4.2   Extending the original complex channel to include this comparison process

Next we need to add an adaptable contrast comparison process (like that in Figure 2.20)
to the original complex channel (Figure 2.9). The resulting Buffy channel (as we will
call it for this chapter) is sketched in Figure 2.22.

A Buffy channel has three linear filters with two nonlinearities sandwiched between
(a $FNFNF$ structure). The first three stages ($F1 - N1 - F2$) have a structure identical
to that in Figure 2.21. The output from $F2$ – called $O_1(x, y, t)$ in Figure 2.22 – is a
measure of local contrast for a particular range of spatial frequency and orientation. It is
fed into a second nonlinearity $N2$ that acts at every spatial position. Very importantly,

A Buffy Channel

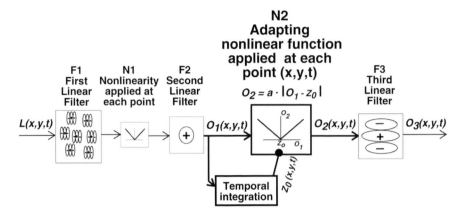

Figure 2.22. Diagram of a new kind of complex channel – a Buffy channel. It contains an embedded contrast adaptation process. The first three processes in the Buffy channel are a repeat of the structure shown in Figure 2.21. Their output, labeled $O_1(x, y, t)$ or O_1, is a measure of the local contrast at position (x, y) and time t. The zero-point (or comparison level) of the second nonlinearity $N2$ (the adapting nonlinearity) is denoted by the symbol $Z_0(x, y, t)$ or Z_0. This zero-point is set equal to the output of the temporal integration box, that is, to the recent time-averaged output of the second filter $F2$. The zero-point thus reflects the recent time-averaged local contrast. Thus $O_2(x, y, t)$ or O_2 (the output of the second nonlinearity $N2$) is zero whenever the current stimulus contrast is the same as the recent time-averaged contrast. And the output becomes larger as the current contrast becomes further (either increasing or decreasing) from the time-average contrast. The nonlinear function in $N2$ is shown here as a full-wave rectification (with a constant of proportionality a), but see Figure 2.23 for more information. The output $O_3(x, y, t)$ of the third filter $F3$, which is also the output from the whole Buffy channel, depends on the arrangement of the two elements types in the pattern. The third filter $F3$ shown in the illustrated Buffy channel will respond to contrast-defined horizontal stripes at a spacing corresponding to the spacing between the excitatory and inhibitory parts of the receptive field shown for $F3$. See text for further description.

this second pointwise nonlinearity $N2$ is *not* stable across time but instead adapts. In fact, it will play the role of the comparison process that was sketched in Figure 2.20. So let's look at this adaptable nonlinearity $N2$ more carefully.

The form of the nonlinear function $N2$ at any point (x, y, t) is some type of rectification. (An approximately symmetric full-wave rectification is shown in Figure 2.22.) Note the temporal-integration box in the figure: it integrates the measure of local contrast $O_1(x, y, t)$ where the integration is primarily over time although there could be some spatial integration as well. Thus the output of the temporal integration box $O_2(x, y, t)$ represents the average contrast over the recent past at position (x, y). This output is then connected (by a funny round-headed "arrow") to the second nonlinearity $N2$, in particular, to its zero-point Z_o which is the level of input into $N2$ that leads to an output of zero. The round-headed "arrow" is meant to indicate that the output from the temporal-integration box directly sets the value of the zero-point, and thus the zero-point Z_o at each position (x, y) acts like the comparison level in Figure 2.20. It adapts to reflect the average recent contrast at that position. Therefore, if the current contrast at a particular position equals the recent averaged contrast at that position, the output of the second nonlinearity $N2$ will be (approximately) zero there. But if the current contrast differs from the recent averaged contrast (either above or below it), the output from $N2$ will be positive with a magnitude reflecting the difference between the current contrast and the recent averaged contrast.

The output from the second nonlinearity $N2$ is fed into a third filter $F3$. This third filter in the Buffy channel performs the function of the second filter in the original form of complex channel (Figure 2.9). It is able to respond to the striped arrangement in an element-arrangement texture when the stripes have the right spatial period and orientation to match the characteristics of its receptive field and the elements are matched to the characteristics of the first-stage receptive fields.

Figure 2.22 shows one Buffy channel. Of course, we are assuming the existence of many Buffy channels sensitive to many different ranges of spatial frequency and orientation at the first and third stage filters. The excitatory center in the second filter is always approximately matched in size to the receptive field of the first filter.

As it turns out, we will also have to assume that the kind of rectification in the adapting nonlinearity $N2$ can vary depending on the observer. It is usually not a standard full-wave or half-wave rectification but something intermediate.

And, further, for a half-wave or intermediate case, we will need to assume a pair of Buffy channels, identical to one another except for the exact form of their second nonlinearities. Figure 2.23 shows an example of the $N2$ functions for such a pair of channels. In each such pair, one channel's second nonlinearity has an asymmetry favoring increases or onsets in contrast relative to the comparison level (called here the "On" member of the pair); the other's second nonlinearity has an asymmetry favoring decreases or offsets in contrast (the "Off" member of the pair). We are using "On" and "Off" here to refer to contrast in analogy to the way they have often been used to refer to increases (onsets) and decreases (offsets) of luminance.

Before moving on to predictions for experimental results, let's note one general aspect of the change in the second nonlinearity $N2$, that is, the resetting of the zero-point (i.e. comparison level) based on recent average contrast. This change is of an additive/subtractive sort rather than multiplicative/divisive. The zero-point that is changed is *subtracted* from the current contrast. This change is not in a multiplicative or divisive "gain" parameter, which is the kind of change in most contrast-gain processes that people talk about (including the normalization process that was the beginning point of our interest in these experiments).

N2 functions from a pair of otherwise-identical Buffy channels

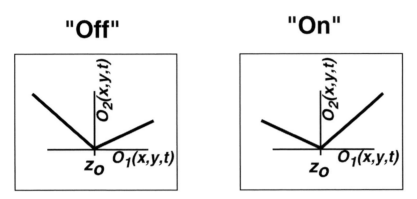

Figure 2.23. A possible pair of $N2$ functions for a pair of Buffy channels. For most observers, the static form of $N2$ does not seem to be either precisely a full-wave or half-wave rectification but rather something intermediate. And, further, one needs to assume that there will be a pair of channels where one channel has an asymmetry favoring increases in contrast (the "On" member of the pair) and the other has an asymmetry favoring decreases in contrast (the "Off" member of the pair). The $N2$ functions from such a pair are what is shown in this figure.

The next figure (Figure 2.24) shows the full model framework that appeared earlier in Figure 2.8 but now with the original complex channels replaced by Buffy channels.

2.4.3   Predictions from Buffy channels

Figure 2.25 compares experimental results (filled diamonds) with predictions from Buffy channels (thick gray smooth curves). The results shown are from the Buffy Steady-State conditions for four observers (including JW and SH from earlier figures). The predictions are from a model containing Buffy channels and little else except the necessary rule relating the observer's response to the outputs of the channels. (We will get back to other processes in Figure 2.24 – e.g. normalization – below.) And we made one important further assumption for the predictions shown in Figure 2.25: We assumed that the integration time of the temporal-integration box was shorter than the approximate 1 s of steady-state background before the probe was presented. Thus, the zero-point of $N2$ for these predictions always corresponded to the Buffy Steady-State

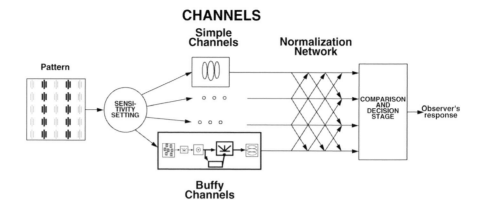

Figure 2.24. The full model from Figure 2.8 with Buffy channels replacing the original complex channels.

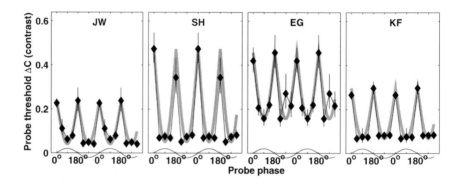

Figure 2.25. The solid diamonds show results from the Buffy Steady-State experiments for four observers (in different panels). The thick gray curved lines are predictions from a simplified model containing only Buffy channels. The predictions describe the experimental results well.

background contrast level C_0 (which was a contrast of 0.5 or 50% in these experiments).

The predictions in Figure 2.25 can be described quite easily as follows (although we will not derive them here). You take a sinusoidal function of the same frequency as the background flicker and in phase with it. You full-wave rectify this sinusoidal function. You turn it upside down. You move it up and down (an additive parameter) and stretch it or compress it uniformly (a multiplicative parameter). There is another possible degree of freedom in the predicted functions, although we didn't use it here: It allows you to cut off the rounded bottom of the predictions with a flat horizontal line at an arbitrary height. In principle, you do all of these things simultaneously until you get a best fit. Here we have just settled for a satisfactory fit by eye since that fit is already better than the experimental results collected to date could reject.

For the interested reader, the next subsection will pursue somewhat further the effect of changing various characteristics of the Buffy channels on the exact predictions. But a reader can skip this next subsection with no loss of continuity.

2.4.4   The parameters of predictions like those in Figure 2.25

Collectively the freedom in the manipulations described above for fitting the predictions to the results in Figure 2.25 come from three parameters in the simplified Buffy channel model. These are (1) a parameter representing the observer's visual sensitivity to these patterns, (2) a parameter representing properties of the decision stage, and (3) a parameter indicating the exact form of the functions characterizing $N2$.

This last parameter is most interesting. If these $N2$ functions are exactly conventional full-wave functions, the maximum thresholds (those for the STRADDLING test stimuli – phases $0°$ and $180°$) would be infinite. This is unlike any of our observers so far. If the $N2$ functions are exactly conventional half-wave functions, the ratio between the maximum thresholds (for STRADDLING test stimuli) and the minimum thresholds (for ABOVE and BELOW test stimuli at phases $90°$ and $270°$) would be at most equal to 2. The exact ratio depends on factors other than the functions in $N2$. Conventional half-wave functions may predict the results for observer EG for whom the ratio of maximum to minimum is the smallest of all the observers (and not significantly different from 2). For the other observers we have studied so far, however, the $N2$ functions need to be intermediate between half-wave and full-wave (like those in Figure 2.23). Alternately, although we have not yet explored this formally, the results might also be predictable by mixtures of different kinds of channels, where some channels have half-wave and some have full-wave $N2$ functions.

Still other degrees of freedom in the model are connected with other variations in the form of the $N2$ functions. For the predictions in Figure 2.25, we considered only piecewise-linear functions and assumed that the two functions in a pair are mirror images of each other (as in Figure 2.23). However, some previous evidence (Graham and Sutter, 1998) suggests that either these $N2$ functions – or else the functions in $N1$ – need to be power functions with an exponent between 3 and 4 rather than piecewise-linear (an exponent of 1) as shown here. If the $N2$ functions are such power functions, the predictions in Figure 2.25 would be somewhat differently shaped but they would still fit the results well. Or to put it another way, the results shown here cannot discriminate among different powers (unlike the results in Graham and Sutter, 1998).

There is another variation in the exact form of the $N2$ functions which results like those in Figure 2.25 could discriminate among. The pairs of functions we have considered so far have contained mirror-image members (as in Figure 2.23). If the two members of a pair are not mirror images, the thresholds for the peak ($90°$) and trough ($270°$) phases may differ from one another. There is a hint of such asymmetry in the data of JW (Figure 2.25) but that result is not reliable, and we have not seen any observers showing a reliable difference.

2.5   Where are we now?

Overall, the fits in Figure 2.25 – which assume the contrast-adaptation process embedded in Buffy channels – are very good. This successful prediction of experimental results suggests that such an adaptation process exists. But that leaves us with a number of questions.

2.5.1   Do we know anything yet about the dynamics of the contrast-adaptation process in the Buffy channels?

First, let's look at the following question. Can we use the experimental results on flickering backgrounds (Figure 2.10) to give us some indication of the dynamics of the adaptation process in the Buffy channel (the process that resets the comparison level Z_o in the adapting nonlinearity $N2$)?

Remember that the results from the Buffy Steady-State condition are presumed to be the results on an infinitely high frequency flickering background (assuming the existence of a temporal-integration process). Notice also the results on a 5.3 Hz flickering background (lower right panel Figure 2.10) show strong indications of the same process that is shown in the observer's results in the Buffy Steady-State condition (Figure 2.16, right panel); in particular, there is dramatic frequency doubling in both. This similarity of results suggests that 5.3 Hz is approximately equal to an infinitely-high frequency (only for our purposes here, of course). Or to put it another way, first noting that one cycle of 5.3 Hz occupies 190 ms, the similarity suggests that most (although perhaps not all) of the temporal integration in the Buffy channels extends for at least 190 ms.

Can we estimate an upper limit on how long the temporal integration window might be? For some observers (but not JW), there is also some obvious frequency doubling in the results for a frequency of 2.7 Hz or even lower. And even when you cannot see frequency doubling in the results, there may be some effect of the contrast-adaptation process in the Buffy channels nonetheless. (The frequency-doubling effect of a Buffy channel's adaptation process may be counteracted by effects of some other process controlled by contrast, for example the normalization which was ignored in the predictions of Figure 2.25. We will return to that normalization process below.) However, we think it is probably reasonable to say the following, first noting that one cycle of 2.7 Hz is 380 ms. Although there may be some effect of temporal integration in the Buffy channels that extends for as long 380 ms or even longer, most of the temporal integration is over before then. So the effective integration time of the adapting nonlinearity in the Buffy channels might be something like 250 ms.

It is interesting to consider the relationship of this timing to that of eye movements. The integration time here is probably short enough that the comparison level (zero-point) in the Buffy channel is totally reset by the end of most fixations of the eye. And resetting a contrast comparison level within each eye fixation may be important since the contrast (in the image stimulating any one receptive field) is almost completely uncorrelated from one fixation to the next (Frazor and Geisler, 2006).

But more work – both empirical and modeling – is certainly required to tie this estimate down. Some of the complications are discussed next.

2.5.2 What about the dynamics of the normalization process?

As mentioned before, the predictions in Figure 2.25 were done assuming the existence of Buffy channels but ignoring the possibility of any kind of process like normalization. Yet we have good reason to suppose that a normalization-type contrast-gain control process is operating on these patterns. In the interest of closure, although more empirical and modeling work needs to be done before we have any good basis for believing anything, let us say what is our current opinion is. We think that some of the changes in probe threshold as we change the phase of the probe and the frequency of the flickering background (especially at very low frequencies) may reflect the dynamics of the normalization process (the process that we intended to study when we began these experiments). Whether it will ever be possible to disentangle the dynamics of normalization from those of the adaptation process in the Buffy channel is unclear to us.

2.5.3 What about the original form of complex channels?

When one finds a new result, that requires for its explanation the addition or modification of a process in a model that has already successfully predicted many other experimental results, one needs to go back and think carefully about the previous successful predictions.

One very important issue is whether the new entity – in this case the Buffy channel – is still consistent with successful predictions for the older experiments. In our case, the answer is quite easy. Since all our older experiments had the observer adapted to zero contrast (a plain gray field) before each test stimulus, that is the only condition we need to consider. The Buffy channels, after adaptation to zero contrast, act exactly like the original form of complex channel. Since the original form led to successful predictions, so will the Buffy form.

A more subtle question is whether the human visual system might contain both the original *un*-adaptable type of complex channel and also the adaptable Buffy channels. For reasons that are not worth the space to explain here, we think the answer is yes. We think we can design experiments that will test the possibility that both exist, but have not done so yet.

2.5.4 Why should there be a contrast-adaptation process like that in the Buffy channels?

Let's go now to the evolutionary "why" question. Why does a process exist that produces results like those in Figures 2.17 and 2.19, results that can be predicted by the Buffy channels shown in Figure 2.22? Why should there be a process like this at all? Why has evolution led to this? Getting definitive evidence about any evolutionary "why" question is difficult if not impossible. But thinking about the functionality –

about the evolutionary history – of visual processes has led to many interesting insights and ideas for further research. So we will do a bit here.

Adaptation to many different characteristics of visual stimuli occurs. We have discussed adaptation both to luminance and to contrast in this chapter, but there are a very large number of others. A number of different reasons why such adaptation might exist (functions that such adaptation might perform) have been suggested, most of which can be grouped within two general classes. First let's briefly look at these two classes and then go on to ask whether either class of explanation can help make sense of the experimental results here.

(1) *Re-centering the operating range of a process to enhance its ability to discriminate among stimuli within that operating range.*

A system can usually only respond in a well-differentiated way to stimulus values within an operating (or dynamic) range, that is, within a limited portion of the possible range of stimulus values in the environment. The responses to values below and above that operating range are all at the minimum or all at the maximum response level, respectively. Thus the observer can discriminate very well between two values that are within the operating range, but cannot discriminate at all well between two values that are either both below or both above that range. But if the placement of that range on the stimulus dimension can be adjusted by a process of adaptation to match the environment, then this limit in dynamic range may not be a large deficit because the range might be approximately in the right place for whatever stimulus comes next. Thus one common idea is that: the function of adaptation is to re-center the operating range of the system to be centered near or at the current adaptation level (the average level in the recent past of whatever kind of input is at issue). The function of light adaptation is widely believed to be of this sort.

(2) *Responding to changes in the visual field (because changes signal important events in the environment, and/or to make neural coding more efficient).*

An alternate view is that the important function of adaptation is to suppress the response to unchanged visual stimuli and thereby highlight the responses to changes in stimuli. Two different classes of supporting arguments seem to be given. One is that a change in the visual stimulus is likely to mean an important change in the environment. The arrival of a predator is a common and dramatic example. Alternatively, people sometimes argue that physiology places serious constraints on how much information can be transmitted by the visual system. They argue that a coding scheme that suppresses the amount of information transmitted about unchanged things and only transmits information about changes can be more efficient in various ways. Either of these two classes of supporting argument suggest that evolutionary pressures might tend to produce visual processes that respond best to changes in stimulation rather than to continuation of unchanged stimulation. Or, as sometimes said, the visual system responds best to transients.

Let's look now at whether either of these classes of proposed explanations of adaptation's function helps us make sense of our results here.

The first class of explanation – re-centering the dynamic range at the recent average level in order to keep discriminability high there – does not seem to help us at all. In particular, as mentioned earlier, performance in the Buffy Steady-State condition is worse for a test stimulus that STRADDLES the background level (the recent average level) than for test stimuli containing contrasts further away from the background (the ABOVE and BELOW test stimuli). Being worst near the adaptation level is exactly the opposite of what you would expect from the first class of explanation.

The second class of explanation may provide some insight although it still leaves us wondering. The adaptation process we are suggesting resets the comparison level in the Buffy channel to represent the recent average level of contrast. Or, to say this in slightly different words: the zero-point of the Buffy channel's second nonlinearity $N2$ (at any particular spatial position) resets during the course of a steady background so that the second nonlinearity $N2$ produces zero response to a continuation of the steady background. But when a test stimulus comes on, producing a sudden transient in the contrast (at that spatial position), the second nonlinearity $N2$ (at that spatial position) now can easily signal that transient change by responding above zero. So the desirability of responding only to changes (and not responding at all to ongoing stimuli), as assumed by the second class of explanation, does seem illuminating up to this point. The adaptation of the zero-point Z_0 in the second nonlinearity $N2$ could be a process whose function is to signal transients.

A puzzle remains, however. The experimental results show that the STRADDLING test pattern is very hard to see. In other words, they show that increases and decreases in contrast do not produce diffferent enough results to allow the observer to perceive a pattern made up of these increases and decreases (e.g. our STRADDLING test pattern). To put it still another way, although the fact of a change of contrast can be well signaled in each local area of the pattern, the direction of that change is not signaled well. In terms of our model, increases and decreases in contrast lead to such similar responses by the second nonlinearity $N2$ that the contrast-defined arrangement in the test pattern is very hard to perceive.

This last aspect of the Buffy channel and its embedded contrast adaptation seems odd. Why would evolution have led to this result? Was it something that had some particular functional value in and of itself that led to it being actively selected-for by evolutionary pressures? We cannot imagine what that functional value would be, but perhaps someone else can. Or was its evolution a side-effect of the selection of some other thing? That seems a bit more likely to us. The thing that might have been so useful that it drove evolution might well have been the fact of signaling a change, any change, as quickly as possible. And then the following seems plausible to us. Perhaps wiring a neural system so that it can signal a change quickly without regard to direction of the change is much less costly (in terms of whatever kinds of costs limit evolution of neural tissue) than wiring a system to signal quickly both a change and its direction. We wish we had some idea of what the constraint producing that cost might be.

2.5.5 Ending comment

And so ends the first episode of a story that began with some experimental results that we did not believe and that might have halted our investigation into the dynamics of contrast-controlled adaptation processes. But we were saved by the expectancy-overcoming effects of watching *Buffy the Vampire Slayer*. This story ends, for now, with the introduction of Buffy channels, a suggested new form of channel that contains a nonlinearity showing fast contrast adaptation. This contrast adaptation changes an additive constant, a constant you might call "a comparison level." The integration period for this adaptation may be something like 250 ms. We still find this proposed channel somewhat puzzling. In the near future we plan to investigate it further, empirically and theoretically. We will perhaps find a more descriptive name for it once we understand better its characteristics and function, but for the moment we are happy to give Buffy the credit she deserves.

Acknowledgements

This work was supported in part by National Eye Institute grant EY08459. Some of these results were presented at the Spring 2005 VSS meeting (Wolfson and Graham, 2005b). We thank our observers for their hours of effort, and we thank Alisa Surkis and Jiatao Wang for computing predictions from the models of contrast-gain processes mentioned in Section 2.2. Finally, we would also like to thank the colleagues who spent time and energy talking to us about these results and ideas.

References

Beck, J., Prazdny K. and Rosenfeld, A. (1983). A theory of textural segmentation. In J. Beck, B. Hope and A. Rosenfeld, eds. *Human and Machine Vision*. New York: Academic, pp. 1–38.

Carandini, M., Heeger, D. J. and Movshon, J. A. (1997). Linearity and normalization in simple cells of the macaque primary visual cortex. *J. Neurosci.*, **17**, 8621–8644.

Frazor, R. A. and Geisler, W. S. (2006). Local luminance and contrast in natural images. *Vis. Res.*, **46**, 1585–1598.

Graham, N. (1989). *Visual Pattern Analyzers*. New York: Oxford University Press.

Graham, N. (1992). Breaking the visual stimulus into parts. *Cur. Direct. Psycholog. Sci.*, **1**, 55–61.

Graham, N., Beck, J. and Sutter, A. (1992). Nonlinear processes in spatial-frequency channel models of perceived texture segregation. *Vis. Res.*, **32**, 719–743.

Graham, N. and Hood, D. C. (1992). Modeling the dynamics of light adaptation: The merging of two traditions. *Vis. Res.*, **32**, 1373–1393.

Graham, N. and Sutter, A. (1998). Spatial summation in simple (Fourier) and complex (non-Fourier) texture channels. *Vis. Res.*, **38**, 231–257.

Graham, N. and Sutter, A. (2000). Normalization: Contrast-gain control in simple (Fourier) and complex (non-Fourier) pathways of pattern vision. *Vis. Res.*, **40**, 2737–2761.

Graham, N. and Wolfson, S. S. (2001). A note about preferred orientations at the first and second stages of complex (second-order) texture channels. *J. Opt. Soc. Am. A*, **18**, 2273–2281.

Graham, N., Wolfson, S. S. and Chowdhury, J. (2001). A comparison of light adaptation results from 40 years of the probed-sinewave paradigm. *Invest. Ophth. Vis. Sci.*, **42**, S157, abstract #840.

Hayhoe, M. M., Levin, M. E. and Koshel, R. J. (1992). Subtractive processes in light adaptation. *Vis. Res.*, **32**, 323–333.

Hood, D. C. and Graham, N. (1998). Threshold fluctuations on temporally modulated backgrounds: A possible physiological explanation based upon a recent computational model. *Vis. Neurosci.*, **15**, 957–967.

Hood, D. C., Graham, N., von Wiegand, T. E. and Chase, V. M. (1997). Probed-sinewave paradigm: A test of models of light-adaptation dynamics. *Vis. Res.*, **37**, 1177–1191.

Landy, M. and Graham, N. (2003). Visual perception of texture. In L. M. Chalupa and J. S. Werner, eds., *The Visual Neurosciences*. MIT Press: Cambridge, MA, pp. 1106-1118.

Lennie, P. (1998). Single units and visual cortical organization. *Percept.*, **27**, 889–935.

Snippe, H. P, Poot, L. and van Hateren, J. H. (2000). A temporal model for early vision that explains detection thresholds for light pulses on flickering backgrounds. *Vis. Neurosci.*, **17**, 449–462.

Snippe, H. P., Poot, L. and van Hateren, J. H. (2004). Asymmetric dynamics of adaptation after onset and offset of flicker. *J. Vis.*, **4**, 1–12.

Wilson, H. R. (1997). A neural model of foveal light adaptation and afterimage formation. *Vis. Neurosci.*, **14**, 403–423.

Wilson, H. R. and Humanski, R. (1993). Spatial frequency adaptation and contrast gain control. *Vis. Res.*, **33**, 1133–1149.

Wolfson, S. S. and Graham, N. (2000). Exploring the dynamics of light adaptation: The effects varying the flickering background's duration in the probed-sinewave paradigm. *Vis. Res.*, **40**, 2277–2289.

Wolfson, S. S. and Graham, N. (2001a). Comparing increment and decrement probes in the probed-sinewave paradigm. *Vis. Res.*, **41**, 1119–1131.

Wolfson, S. S. and Graham, N. (2001b). Processing in the probed-sinewave paradigm is likely retinal. *Vis. Neurosci.*, **18**, 1003–1010.

Wolfson, S. S. and Graham, N. (2005a). Element-arrangement textures in multiple objective tasks. *Spatial Vis.*, **18**, 209–226.

Wolfson, S. S. and Graham, N. (2005b). Dynamics of contrast-gain controls in pattern vision. *Vis. Sci. Soc.*, **5**, 760a.

Wu, S., Burns, S. A., Elsner, A. E., Eskew Jr., R. T. and He, J. (1997). Rapid sensitivity changes on flickering backgrounds: Tests of models of light adaptation. *J. Opt. Soc. Am. A*, **14**, 2367–2378.

3 Image comparison and motion detection by *a contrario* methods

Frédéric Cao, Thomas Veit and Patrick Bouthemy

3.1 Introduction

One of the main problems in computer vision is to make decisions automatically, since the visual interpretation of a scene may be viewed as the answers to a series of questions. These questions can often be turned into binary ones, in which case the answer can often be formulated in terms of thresholding. Since a complete system will raise many questions, many thresholds have to be fixed. Such a system is usable only if those thresholds are robust, or/and can be set automatically. Many recent developments make the assumption that there is a "ground truth" and that this ground truth can be learned. This is the point of view of machine learning theory and most methods use Bayesian approaches: given some prior knowledge, what is the best interpretation of the scene? Although this point of view is very rich and allows one to introduce high-level information, the scope of applications has to be precise enough, since the learning database must cover all the possible cases. We believe that for low-level vision tasks, prior knowledge is not always mandatory and learning is not always necessary. On the contrary, we will use a general theory, discovered a few years ago (Desolneux *et al.*, 2000), that enables to answer simple questions in a fully unsupervised way. More precisely, this chapter focuses on two questions.

- Given two images, can we say that they have a strong similarity?

- Given a sequence of images, are there some regions with a motion significantly different from the apparent background motion?

Computational Vision in Neural and Machine Systems, ed. L. Harris and M. Jenkin. Published by Cambridge University Press. © Cambridge University Press 2007.

We will see that exactly the same principle can be applied to solve those apparently very different problems. This principle has been introduced a few years ago by Desolneux and others (Desolneux *et al.*, 2000, 2001, 2005) who aimed at applying some of the principles of Gestalt Theory to computer vision. The idea is very simple and had already been somehow found by Helmholtz (1867). It says that an event is conspicuous (and can therefore be perceived) if it has a very small probability to occur "by chance". Of course, "by chance" here refers to a probabilistic model of randomness that must be defined before any calculation. Instead of trying to formulate this principle in full generality (this would be abstract and actually inapplicable), an instantiation in several simple cases will be given, with applications to computer vision.

3.1.1 Number of false alarms and the birthday problem

Let us first consider the following toy example, known as the birthday problem. In a group of N people, we remark that k of them have the same birthday. Is this is a pure coincidence, or there is another unknown reason to explain this observation? A classical way to answer this question is to make the *a contrario* hypothesis that all birthdays are independent and uniformly distributed in the year. Under this assumption, it is possible to compute the probability P_k^N of the event E_k^N defined by: "there is at least a k-tuple of people (out of N) born on the same day." A classical result gives

$$P_2^N = 1 - \frac{1}{365^N} \prod_{i=0}^{N-1} (365 - i). \tag{3.1}$$

Indeed, it is easy to compute the probability that all people have different birthdays. The birthday of the first person is arbitrarily chosen. This leaves 364 possible days for the second birthday, then 363 for the third one, etc. Numerical computation leads to $P_2^{23} = 0.5073$. Hence a classical answer is that if $N \geq 23$ (which may seem very low), it should not be a surprise to observe two common birthdays, since this happens 50% of the time. Of course, this model is very simplistic since it neglects leap years, and it is also well known that birthdays are not uniformly spread over the year.

A less obvious calculation leads to P_3^N, the probability that at least 3 people are born on the same day:

$$P_3^N = P_2^N - \frac{1}{365^N} \sum_{i=0}^{\lfloor N/2 \rfloor} \frac{\prod_{j=1}^{i} \left(\dfrac{N - 2j + 2}{2} \right)}{i!} \prod_{j=0}^{N-i-1} (365 - j). \tag{3.2}$$

The numerical evaluation is also quite difficult. For $k \geq 3$, the calculation of P_k^N by induction is still feasible but it gets worse and the numerical evaluation is also more difficult. The difficulty of the calculation comes from the non-independence of all the k-tuples (since they may have a non-empty intersection). A much more easy calculation is the following. Consider the expectation of the number of k-tuples of people born on the same day. We call number of false alarms of E_k^N this expectation, and denote it by $NFA(E_k^N)$. This terminology is motivated by the following argument.

The situation is completely random; hence, each time an event is observed, the only explanation is chance, and detecting it is irrelevant. It is elementary to prove that

$$NFA(E_k^N) = \binom{N}{k} \frac{1}{365^{k-1}}. \tag{3.3}$$

Indeed, for a given k-tuple $(i_1, \ldots, i_k)$, let $Y(i_1, \ldots, i_k)$ be the binary random variable equal to 1 if the i_1th, ..., i_kth persons are born on the same day and 0 else. Then $Y(i_1, \ldots, i_k) = 1$ with probability 365^{1-k}, yielding $\mathbb{E}(Y(i_1, \ldots, i_k)) = 365^{1-k}$. But

$$NFA(E_k^N) = \mathbb{E}\left(\sum_{(i_1, \ldots i_k)} Y(i_1, \ldots i_k) \right), \tag{3.4}$$

the sum being taken on all k-tuples. Since there are exactly $\binom{N}{k}$ k-tuples in a set of N elements, (3.3) follows by linearity of the expectation.

What is the interest of the NFA? First, let us remark that $\log(NFA(E_k^N))$ is not very hard to approximate even for large values of k and N. Moreover, $NFA(E_k^N) \geq 1$ means that, in average, we can expect at least one k-tuple of common birthdays. Hence, this is definitely not surprising to observe such an event. On the contrary, if $NFA(E_k^N)$ is less than 1, then we should not observe E_k^N. More generally, we will say that E_k^N is ε-meaningful if $NFA(E_k^N) < \varepsilon$. The lower ε, the less likely E_k^N is produced by chance, hence the more meaningful it is. Making the decision amounts to choose a value to ε. We will see in the following that this value only has a logarithmic influence and it can be set to 1 in all applications.

3.1.2 Outline of the chapter

Section 3.2 is dedicated to image comparison. After introducing the general framework in Section 3.2.1, a number of false alarms (NFA) is defined in Section 3.2.2. It will be seen that the decision can only be based on this number, and that decision is robust (Section 3.2.3). The relation with classical hypothesis testing will be discussed in Section 3.2.4. Section 3.2.5 gives some experiments. Section 3.3 deals with motion detection. In Section 3.3.2, the formulation of the problem will lead to the very same calculations as for image comparison. Section 3.3.3 points out some possible extensions and improvements. Section 3.3.4 gives experiments on real sequences.

3.2 Image comparison

3.2.1 Problem statement

Let us now apply the same ideas for image comparison. Assume that a database of N_B images is given. We now consider an image and want to know whether or not the database contains a "very similar" image. What "similar" does really mean is highly contextual: are we talking about colors, about geometrical shapes, or semantical objects? The following theory definitely does not cope with semantics, which is much more difficult and requires prior knowledge.

We shall only be interested in very strong hints of common geometrical content. The problem is that the original image can undergo deformations including scaling, contrast change, transmitting or compression noise, partial occlusion. The purpose is to detect geometrical similarity, possibly modulo a class of geometrical and radiometric transformations.

Most comparison methods use two steps: the extraction of robust, local, invariant parts of the images, and a distance between parts of the image. In this chapter, we do not cope with the first part (normalization), and refer the reader to Mikolajczyk *et al.* (2005) where parts of images are extracted from local characteristics as key points, to Lisani *et al.* (2003) and Rothwell (1995) where stable directions are used to compute local frames. Instead, we focus on the second part which is the comparison phase.

Hence, the starting point is a pair of normalized (i.e. set in an intrinsic frame) images u and v of size $N \times N$. Geometrical distortion (translation, rotation and scaling) is assumed canceled by the normalization. (Let us remark that we cannot talk about registration for now, since we do not know whether u and v correspond to the same scene.) On the other hand, contrast change may not be corrected at this point. However, the criterion which is described in the following is invariant with respect to contrast change. The aim is to decide if yes or no, u and v are similar images, and likely to have shapes or geometrical contents in common.

The statistical arguments we introduce can be related to the work of Lisani and Morel (2003). Their approach uses the direction of the spatial gradient of a grey level image, and they detect local changes in registered stereo pairs of satellite images. Our method is dual since, on the contrary, we use the gradient direction in both images to decide that they have much spatial information in common. Older work (Venot *et al.*, 1982) used the same kind of ideas but detection thresholds were not precisely computed. Other widely used image features are SIFT descriptors (Lowe, 1999, 2004) which are basically local direction distributions. Nevertheless, the indexing and comparison of descriptors is achieved by a nearest-neighbor procedure. Hence, there are no automatic decision thresholds, which is precisely our main concern. On the other hand, we think that our methodology can be adapted to the comparison of SIFT features. Basically, our method consists in sampling random points in two images and counting the number of points such that the difference of the gradient direction is "small". If this number is large enough, then images have certainly a common cause. Let us remark that contrarily to methods as RANSAC (Fischler and Bolles, 1981), we do not try to estimate any registration parameters, because probabilities will be computed in a model representing the absence of similarity (background model, in the statistical meaning). Some similar idea can be found in (Grimson and Huttenlocher, 1990) where the authors study the influence of "conspiracy of random."

3.2.2   Image comparison criterion

We assume that u and v are grey level images, and $u(x)$ and $v(x)$ denote the grey level of u and v at position x. For any point x, let us denote by $\theta_u(x)$ and $\theta_v(x)$ the directions of the gradient of u and v at point x. Let us denote by $D_{u,v}(x)$ the angular difference between $\theta_u(x)$ and $\theta_v(x)$). It is a real value in $[0, \pi]$, and to simplify the notations, it will be denoted by $D(x)$. Since this measure is to be fairly accurate, only points where both image gradients are large enough (larger than 5 in practice) are taken into account. Now, two images differing from a contrast change have the same gradient direction everywhere. Indeed, if $v = g(u)$ where $g : \mathbb{R} \to \mathbb{R}$ is a nondecreasing function, $Dv(x) = g'(u)Du(x)$, implying that Du and Dv point in the same direction.

Let us fix $\alpha \in (0, \pi)$. Consider M distinct points $\{x_1, \ldots, x_M\}$ and make the hypothesis that the M values $D(x_i)$ are independent and uniformly distributed in $(0, \pi)$. This hypothesis is certainly false if u and v are the same image, but it is sound if u and v are not related. Hence, it will be called *a contrario* hypothesis. Under this hypothesis, the probability that at least k among the M values $\{D(x_1), \ldots D(x_M)\}$ are less than α is given by the tail of the binomial law

$$B\left(M, k, \frac{\alpha}{\pi}\right) = \sum_{j=k}^{M} \binom{M}{j} \left(\frac{\alpha}{\pi}\right)^j \left(1 - \frac{\alpha}{\pi}\right)^{M-j}. \tag{3.5}$$

This leads to the following definition.

Definition 3.1 *Let $0 \leq \alpha_1 \leq \cdots \leq \alpha_L \leq \pi$ be L values in $[0, \pi]$. Let u be a real valued image, and $x_1, \ldots x_M$, M distinct points. Let us also consider a database $\mathcal{B}$ of $N_\mathcal{B}$ images. For any $v \in \mathcal{B}$, we call number of false alarms of (u, v) the quantity*

$$NFA(u, v) = N_\mathcal{B} \cdot L \cdot \min_{1 \leq i \leq L} B\left(M, k_i, \frac{\alpha_i}{\pi}\right), \tag{3.6}$$

where k_i is the cardinality of

$$\{j, 1 \leq j \leq M, D(x_j) \leq \alpha_i\}.$$

We say that (u, v) is ε-meaningful, or that u and v are ε-similar if $NFA(u, v) < \varepsilon$. The NFA is clearly monotonically decreasing in k_i. If u and v are similar, then their gradient have the same direction, and k_i is large. Hence, the NFA is a measure of similarity between two images. The lower the NFA, the more similar the images, and vice versa. Actually, the NFA is up to a normalization constant, related to the probability to observe at least k_i points with equal gradient direction (up to an error α_i). This normalization is explained by the following result.

Proposition 3.2 *For a database of $N_\mathcal{B}$ images such that the gradient direction difference with a query u has been generated under the a contrario hypothesis, the expected number of images v such that (u, v) is ε-meaningful is less than ε.* Proof. For a random image v, and a given i, $1 \leq i \leq L$, let us denote by K_i the random number of points among the x_j, $1 \leq j \leq M$ such that $D(x_j) \leq \alpha_i$. The pair (u, v) is ε-meaningful, if there exists $1 \leq i \leq L$ such that $N_\mathcal{B} \cdot L \cdot B(M, K_i, \alpha_i/\pi) < \varepsilon$. Let us denote by $E(v, i)$ this event. Its probability is

$$P(E(v, i)) = P\left(B\left(M, K_i, \frac{\alpha_i}{\pi}\right) < \frac{\varepsilon}{L \cdot N_\mathcal{B}}\right). \tag{3.7}$$

By definition of the *a contrario* hypothesis, K_i follows a binomial law, with parameters M and α_i/π. It is a classical result that if H is the survival function of a real valued random variable X (*i.e.* $H(t) = P(X > t)$), then $P(H(X) < t) \leq t$ for all $t \in (0, 1)$. Hence,

$$P\left(B\left(M, K_i, \frac{\alpha_i}{\pi}\right) < \frac{\varepsilon}{L \cdot N_\mathcal{B}}\right) \leq \frac{\varepsilon}{L \cdot N_\mathcal{B}}. \tag{3.8}$$

The event $E(v)$ defined by "(u, v) is ε-meaningful" is $E(v) = \cup_{1 \leq i \leq L} E(v, i)$. Let us denote by $\mathbb{E}$ the mathematical expectation under the *a contrario* hypothesis. Then,

$$
\begin{aligned}
\mathbb{E}\left(\sum_{v \in \mathcal{B}} \mathbf{1}_{E(v)}\right) &= \sum_{v \in \mathcal{B}} \mathbb{E}(\mathbf{1}_{E(v)}) \\
&= \sum_{v \in \mathcal{B}} P(E(v)) \\
&\leq \sum_{\substack{v \in \mathcal{B} \\ 1 \leq i \leq L}} P(E(v, i)) \\
&\leq \sum_{\substack{v \in \mathcal{B} \\ 1 \leq i \leq L}} \frac{\varepsilon}{L \cdot N_\mathcal{B}} = \varepsilon. \qquad \square
\end{aligned}
$$

Thus, Definition 3.1 together with Proposition 3.2 mean that, on average, there are less than ε images in the database $\mathcal{B}$ that match with u "by chance", that is to say, when the *a contrario* hypothesis holds. Under this hypothesis, any detection must be considered as a false alarm (hence the denomination). For instance, if $\varepsilon = 1$, we can expect in average one match between u and a database of white noise images. When less than a false alarm is required, we can simply set $\varepsilon < 1$. Let us note that the dependence upon the size of the database is automatically set in the definition of the NFA.

3.2.3 Numerical consideration on the NFA

The algorithm is actually simple, since it is mainly a mere counting after quantization of the observed angle values.

(1) Choose M random positions.

(2) Compute the direction of the gradients at these points.

(3) For each value of α_i:

   - count the number of points k_i such that the difference of gradient direction is less than α_i;
   - compute the values $N_\mathcal{B} \cdot L \cdot B\left(M, k_i, \alpha_i/\pi\right)$.

(4) If one of the computed values is less than ε, detect (u, v) as meaningful.

Now, there is a natural question: how to choose ε, M and L? We could take $L = 1$, that is choose a single quantization step. Since this choice is arbitrary, we prefer to test several hypotheses. The number of tested values is given by the accuracy we can expect on the angles, which is about $10°$. Hence L does not need to be very large. The price to pay for this multiple test is to multiply the NFA by L or, equivalently, divide ε by L. Actually, this has hardly any incidence. Indeed, let $r = k/M$ and $H(r, p) = r \ln(r/p) + (1-r) \ln[(1-r)/(1-p)]$. Classical asymptotic results (Hoeffding, 1963) yield

$$\ln(B(M, k, p)) \sim -M \cdot H(r, p),$$

when $k = rN$ for a fixed value $r \in (p, 1)$, and M goes to $+\infty$. The only observed value in this expression is r. Thus, it turns out that asymptotically, the threshold value on r (i.e. the ratio of points passing the test) depends on $\ln \varepsilon$. If we now assume that $r = k/M$ is fixed, it is clear that the NFA decreases when M gets larger. However, M should not be taken arbitrarily large, for two reasons.

(1) Large M need more computations.

(2) If two unrelated images have an alignment in common, and if many points are on the aligned segments, the image may be classified as similar because the *a contrario* hypothesis is (rightly) rejected. However, this simply detects that images are not random and contain alignments. Hence the sampled points have to be sparse enough.

Necessary and sufficient bounds on M can be derived from a more careful examination of the NFA (see Cao and Bouthemy, 2005). It turns out that values of M around 200 are sufficient even with a large amount of noise (e.g. Gaussian noise with standard deviation 20 for images with 256 gray levels). The experiments validate this estimate.

3.2.4 Relation with hypothesis testing

This section aims at comparing the *a contrario* decision with a more classical hypothesis testing approach. A usual way to solve the problem raised in the previous sections is to define the two hypotheses:

- $\mathcal{H}_0$: u and v are not related,

- $\mathcal{H}_1$: u and v are similar images.

As above, M pixels are randomly selected in the images and the directions of the grey level gradient are compared. To simplify, assume that we set only one threshold for the difference of the direction, that is to say $L = 1$. Let E_k^M be the event: "for at least k points out of M, the difference of the gradient direction is less than α." Two quantities are of particular interest:

- the probability of false alarm defined by $P(E_k^M | \mathcal{H}_0)$,

- and the probability of detection defined by $P(E_k^M | \mathcal{H}_1)$.

The decision rule (for instance the optimal Neyman–Pearson test; see Poor, 1994) is often obtained by thresholding the ratio between those probabilities. To compute them, it is necessary to analytically define $\mathcal{H}_0$ and $\mathcal{H}_1$. When the images are not related, it is quite natural to assume that the directions of the gradient are independent and that the differences are uniform. This is precisely the *a contrario* hypothesis of the previous section. Now, defining $\mathcal{H}_1$ is far less obvious since it would imply to know the dependencies between the samples or the noise amount. If $L > 1$ (multiple thresholds), the computation is even less feasible, since all the events with different angle thresholds are not independent. Definition 3.1 and Proposition 3.2 show that a decision rule can be defined only by using the probability of false alarms. It simply consists in thresholding this probability, by taking the number of observations into account, by a Bonferroni correction.

3.2.5   Experiments on image comparison

We first consider the following experiment. We select a single image in a sequence containing about one hour of video (86 096 images). A white Gaussian noise with standard deviation $\sigma = 30$ is added to this image, and will be taken as the query. The proposed criterion is applied with $M = 500$ random sample points in the images. The true image is detected with an *NFA* equal to 10^{-7}. The same view of the stadium appeared three other times, all of which are detected with the same magnitude of *NFA*. About 20 images (belonging to the same static shot) are detected around the query. There is a single true false alarm (unrelated images) with an *NFA* equal to $10^{-0.73}$, which is probably caused by the presence of the logo, on the top-right. This is a success since the theory predicts in average one casual detection. Moreover, the *NFA* of this detection is very close to 1. No false alarms are obtained for an impulse noise of 50%. Extreme JPEG compression (quality less than 10) may lead to false detections since gradient orientation is constrained by the blocking effect. For usual compression ratios, this effect was not observed.

In Figure 3.2, two images exhibiting a strong transparency effect are compared. In this case, the grey level is not reliable at all. However, the images clearly show some similarity. The comparison of the gradient direction proves that these images are similar, and explained bby the *a contrario* model. The NFA is extremely small (less than $10 - 58$ for 200 random points).

Figure 3.3 shows the robustness to occlusion. The score panel occludes a large part of the image in this tennis match video. The two images are detected as very similar since their number of false alarms is about 10^{-50}. Since an hour of video contains about 10^5 images, the match remains meaningful for any database size. The threshold on the gradient norm is equal to 5 in this experiment. The same experiment (still with 200 sample points) was performed for a gradient threshold equal to 0.2. The *NFA* increases, since points are selected where the gradient orientation is dominated by quantization. However, with an equal probability, points with larger gradients are also chosen, and the directions then match very well. Therefore, the *NFA* is still very low, and about 10^{-32}.

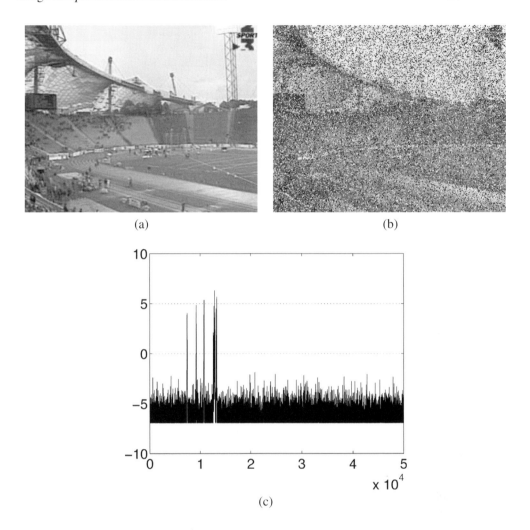

Figure 3.1. Image (b) is a 50% impulse noise version of image (a). In a database of 10^5 images, they still match with an *NFA* close to 10^{-5}. Image (c) shows $-\log_{10}(NFA)$ for the first 50 000 images of the sequence, the query being the noisy image. The peaks indeed correspond to exactly the same view of the stadium. The same views, but translated by 10 pixels, are not detected, since no prior registration has been performed in this experiment.

3.3 Motion detection

Another application of the same principle is early motion detection. By this, we mean that detection is performed on a very small temporal neighborhood, typically two or three frames, and no motion coherence is used.

Most motion detection algorithms decide for each image pixel if it belongs to a

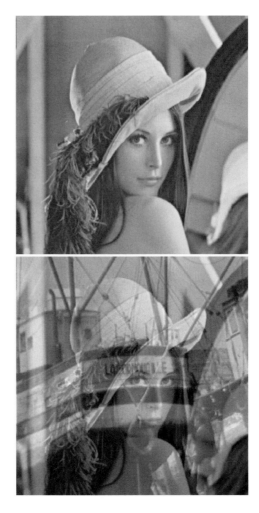

Figure 3.2. Robustness to transparency. The second image is the superposition of the first one and another image. With 200 sample points, the resemblance is easily detected and $\log_{10}(NFA) = -58.68$.

moving part of the image or to the static background. The decision is based on the thresholding of difference images according to an appropriate statistical model (Hsu *et al.*, 1984; Konrad, 2005; Rosin, 2002). The result is usually a binary map. Each pixel is labeled either as moving or static. A motion detection mask provided by a decision for each image pixel usually contains holes, owing to the lack of motion information inside the object and spots of false detection in static regions due to noise. These errors are attenuated (but not eliminated) by introducing regularization constraints and contextual information via Markov Random Fields (Aach and Kaup, 1995; Odobez and Bouthemy, 1997). The boundaries of the sets of detected pixels only approximately correspond to the contours of the moving objects.

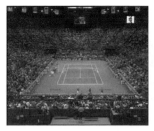 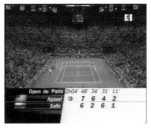 

Figure 3.3. Robustness to occlusion. Despite the large occlusion, the two images are detected as very similar with $\log_{10}(NFA) = -50.1$. The right plot gives the position of the 200 sample points. No points are selected in uniform areas (because of the gradient threshold). However, some points are selected in the non-matching area (scores banner), but the *NFA* is still very low.

A higher level of spatial structure can be reached using active contours. For instance the approach described by Paragios and Deriche (2000) applies active contours for detection and tracking of moving objects. It relies on the gray level intensities for providing object boundaries. Two methods using level sets implementation are introduced by Mansouri and Konrad (2003): one purely based on motion and another enforcing correspondence between motion boundaries and intensity boundaries. Besides, they can distinguish between different moving objects. However, the presence of moving objects is implicitly assumed by this kind of approach. Moving objects are segmented but the detection question is not answered.

Region-based motion detection based on spatial segmentation were proposed by Fablet *et al.* (1999) and Moscheni *et al.* (1998). The method in Moscheni *et al.* (1998) resorts to a graph-based region procedure controlled by several user-set parameters. In Fablet *et al.* (1999) a region-level graph is embedded in a Markovian framework. Again, the energy term involved in the definition of the Markov Random Field includes several parameters.

Variational Segmentation methods are often accurate but they do not solve the final decision step. This is precisely the aim of the following sections. A more detailed presentation of this work can be found in Veit *et al.* (2005a).

3.3.1   Problem setting and prerequisites

The camera motion is compensated for so that camera may be supposed static. Consider a set of N given regions of the image. Assume that a qualitative measure of motion is observed on the image; it is a scalar quantity, observed at each point taking a large value when the intensity varies much between consecutive instants. The question is: among the N candidate regions, are there some exhibiting a meaningful movement between consecutive instants?

Before answering this question, three prerequisites in the previous paragraph have to be fulfilled.

(1) The camera motion can be estimated. There exists very efficient methods com-

puting a global parametric motion, that mostly compensate the camera motion. For instance, Odobez and Bouthemy (1995) propose a fast robust multiresolution method to estimate the parameters of a polynomial motion field (up to 12 scalar parameters). In the following, this algorithm is used to estimate a quadratic 8 parameters model, whose expression is

$$\mathbf{w}_\theta(x) = \begin{pmatrix} a_1 \\ a_2 \end{pmatrix} + \begin{pmatrix} a_3 & a_4 \\ a_5 & a_6 \end{pmatrix} \cdot \begin{pmatrix} x_1 \\ x_2 \end{pmatrix} + \begin{pmatrix} a_7 & a_8 & 0 \\ 0 & a_7 & a_8 \end{pmatrix} \cdot \begin{pmatrix} x_1^2 \\ x_1 x_2 \\ x_2^2 \end{pmatrix} \tag{3.9}$$

with $\theta = (a_1, \ldots, a_8)$, and $x = (x_1, x_2)$. As all 2D-parametric motion models, this one cannot handle strong depth disparities (parallax), but it is a good compromise between accuracy and efficiency. It is exact for a rigid 3D-motion (as camera motion) undergone by a planar surface. The result of this step is an optimal set of parameters $\hat{\theta}$.

(2) A simple measure of change would be the so-called displaced frame difference (DFD) which is the difference of the grey level at each position, after motion compensation by $\mathbf{w}_{\hat{\theta}}$, i.e.

$$DFD_{\hat{\theta}}(x, t, t+1) = u(x + \mathbf{w}_{\hat{\theta}}(x), t+1) - u(x, t), \tag{3.10}$$

$u(x, t)$ and $u(x + \mathbf{w}_{\hat{\theta}}(x), t+1)$ being the image intensity at time t and $t+1$, respectively at point x and $x + \mathbf{w}_{\hat{\theta}}(x)$. (It is also usual to take the time unit equal to the interval between two frames.) However, this quantity is extremely sensitive to spatial intensity gradient. Pixels on or in the vicinity of image contours may display large DFD values, even if the residual motion is low. Indeed, small errors in the dominant motion estimation are enhanced along highly contrasted edges. On the contrary, uniform regions where the spatial intensity gradient is low obviously have low DFD whatever the magnitude of the residual motion.

For this reason, a more appropriate measure is the residual normal flow magnitude $w_{\hat{\theta}}^{res}$ defined by

$$w_{\hat{\theta}}^{res}(x, t, t+1) = \frac{|DFD_{\hat{\theta}}(x, t, t+1)|}{|Du(x, t)|}, \tag{3.11}$$

where $Du(x, t)$ is the *spatial* image intensity gradient. Remark that this quantity is indeed homogeneous to a velocity. Moreover, a straightforward calculation shows that it is an approximation of $1/|Du| \left(\frac{\partial u}{\partial t} + Du \cdot w_{\hat{\theta}} \right)$, which is contrast invariant (i.e. invariant to the transformation $u \rightarrow g(u)$ where g is smooth and nondecreasing). In order to deal with occlusion and disocclusion of the scene background by moving objects, a three-image scheme on images $u(t-1)$, $u(t)$ and $u(t+1)$ is considered. The reference image remains $u(t)$. Two dominant motions are estimated: a forward one from $u(t)$ to $u(t+1)$, leading to a set of parameters $\hat{\theta}_t^{t+1}$, and a backward one from $u(t)$ to $u(t-1)$, leading to $\hat{\theta}_t^{t-1}$. The considered measure is

$$C(x) = \min(w_{\hat{\theta}_t^{t+1}}^{res}(x, t, t+1), w_{\hat{\theta}_t^{t-1}}^{res}(x, t, t-1)) \,. \qquad (3.12)$$

Figure 3.8 shows the map of residual $C(x)$ for an image sequence.

(3) The last prerequisite is a set of candidate regions. These regions may be obtained by a simple quad-tree decomposition of the image. This choice is easy, fast, multiscale, but not accurate, since it is completely independent of the image. In the following, the interior of meaningful level lines (Desolneux *et al.*, 2001) will be used instead. It provides a set of nested regions and thus a hierarchy of segmentations. The interesting point is that they are also detected by an *a contrario* decision. These level lines often locally coincide with object contours. However, the motion detection below is not limited to this particular set of regions and can be applied to any type of spatial segmentation.

3.3.2 *A contrario* motion detection test

In an image where no moving object is present, the local residual motion measures C are only temporal noise. It is sound to assume that they are uncorrelated when considering sufficiently distant pixels. The computation of C requires the computation of the spatial gradient. This last one is computed by a 2×2 finite difference scheme. Hence, it cannot be assumed that points at distance less than 2 lead to independent values of C. Therefore, it is assumed that a region containing n pixels actually contains $n/4$ independent pixels. Moreover, since nothing is known about the location of the dynamical content of the scene, in the absence of motion, the local residual motion measures are supposed to be distributed identically upon the whole image according to the same probability distribution. This probability distribution can be learned empirically on the whole image. The accuracy of the learned distribution is not of the highest importance in this framework.

Now, that the *a contrario* model is specified, let us detail which events are considered under this model.

Let F denote the survival function of C. This function is defined by $F(\mu) = P(C > \mu)$, the probability that the local residual motion measure exceeds a given threshold μ. Let $\mu_i, i \in \{1, ..., N_t\}$ bet a set of N_t thresholds. Consider a region R containing n independent pixels, let k_i denote the observed number of independent pixels at which the motion measure exceeds the threshold μ_i. According to the *a contrario* model, the probability that at least k_i independent values of C among the n exceed the threshold μ_i is exactly the tail of a binomial distribution,

$$B(n, k_i, F(\mu_i)) = \sum_{j=k_i}^{n} \binom{n}{j} F(\mu_i)^j (1 - F(\mu_i))^{n-j}. \qquad (3.13)$$

This problem is exactly analogous to the problem of image comparison, and naturally leads to the following definition.

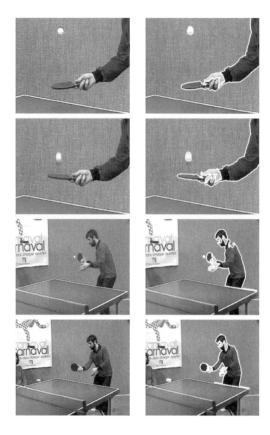

Figure 3.4. Table tennis sequence. Original images in the left column. The boundaries of the detected moving regions appear in white in the right column. Both the player and the ball are accurately detected in the four images. The values of the *NFA* for the detected regions are detailed in the text.

Definition 3.3   *Given a set of N_t values μ_i, $i = 1, \dots, N_t$, and a set of N_R regions, the Number of False Alarms (NFA) of a region R containing n independent pixels is*

$$NFA(R) = N_R \cdot N_t \cdot \min_{i=1,\dots,N_t} B(n, k_i, F(\mu_i)). \tag{3.14}$$

A region is an ε-meaningful (moving) region if $NFA(R) < \varepsilon$.   This definition is motivated by the following proposition.

Proposition 3.4   *The expected number of ε-meaningful moving regions under the a* contrario *hypothesis is less than ε.*   The proof is exactly the same as for Proposition 3.2.

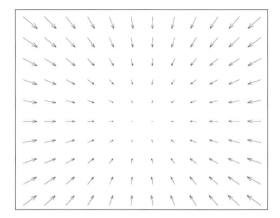

Figure 3.5. Estimated dominant motion for the second part of the table tennis sequence. The camera is zooming out. The computed quadratic motion model is represented by the velocity vectors evaluated at a given sampling rate over the image grid and magnified (with a scale factor of 5). Values of the parameters are $a_1 = 0.0386$, $a_2 = 0.0604$, $a_3 = -0.0181$, $a_4 = -0.0003$, $a_5 = -0.00171$, $a_6 = -0.01945$, $a_7 = 0.00001$, $a_8 = 0.00001$. The camera motion has been correctly estimated despite the presence of the moving player.

3.3.3 Extensions and improvements

It may happen that small and/or slowly moving regions are not detected, since their NFA may be too large. It may be necessary to integrate more than three images. This can be done very easily with the NFA since it is an additive measure. (It relates to an expectation.) More hypotheses can indeed be integrated in the definition of the NFA, which is a linear function of the number of tested hypotheses. The price to pay is a larger multiplicative constant. However, from Section 3.2.3, it is not a hard penalization (since detection depends on the logarithm of this multiplicative constant) and it usually improves the results. Another interesting extension can be achieved when the candidate regions are nested. In this case, they form a tree, and their "most meaningful" representation can be defined. The key point is to define a merging criterion choosing between a single large region and disjoint regions contained in it. The output of this algorithm is a set of *maximal meaningful regions*. All details can be found in Veit *et al.* (2005b).

3.3.4 Experimental results

The proposed method was tested on several outdoor and indoor image sequences. These sequences involve both rigid and articulated motions, static and moving cameras. The threshold ε on the number of false alarms was set to 1 for all experiments. The maximality principle cited in the previous section has been applied to select the

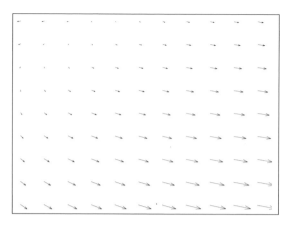

Figure 3.6. Estimated dominant motion for the road sequence. The camera is placed on a helicopter. It is rotating and translating in order to track the cars. Parameter values for the motion model are $a_1 = 7.1745$, $a_2 = 2.0394$, $a_3 = 0.02849$, $a_4 = 0.04075$, $a_5 = -0.0016$, $a_6 = 0.0122$, $a_7 = -0.00002$, and $a_8 = 0.00002$.

most meaningful regions. Let us emphasize that the NFA can directly be interpreted as a confidence level: the lower the NFA, the higher the confidence in the detection decision. An NFA of 10^{-10} means that, on average, 10^{10} images distributed according to the *a contrario* distribution have to be generated in order to observe such an accumulation of high residual velocity values.

The first video sequence depicts a table tennis player (see Figure 3.4). In the first part of this video (two upper rows of Figure 3.4), the camera is almost static and only the forearm of the player appears. The ball, the arm and the racket are correctly detected. The detected moving regions closely fit the contours of the moving object. The regions detected on the ball are associated with $NFAs$ of 10^{-20}. $NFAs$ on the arm are even much lower, about 10^{-150}. This reflects that the motion of the arm is perceptually much more meaningful.

In the second part of the video (two lower rows of Figure 3.4), the camera is zooming out. The global dominant motion estimation performs well (Figure 3.5), although the assumption of a planar background is not valid because the scene background (table + wall) is not planar. Both the ball and the body of the player are accurately detected. The NFA on the ball is about 10^{-1} on the third row. This means that the residual motion observations on the ball hardly distinguish from noise. Indeed, the velocity of the ball reaches a minimum before being hit by the racket. On top of that, the size of the ball is only about 30 pixels. It is hardly possible to gather enough motion evidence on such a small region with a slow motion. On the last raw, the velocity of the ball increased dramatically. This is reflected by an increase of the confidence in the detection and the NFA of the region corresponding to the ball decreases to 10^{-15}. The velocity of the player varies inversely to that of the ball. It is maximal just before hitting the ball. The NFA is about 10^{-80} on the player on the third row. The velocity of the player decreases afterward and the associated NFA raises to 10^{-30} in the last row.

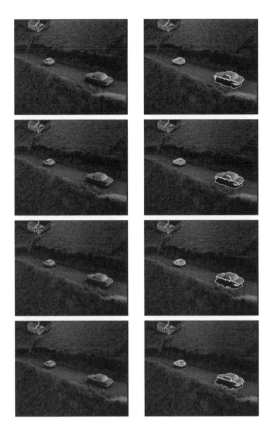

Figure 3.7. Four consecutive images of the road sequence. Original images in the left column. Outline of detected regions in white in the right column. NFAs are about 10^{-10} on the white car on the left of the scene. Two regions are detected on the darker car on the right. The upper region corresponding to the more contrasted part has an NFA about 10^{-70} in the four images. The lower region has an NFA of 10^{-15}. The higher NFA (lower confidence) is explained by the saturated gray levels on the lower region.

The second video sequence contains two cars driving down a road. The scene is shot from a helicopter and the camera tracks the cars. Camera motion is complex and combines translation and rotation. The global motion estimation using the 2D quadratic motion model, Figure 3.6, performs well again. (It can only be checked by registering the two images and compare them, by sight, or of course by the method described in Sect. 3.2.) Let us remind that the 8-parameter motion model is exact for a planar surface undergoing rigid motion. The planar assumption on the scene background is valid here. From Figure 3.8 it appears that the residual motion observations are sparse on the moving objects.

The two moving cars are detected over the four images (Figure 3.7). Let us note

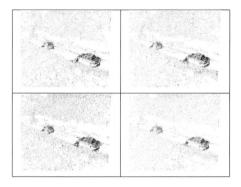

Figure 3.8. Road sequence. Maps of residual motion as defined by expression (3.12) for the four successive images displayed in Figure 3.7. On the lower part of the right car, the low contrast prevents from extracting motion measures.

the important stability of the detected moving regions over time. Let us stress that the algorithm works only with three frames and that no temporal regularization is applied on the detected regions. The stability of the detected moving regions is also due to the stability of the image segmentation provided by the maximal meaningful level line method. The level line segmentation preserves shape information over time.

NFAs are about 10^{-10} for the regions corresponding to the small car on the left. On the larger car on the right two regions are detected. The region corresponding to the upper part of the car has an NFA of 10^{-70}. The higher confidence is explained by the size of the region. The region corresponding to the lower part of the car has an NFA of 10^{-15}. This lower confidence is explained by the sparseness of high values of the residual motion measure (Figure 3.8). The lower part of the darker car has very low contrast and the grey level are saturated. Therefore, high values of the residual motion measure appear only on the edges.

The street sequence (Figure 3.9) is shot from a static camera. Two pedestrians, one in the foreground and another in the background, walk parallel to the image plane. The detection algorithm manages to select the correct regions, with no false alarms. The NFAs are about 10^{-80} for the pedestrian closer to the camera and about 10^{-18} for the pedestrian in the background. Again the NFAs on the detected regions are extremely low. This means that the detection is absolutely certain. The confidence in the detection of the pedestrian closer to the camera is higher since it is larger and moving faster.

3.4   Conclusions and perspectives

A detection principle was described. It is very general and was applied to two different applications of low-level video-processing. It allows us to automatically compute very robust detection thresholds, based on a single quantity: the number of false alarms. The examples presented in this chapter need some further work: a more general image comparison application needs to involve local windows and intrinsic local frames in

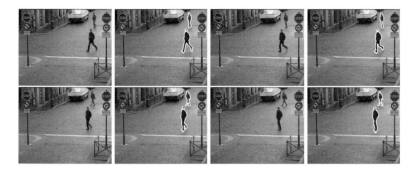

Figure 3.9. Four images of the street sequence. Original images on the left. Detected regions are outlined in white on the right. $NFAs$ are about 10^{-80} on the pedestrian closer to the camera and about 10^{-18} for the pedestrian in the background

the images. Motion detection should be considered as a very basic task in video analysis, although it is not easy. More useful applications are the analysis of trajectories. We are currently studying *a contrario* approaches for the definition of spatio-temporal coherence of detected moving regions.

Acknowledgements

This work was partially funded by the Rgion Bretagne, the IST European project LAVA, and the Network of Excellence Muscle.

References

Aach, T. and Kaup, A. (1995). Bayesian algorithms for change detection in image sequences using Markov random fields. *Signal Processing: Image Communication*, **7**(2), 147–160.

Cao, F. and Bouthemy, P. (2005). A general criterion for image similarity detection. *Technical Report 1732*, IRISA.

Desolneux, A., Moisan, L. and Morel, J. M. (2000). Meaningful alignments. *Int. J. Comput. Vision*, **40**, 7–23.

Desolneux, A., Moisan, L. and Morel, J. M. (2001). Edge detection by Helmholtz principle. *J. Math. Imag. Vision*, **14**, 271–284.

Desolneux, A., Moisan, L. and Morel, J. M. (2003). A grouping principle and four applications. *IEEE PAMI*, **25**, 508–513.

Fablet, R., Bouthemy, P. and Gelgon, M. (1999). Moving object detection in color image sequences using region-level graph labeling. *IEEE Int. Conf. Image Proc.*, Kobe, Japan.

Fischler, M. A. and Bolles, R. C. (1981). Random sample consensus: a paradigm for model fitting with applications to image analysis and automated cartography. *Comm. ACM*, **24**, 381–395.

Grimson, W. E. L. and Huttenlocher, D. P. (1990). On the sensitivity of the Hough transform for object recognition. *IEEE PAMI*, **12**, 255–274.

Helmholtz, H. (1867). *Handbuch der Physiologischen Optik*. Allgemeine Encyklopädie der Physik.

Hoeffding, W. (1963). Probability inequalities for sum of bounded random variables. *J. American Statistical Association*, **58**, 13–30.

Hsu, Y. Z., Nagel, H. H. and Rekers, G. (1984). New likelihood test methods for change detection in image sequences. *Comp. Vis. Graph. Image Proc.*, **26**, 73–106.

Konrad, J. (2005). Motion detection and estimation. In A. C. Bovik (ed.), *Handbook of Image and Video Processing*, 2nd edition, San Diego: Academic Press.

Lisani, J. L. and Morel, J. M. (2003). Detection of major changes in satellite images. *IEEE Int. Conf. on Image Proc.*, pp. 941–944.

Lisani, J. L., Moisan, L., Monasse, P. and Morel, J. M. (2003). On the theory of planar shape. *SIAM Multiscale Modeling and Simulation*, **1**, 1–24.

Lowe, D. (1999). Object recognition from local scale-invariant features. *Int. Conf. Comp. Vis.*, Corfu, pp. 1150–1157.

Lowe, D. (2004). Distinctive image features from scale-invariant keypoints. *Int. J. Comp. Vis.*, **60**, 91–110.

Mansouri, A. R. and Konrad, J. (2003). Multiple motion segmentation with level sets. *IEEE Trans. Image Proc.*, **12**, 201–220.

Mikolajczyk, K., Tuytelaars, T., Schmid, C.*et al.* (2005). A comparison of affine region detectors. *Int. J. Com. Vis.*, **65**, 2005.

Moscheni, F., Bhattacharjee, S. and Kunt, M. (1998). Spatiotemporal segmentation based on region merging. *IEEE PAMI*, **20**, 897–915.

Odobez, J. M. and Bouthemy, P. (1995). Robust multiresolution estimation of parametric motion models. *J. Visual Comm. Image Rep.*, **6**, 348–365. Software available at http://www.irisa.fr/Vista/Motion2D.

Odobez, J. M. and Bouthemy, P. (1997). Separation of moving regions from background in an image sequence acquired with a mobile camera. In H. H. Li, S. Sun and H. Derin, eds., *Video Data Compression for Multimedia computing*. Norwell, MA: Kluwer Academic Publisher. pp. 283–311.

Paragios, N. and Deriche, R. (2000). Geodesic active contour and level sets for the detection and tracking of moving objects. *IEEE PAMI*, **22**, 266–280.

Poor, H. V. (1994). *An Introduction to Signal Detection and Estimation* 2nd edition. Springer Texts in Electrical Engineering. New York: Springer Verlag.

Rosin, P. L. (2002). Thresholding for change detection. *Comp. Vis. Image Understand.*, **86**, 79–95.

Rothwell, C. A. (1995). *Object Recognition Through Invariant Indexing*. Oxford: Oxford Science Publications.

Veit, T., Cao, F. and Bouthemy, P. (2005a). An *a contrario* decision framework of region-based motion. *Int. J. Comp. Vis.*, **68**, 163–178, 2005.

Veit, T., Cao, F. and Bouthemy, P. (2005b). A maximality principle applied to a contrario motion detection. *Proc. IEEE Inter. Conf. on Image Processing*, Genova, Italy.

Venot, A., Lebruchec, J. F. and Roucayrol, J. C. (1982). A new class of similarity measures for robust image registration. *Comp. Vis. Graph. Image Proc.*, **28**, 176–184.

4 Computer vision in the Mars Exploration Rover (MER) mission

Larry Matthies, Mark Maimone, Yang Cheng, Andrew Johnson and Reg Willson

4.1 Introduction

The planet Mars has seen the most extensive unmanned exploration activity in the Solar System for several reasons, including its proximity to Earth, its relative ease of exploration (compared to Venus, for example), and, probably most importantly, the tantalizing prospect that it may have had a climate early in its history that may have enabled the development of microscopic life. Whether life actually developed there is still unknown and will take more missions and many years to decipher (Squyres and Knoll, 2005). Answering this question requires examining the geological record in rocks on the surface, which in turn requires surface mobility to maximize the extent of the record that can be examined. Mars rovers provide that surface mobility.

Energy and cost issues dictate that missions to Mars be launched when Earth and Mars are close to each other in their orbits, which happens roughly every 26 months. This means that the communication latency time, governed by the speed of light, is smallest at the time of landing; nevertheless, this is still about 10 minutes each way at landing and is about 20 minutes each way when the planets are farthest apart. More-over, for a variety of reasons, only a few communication "windows" are available per day. These factors imply that rovers must have significant autonomy to be able to do useful amounts of exploration and to do that safely.

The first planetary rover to successfully land on and explore the surface of Mars was

Computational Vision in Neural and Machine Systems, ed. L. Harris and M. Jenkin. Published by Cambridge University Press. © Cambridge University Press 2007.

the Sojourner rover in the 1997 NASA/JPL Mars Pathfinder (MPF) mission (Wilcox and Nguyen, 1998). Sojourner's computer system was based on an Intel 80C85 processor that delivered a computing throughput of about 100,000 instructions per second. Autonomous navigation requires 3D perception for obstacle detection; given Sojourner's limited computing power, its 3D perception was provided by a structured light system. Sojourner traveled a total of about 10 m in 83 Mars days ("sols," which are about 40 minutes longer than an Earth day), reaching a maximum distance from the lander of about 12 m. Sojourner was solar powered, 68 cm long, with a mass of 10.5 kg. The mission ended when communication was lost with the lander, which was the only communication link to the rover.

The MER mission landed two rovers, Spirit and Opportunity, on Mars in January, 2004. Spirit landed in the 150 km diameter Gusev Crater, which was considered to have possibly held an ancient lake. Opportunity landed in a large, very flat and featureless plain called Meridiani Planum, which had been seen from orbit to contain large amounts of the mineral grey hematite, that on Earth often forms in association with water. These rovers were also solar powered, but much larger, at 1.6 m long and a mass of 174 kg. Their onboard computer used a "RAD6000" processor that delivered a throughput of about 2 MIPS. Although this is two orders of magnitude less than what is available on desktop computers today, it is still enough to do some onboard computer vision. In order to get a richer 3D scene description and to enable other functions, the primary 3D perception mechanism was switched from structured light to stereo vision. The original objective for this mission was to be able to traverse up to 100 m per day over a 90 day primary mission, with a maximum distance from the landers of on the order of 1 km. As of December 2005, both rovers were still operating, having traveled a combined total of about 12 km and each having moved several kilometers from their landing sites.

The rovers were designed from the outset to use stereo vision for obstacle detection. Stereo vision-based visual odometry was included in the flight software as an optional capability, without a firm commitment to use it; experience after landing led this to be used frequently, especially on slopes and among sand drifts. Part way through development of the spacecraft, a new requirement emerged for a horizontal velocity sensor for the lander to use in controlling retro-rocket firing in terminal descent. A third vision algorithm, called the Descent Image Motion Estimation System (DIMES), was added to serve this function.

Section 4.2 gives an overview of the rover hardware architecture and mission operations. Sections 4.3, 4.4, and 4.5 describe the stereo vision, visual odometry, and DIMES algorithms respectively, including results from operation in the mission. Section 4.6 summarizes key lessons learned from this mission and notes important avenues for further work.

4.2 Overview of rover hardware and mission operations

Figure 4.1 shows one of the rovers during clean room testing; Figure 4.2 is an artist's sketch of one of the rovers annotated with major components. Details about the hardware and the mission are available in press release material on the web (see

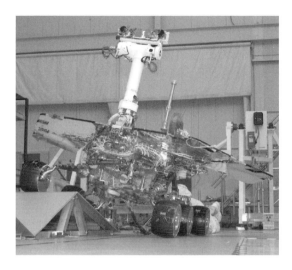

Figure 4.1. One of the MER rovers in clean room testing. See the accompanying CD-ROM for color versions of the figures.

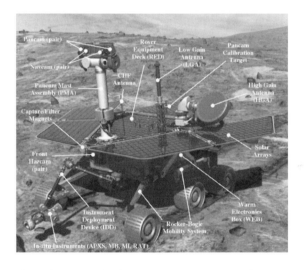

Figure 4.2. Artist's sketch of rover annotated with major components.

http://marsrovers.jpl.nasa.gov). Each vehicle weighs about 174 kg, is 1.6 m long, has a wheelbase of 1.1 m, and is 1.5 m tall to the top of the camera mast. Locomotion is achieved with a rocker bogie system very similar to that used in the 1997 Mars Pathfinder mission, with six driven wheels that are all kept in contact with the ground by passive pivot joints in the rocker bogey suspension. The outer four wheels are steerable.

The rovers are solar powered, with a rechargeable lithium ion battery for nighttime science and communication operations. The onboard computer is a 20 MHz RAD6000, which has an early PowerPC instruction set, with a very small L1 cache, no L2 cache, 128 MB of RAM, and 256 MB flash memory. Navigation is done with three sets of stereo camera pairs: one pair of "hazcams" (hazard cameras) looking forward under the solar panel in front, another pair of hazcams looking backward under the solar panel in the back, and a pair of "navcams" (navigation cameras) on the mast. All cameras have 1024×1024 pixel CCD arrays that create 12 bit grayscale images. The hazcams have a 126° field of view (FOV) and baseline of 10 cm; the navcams have a 45° FOV and baseline of 20 cm (Maki *et al.*, 2003). Each rover has a five degree of freedom arm in front which carries a science instrument payload with a microscopic imager, Mossbauer spectrometer, alpha/proton/X-ray backscatter spectrometer (APXS), and a rock abrasion tool (RAT). The camera mast has two additional science instruments: a stereo pair of "pancams" (panoramic cameras) and the "mini-TES" (thermal emission spectrometer). The pancams have filter wheels for multispectral visible and near-infrared imaging for mineral classification. They have the highest angular and range resolution of all cameras on the rover, with a 16° field of view and 30 cm baseline. The mini-TES acquires 167 bands between 5 and 29 μm in a single pixel. All instruments on the mast are pointable by one set of pan/tilt motors.

Because of constraints on solar power, the rovers drive for 3 to 4 h/sol, followed by a downlink telemetry session of up to 2 h/sol. A large team of people plans the next day or several days mission in the remaining hours per sol. The rovers' top driving speed is 5 cm/s. The basic traverse cycle involves acquiring hazcam stereo images and planning a short drive segment while standing still, then driving one half to one vehicle length, then stopping and repeating the process. With computing delays, this results in a net driving speed on the order of 1 cm/s or 36 m/h. Because the a priori 3-sigma landing uncertainty ellipse was about 80×10 km, exact targets for exploration could not be identified before landing. After landing, the science team concluded that the desirable investigation sites required the rovers to travel more quickly in order to reach them within tolerable time limits. This led to a new operational mode for long distance drives in which navcam or pancam stereo pairs acquired at the end of each sol are used by human operators to identify hazard-free paths several tens of meters ahead for the next sol's traverse. The rovers drive these initial segments with little or no obstacle detection and avoidance processing, then switch to "autonav" mode with complete obstacle detection and avoidance. This has enabled drives of up to about 350 m/sol in the most flat, safe terrain.

4.3 Stereo vision-based obstacle detection and avoidance

Owing to budget and schedule constraints, the baseline autonomous navigation system included only local obstacle avoidance with stereo vision; that is, there were no on-board global mapping, global path planning, or global localization functions. Stereo vision is used as the range sensor for obstacle avoidance because mature algorithms and reasonably compact, low-power, flight-qualified cameras were available for this, whereas flight-qualified versions of alternate sensors (e.g. ladar) with acceptable performance and form factor were not available. Obstacle avoidance is achieved with two major sub-modules: dense range imaging with stereo and local path planning with a system called GESTALT, for Grid-based Estimation of Surface Traversability Applied to Local Terrain. These are described in separate subsections below.

4.3.1 Stereo vision

Details of the stereo algorithm are described in Matthies (1992), Matthies *et al.* (1996) and Goldberg *et al.* (2002); here we give a brief overview of the algorithm, discuss some details that are specific to the MER implementation, and discuss its performance on Mars.

The stereo algorithm is a typical area-based algorithm using the sum of absolute differences (SAD) criterion for matching. Owing to very slow readout from the flight cameras (about 5 s per frame for full resolution, 1024×1024 pixel imagery), images are generally binned vertically within the CCD cameras and read out at 256×1024 pixel resolution. This is reduced by averaging to 256×256 pixels for stereo matching. The images are rectified and bandpass filtered, then correlated with a fast, sliding sums implementation of the SAD operation. A three-point parabolic fit to the SAD minimum at each pixel produces a subpixel disparity estimate for each pixel. Errors are filtered by left–right checking, thresholding the curvature of the parabola fit, and rejecting small, disconnected blobs in the disparity map, where the blob connectivity criterion is a threshold on the directional derivative of disparity. XYZ ranges images are produced as the final result. On the MER flight processor, this takes about 30 s per image pair to compute, when run together with other house-keeping and health check operations that must run in the flight system.

Either the hazcams or the navcams can be used for autonomous navigation. The wide field of view (FOV) of the hazcams was designed to see more than the full width of the rover a short distance ahead of the rover, which is important for obstacle avoidance and to verify the safety of turn-in-place operations. However, the useful look-ahead distance with the hazcams is at most 3–4 m, owing to their wide FOV and narrow baseline. The navcams can see further with their narrower FOV and wider baseline, but the FOV is only wide enough to verify the traversability of one candidate path several meters ahead of the vehicle. The pancams are not used for autonomous navigation.

Spirit uses the hazcams for stereo. Opportunity was unable to get acceptable range data with the hazcams, because the finer texture in the rock-free soil at Meridiani produced inadequate texture in hazcam images for stereo matching. Adequate results could be obtained with the navcams. Since Meridiani is largely obstacle free, it has been sufficient to use navcam stereo to check the traversability of the nominal path forward and stop the vehicle if a hazard is detected.

Figure 4.3 shows sample stereo results from the Spirit navcams looking at a rock that was studied by the science team. Navcam range imagery is typically this dense in the highly textured, relatively simple geometry of the Gusev Crater terrain. Hazcams produce somewhat less dense range imagery, probably owing to slightly poorer image quality and a much higher vertical dispaity derivative due to the low camera height. The small holes in the range image in Figure 4.3 result mostly from the left–right consistency check; we do not interpolate over such holes. The ragged disparity border around

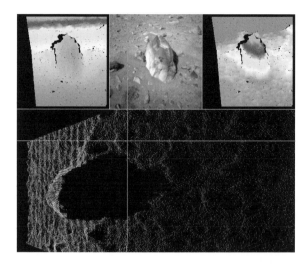

Figure 4.3. Stereo results from the Spirit navcams, looking at Humphrey rock in Gusev Crater. The rock is about 0.5 m tall. Upper left: false color range image (red is closest, magenta is furthest). Upper right: false color height image (red is lowest, magenta is highest). Bottom: elevation plot, seen from above, where the cameras are at the left looking right (same color coding as the height image). Green cross-hairs are not significant in this image.

the edge of the rock is typical of this class of stereo algorithm. We have achieved better borders with more elaborate algorithms, such as the overlapping windows algorithm of Hirschmuller *et al.* (2002); however, these are not in the flight system. This does not noticeably impact obstacle avoidance performance. The rippling visible in the elevation map in Figure 4.3 is the result of pixel-locking artifacts in the subpixel disparity estimation process (Xiong and Matthies, 1997; Shimizu and Okutomi, 2001); there is insufficient computing power onboard to address this within acceptable runtime. Again, however, this does not noticeably affect navigation performance.

4.3.2   GESTALT

The GESTALT obstacle avoidance algorithm is described in detail in Goldberg et al. (2002); here we give a brief overview and discuss implementation and performance issues specific to MER. A higher level description of the overall rover driving software architecture appears in Maimone and Biesiadicki (2005).

Range images from stereo are converted to "goodness" or "traversability" maps with 20 cm cells in a 10×10 m grid centered on the rover. For each range image, the complete set of range points is analyzed for traversability by fitting planar patches centered on each map cell in turn, where each patch is a circle with the diameter of the rover (nominally 2.6 m). The surface normal, RMS residual, and minimum and maximum elevation difference from the best fit plane determine a "goodness" factor for that map cell that characterizes its traversability. Goodness maps from each range image are registered and accumulated over time with the usual modulo map indexing arithmetic to avoid the need to scroll map data to keep the map bounded. Where new data overlap old data, the new data overwrite the old data in the map. The merged goodness map is then used to evaluate traversability of a fixed set of candidate steering trajectories, which are circular arcs of varying radius: 23 forward arcs, 23 backward arcs, and two point turns are evaluated in each driving cycle. Evaluation amounts to adding up the goodness scores along each arc, with nearby cells given higher weight. The result is a set of traversability votes for all arcs. These votes are input to an arbiter, which also takes input from waypoints provided by human operators during mission planning. The rover drives a fixed distance along the winning arc before stopping to acquire new images for the next driving cycle. The distance per cycle is set by human operators at anywhere from 35 cm to 1 m or more depending a variety of operational factors, including terrain difficulty and overall distance goals for the day.

Typical computing time per cycle of GESTALT is around 70 s. While the rover is driving, its peak speed is 5 cm/s, but it is typically operated at less than that (3.75 cm/s) for power reasons. With computing time, the median net driving speed is about 0.6 cm/s. Because this is so slow and the science team desired to cover large distances to Endurance Crater (in Meridiani Planum) and the Columbia Hills (in Gusev Crater), the hybrid daily driving scheme discussed earlier was introduced, with an initial "blind" driving segment planned by human operators on the ground using navcam or pancam imagery, followed by an autonav segment with GESTALT.

After some tuning of the algorithm to overcome excessively conservative behavior at slope changes, GESTALT has performed well. Figure 4.4 shows some results of obstacle avoidance from Spirit. The terrain on the plains at Meridiani was benign enough that the only "obstacles" were occasional hollows from small, in-filled craters. Within Eagle and Endurance Craters at Meridiani, the main navigation issues were slopes and slippage, not obstacles per se. Flight experience with the hybrid and full autonav driving behaviors is discussed at more length in Biesiadecki *et al.* (2005).

4.4 Visual odometry

In routine operation, onboard position estimation is done by dead reckoning with the wheel encoders and IMU, with occasional heading updates by sun sensing with the pancams. Long distance localization is done on Earth using bundle adjustment from manually matched tie points in panoramic imagery (Li *et al.*, 2004). On the plains at Gusev Crater, interpreting the bundle adjustment results as nominal ground truth, dead reckoning errors have been only a few percent of distance over several kilometers of travel. However, both rovers have experienced large slippage on slopes in the Columbia Hills, Eagle Crater, and Endurance Crater; in fact, up to 125% in one case in the Columbia Hills (ie. the rover slipped backwards in an attempted forward drive). Slip became a bigger issue for Spirit when it drove with one wheel locked, due to problems with lubricants in that wheels drive motor. Slip also occurs when the wheels sink in sand drifts, as occurred when Opportunity got stuck in a drift for several weeks. Stereo vision-based visual odometry is part of the flight software, but was not routinely used in early in the mission to maximize driving speed. It has been used to assess

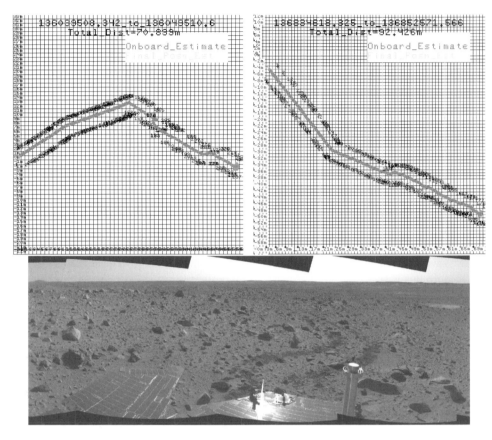

Figure 4.4. GESTALT results from Spirit. Top: two examples of daily traverse plots that started with blind drives and ended with autonomous portions that included some rock avoidance maneuvers, covering total distances of 70.9 m (left) and 92.4 m (right). Bottom: a mosaic of navcam imagery looking back on a day's traverse that ended with some rock avoidance, as can be seen from the rover tracks.

slippage of Opportunity in Eagle Crater and and Endurance Crater, by Opportunity to detect potential sinkage in drifts, by Spirit to measure and counter the effects of slip on slopes in the Columbia Hills.

Our visual odometry algorithm is described in detail elsewhere (Matthies, 1989; Olson *et al.*, 2003; Cheng *et al.*, 2005b). In a nutshell, it selects point features, uses multi-resolution area correlation to match them in stereo to determine their 3D coordinates, tracks them in subsequent stereo pairs get their 3D coordinates relative to subsequent rover positions, and uses the tracking results to estimate the six degree of freedom rover motion between consecutive stereo pairs. This runs in about 160 s in the flight system; for perspective, in Earth-bound applications essentially the same algorithm runs at about 15 frames/s on a 1.6 GHz embedded Pentium-M board. We have evaluated its performance against accurate ground truth on an Earth-based rover testbed

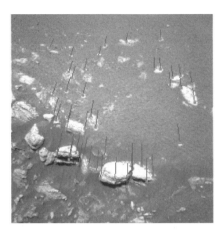 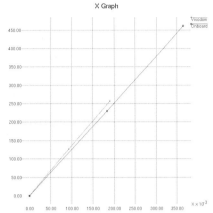

Figure 4.5. Visual odometry results from Opportunity in Eagle Crater. Left: features selected (red dots) in an image near a rock outcrop; blue lines show optical flow to the feature position in the next image. Right: plots of onboard dead reckoned position versus visual odometry (in mm) for a case where visual odometry correctly inferred a 50% slip.

and found that it can achieve 2% or better of distance over 30 m of travel (Helmick *et al.*, 2004). With a high performance embedded Pentium processor in that testbed, we have also integrated visual odometry into a Kalman filter-based position estimator, then used the improved state estimates to control steering to correct slip on slopes (Helmick *et al.*, 2004).

Figure 4.5 shows sample results from Opportunity in Eagle Crater, where visual odometry correctly detected a 50% slip. Additional results from Spirit and Opportunity are shown in Cheng *et al.* (2005b). The combined runtime of autonav (stereo vision plus GESTALT) and visual odometry makes for very slow driving, so autonav and visual odometry are generally not used together, and visual odometry is only used in conditions where slip or sinkage is anticipated. In use on Mars, as of March 2005 visual odometry had been run nearly 1500 times and converged to a solution (presumed correct) 96% of the time. The performance of the algorithm is discussed in much greater detail in Cheng *et al.* (2005b) and Helmick *et al.* (2004).

4.5 Descent Image Motion Estimation System (DIMES)

Both the MPF and MER missions landed on airbags. Both also used retro-rockets to slow the descent before impact, but MPF did not use rockets deliberately to slow horizontal velocity before impact. MER was much heavier, which put more stress on the airbags and more priority on keeping horizontal velocity at impact below a certain threshold so as not to rupture the airbags. Part way through development of the MER spacecraft, an improved understanding of winds on Mars led to the conclusion that explicit sensing and control of horizontal velocity shortly before impact was desirable to improve the probability of safe landing. The retro-rockets already in the design could be adapted to provide horizontal thrust, but no horizontal velocity sensor was in the design and there was neither time nor funding available to add the traditional, radar-based velocity sensor. However, a spare camera and camera interface did exist that could be adapted for this purpose, if software could be developed and shown to have adequate performance in time to be ready for launch. This led to an intense, two-year effort to design, implement, and test such software (Cheng *et al.*, 2004, 2005a; Willson *et al.*, 2005; Johnson *et al.*, 2005). The unique application, the sensor fusion required to achieve the task, some novel vision science drawn upon for the design, and the extensive performance evaluation, both by simulation and by field-testing, all made the resulting Descent Image Motion Estimation System (DIMES) a distinctive vision system and useful case study. We summarize the highlights of DIMES below and refer readers to (Cheng *et al.*, 2004, 2005s; Willson *et al.*, 2005; Johnson *et al.*, 2005) for details.

As shown in Figure 4.6, after dropping the heat shield, the MER descent system consisted of a parachute, the backshell from the interplanetary cruise configuration, which also held the retro-rockets, and the lander itself, which was spooled out on a "bridle" to get it away from the rocket plumes. One set of rockets ("RADs," for Rocket Assisted Descent) were designed to bring the vertical velocity to zero some 10–20 m above the surface, after which the bridle was cut and the lander's fall was cushioned with airbags. A second set of rockets ("TIRS," for Transverse Impulse Rocket System) could fire laterally to ensure that the backshell was vertical before RAD firing, so that the RADs did not add to horizontal velocity. Given a horizontal velocity measurement, TIRS could also be used to tilt the backshell into the wind, so that RAD firing would reduce horizontal as well as vertical velocity.

The lander had an inertial measurement unit (IMU) and a radar altimeter that could measure angular velocity and vertical velocity. Thus, in principle, tracking one feature through two images would add enough information to estimate the entire velocity vector. Using just one feature is not very reliable, of course, but the onboard computer was too slow to do much more than this in real-time during descent. The following scheme was adopted to maximize reliability within the available computing resources. An interest operator picked two features in the first image, acquired at about 2000 m above the surface. A multi-resolution correlation algorithm matched those features in a second image, acquired about 1700 m above the surface. A variety of consistency checks were used to validate the matches. This gave one velocity estimate. Two more features were chosen from this image and matched in a third image, acquired at about 1400 m altitude, to give a second velocity estimate. These two velocity estimates gave an estimate for acceleration for the intervening interval, which was checked against accelerations measured with the IMU as a final consistency check. If all consistency checks passed, the velocity estimate was used to determine whether and how to use the TIRS to offset horizontal velocity. Details of the algorithm are given in Cheng *et al.* (2005a).

From the perspective of vision science, this algorithm embodied knowledge of a surface reflectance phenomenon that is well known in planetary geology but, to our knowledge, has not previously been recognized in the computer vision literature. This is the "opposition effect" (Hapke, 1986), which causes a spike in the reflectance func-

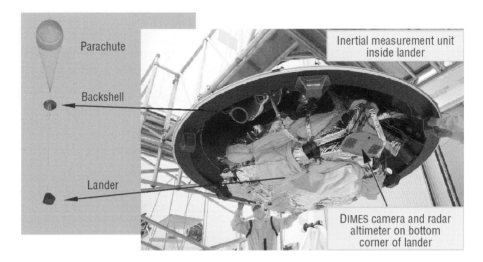

Figure 4.6. MER descent system. Left: artist's illustration of the parachute, backshell, and lander in the last few km of descent. RAD and TIRS rockets were on the backshell. Airbags, when deployed, formed a cocoon around the lander. Right: photo showing the lander stowed inside the backshell during spacecraft assembly, before integrating the heat shield.

tion back toward the observer when the Sun is near zero phase angle (i.e. directly behind the observer). Note that this is distinct from specularity, since the opposition effect is tied to the small phase angle of the point illuminator. For DIMES, it caused a peak in image intensity around the shadow of the lander. Modeling the height and width of this peak allowed an appropriate portion of the image to be ignored in feature selection and tracking and allowed DIMES simulations to better model what real descent imagery would look like (Willson *et al.*, 2005). We have observed that the opposition effect can also have a significant impact on exposure across an image for wide-angle stereo vision systems for ground robots when the Sun is low in the sky.

Performance validation for DIMES involved extensive simulation with a simulation tool called MOC2DIMES (Willson *et al.*, 2005) and extensive field testing with imagery acquired by a manned helicopter (Johnson *et al.*, 2005). MOC2DIMES embodied an elaborate model of the imaging process and noise sources for the descent camera; it used that model together with dynamical simulations of descent trajectories to convert real, orbital imagery of Mars into an ensemble of simulated descent imagery. That is, real orbital imagery was available of terrain near the landing sites, with image resolutions and viewing and illumination geometries not too different from that expected in the mission. MOC2DIMES used the orbital imagery to create high fidelity triples of synthetic descent imagery to test the algorithm described above to estimate the precision of velocity estimates and the probability of failure to produce a valid estimate. These simulations predicted 3-sigma velocity errors of less than 4 m/s for both landing sites.

Field testing used a manned helicopter to acquire imagery at three altitudes over

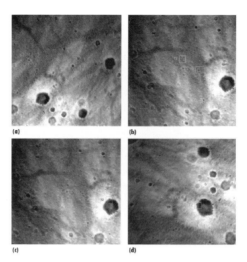

Figure 4.7. DIMES results from the Spirit landing at Gusev Crater: (a) first descent image with selected features shown as the red squares; (b) second descent image with the matched features shown as the green squares; (c) second image again, showing the second set of selected features; (d) third image showing the matched features from the second image. All feature matches were correct.

three test sites in the Mojave Desert (Johnson *et al.*, 2005). An engineering model of the descent camera was mounted with an IMU on motorized gimbals on the helicopter to generate pitch rates for the camera comparable to those expected in the actual Mars landings. Images were selected from each altitude to form an ensemble of triples to test the algorithm. Ground truth was available from ultra-high precision differential GPS. Dispersions of velocity estimates were in good agreement with the precision observed in MOC2DIMES simulations.

In the mission, DIMES determined that TIRS firing was needed for Spirit, but not for Opportunity. After-the-fact reconstructions of landing events showed that, without DIMES, the Spirit impact velocity would have been right on the edge of the tested airbag performance limits; with DIMES, the impact velocity was about half of the airbag limit. Figure 4.7 shows the descent images from Spirit, with the selected and tracked features for each pair of images.

4.6   Discussion

The MER mission was the first use of stereo vision, local map-based obstacle avoidance, and visual odometry for autonomous rover navigation in a planetary exploration mission, as well as the first use of computer vision in an autonomous, real-time function (horizontal velocity estimation) during landing in a planetary mission. The algorithms are competent and emphasize reliability within the constraints of a very slow onboard computer. Algorithms for analogous functions on Earth-based research vehicles can have more sophistication because of the much greater computing resources often available, but are rarely designed or tested to reach the same level of fault tolerance. These algorithms have performed well and contributed to the success of the mission; in particular, DIMES may have saved Spirit from a disastrous landing.

In this mission, the most valuable science results have been found in rock outcrops in sloping, slippery terrain, either inside craters or on hills; moreover, the rovers have had to drive much further than anticipated prior to landing to reach such outcrops. Thus, for future missions, key issues include increasing the speed of the algorithms and integrating visual odometry inside the driving and steering loop to enable safe, efficient traversal on slippery terrain. Incorporating path planning algorithms for longer lookahead and rougher terrain may also be valuable. For landers, the focus of vision algorithm research will switch to enabling precision landing and landing hazard avoidance.

References

Biesiadecki, J., Leger, C. and Maimone, M. (2005). Tradeoffs between directed and autonomous driving on the Mars Exploration Rovers. *Proc. Int. Symp. Robot. Res.*, San Francisco, CA.

Cheng, Y., Goguen, J., Johnson, A. *et al.* (2004). The Mars Exploration Rovers Descent Image Motion Estimation System. *IEEE Intelligent Systems Magazine*, May/June, 13–21.

Cheng, Y., Johnson, A. and Matthies, L. (2005a). MER-DIMES: a planetary landing application of computer vision. *Proc. IEEE CVPR*, San Diego, CA.

Cheng, Y., Maimone, M. and Matthies, L. (2005b). Visual odometry on the Mars Exploration Rovers. *Proc. IEEE Sys. Man Cybern. Conf.*, Waikoloa, HI.

Goldberg, S., Maimone, M. and Matthies, L. (2002). Stereo vision and rover navigation software for planetary exploration. *Proc. IEEE Aerospace Conference*, Big Sky, MO.

Hapke, B. W. (1986). Bidirectional reflectance spectroscopy IV: the extinction coefficient and the opposition effect. *Icarus*, **67**, 264–280.

Helmick, D. M., Cheng, Y., Clouse, D. S. and Matthies, L. (2004). Path following using visual odometry for a Mars rover in high-slip environments. *Proc. IEEE Aerospace Conference*, Big Sky, MO.

Hirschmuller, H., Innocent, P. R. and Garibaldi, J. (2002). Real-time correlation-based stereo vision with reduced border errors. *Int. J. Comp. Vis.*, **47**, 229–246.

Johnson, A., Willson, R., Goguen, J., Alexander, J. and Meller, D. (2005). Field testing of the Mars Exploration Rovers Descent Image Motion Estimation System. *Proc. IEEE International Conference on Robotics and Automation*. Barcelona, Spain.

Li, R., Di, K., Matthies, L., Arvidson, R., Folkner, W. and Archinal, B. (2004). Rover localization and landing site mapping technology for the 2003 Mars Exploration Rover Mission. *J. Photogram. Engin. Remote Sens.*, **70**, 77–90.

Maimone, M. and Biesiadecki, J. (2005). The Mars Exploration Rover surface mobility flight software: driving ambition. *Proc. IEEE Aerospace Conference*, Big Sky, MO.

Maki J., Bell III, J., Herkenhoff *et al.* Mars Exploration Rover engineering cameras. *J. Geophys. Res.*, **108**, E12.

Matthies, L. (1989). *Dynamic Stereo Vision*. PhD thesis, Carnegie Mellon University.

Matthies, L. (1992). Stereo vision for planetary rovers: stochastic modeling to near real-time implementation. *Int. J. Comp. Vis.*, **8**, 71–91.

Matthies, L., Kelly, A., Litwin, T. and Tharp, G. (1996). Obstacle detection for unmanned ground vehicles: a progress report. In G. Giralt and G. Hirzinger, eds., *Robotics Research: the Seventh International Symposium*, London: Springer, pp. 471–486.

Olson, C., Matthies, L. and Schoppers, M. (2003). Rover navigation using stereo egomotion. *Robotics and Autonomous Systems*, **43**, 215–229.

Shimizu, M. and Okutomi, M. (2001). Precise subpixel estimation on area-based matching. *Proc. ICCV*.

Squyres, S. W. and Knoll, A. H. (2005). Sedimentary rocks at Meridiani Planum: origin, diagenesis, and implications for life on Mars. *Earth Planet. Sci. Lett.*, **240**, 1–10.

Wilcox, B. and Nguyen, T. (1998). Sojourner on Mars and lessons learned for future planetary rovers. *28th Int. Conf. on Environmental Systems*, Danvers, MA.

Willson, R., Johnson, A. and Goguen, D. (2005). MOC2DIMES: a camera simulator for the Mars Exploration Rover Descent Image Motion Estimation System. *Proc. 8th International Symposium on Artificial Intelligence, Robotics and Automation in Space (iSAIRAS)*, Munich, Germany.

Xiong, Y. and Matthies, L. (1997). Error analysis of a real-time stereo system. *Proc. IEEE CVPR*.

5 Calibration and shape recovery from videos of dynamic scenes

Marc Pollefeys, Sudipta Sinha and Jingyu Yan

5.1 Introduction

Recovering 3D shape information from images is one of the main challenges in the area of computer vision. A prerequisite for this often consists of recovering the camera calibration. During the past decade tremendous progress has been made in this area. It is now possible to recover both the calibration of a camera and the 3D shape of a rigid object from an uncalibrated video sequence (Pollefeys *et al.*, 2004). There are, however, many remaining challenges. Dynamic scenes are particularly hard to deal with as in this case the rigidity constraint is not available.

In this chapter we present two different approaches that deal with dynamic scenes. The first approach deals with a dynamic scene observed by multiple cameras. Although with many synchronized cameras observing the scene the rigidity constraint might be used between images recorded at the same time, practical systems often only have a few cameras with limited overlap. The approach we propose does not rely on the observation of common feature points between the different cameras, but instead analyzes the silhouettes of the dynamic objects. In a first stage our approach robustly recovers the relative camera placement between pairs of cameras, as well as the temporal offset if the cameras are unsynchronized. Next, this information is combined to recover the complete calibration, relative camera placement and synchronization for the camera network. Finally, an approximate shape of the dynamic object is recovered by computing the visual hull, taking temporal offsets into account.

An even more challenging problem consists of recovering the shape and motion of

---

Computational Vision in Neural and Machine Systems, ed. L. Harris and M. Jenkin. Published by Cambridge University Press. © Cambridge University Press 2007.

dynamic scenes from a monocular video sequence. The second part of this paper studies articulated shapes observed by a single camera. Our approach recovers the 3D shape and motion, as well as the joints of an articulated body observed under orthographic conditions.

Both approaches presented in this paper are based on modified RANSAC algorithms. For the silhouette-based approach the difficulty came from the fact that it is not possible to compute the epipolar geometry directly from silhouettes. Instead, one has to partially randomly generate a hypothesis and then verify it using the silhouettes. We show that it is still possible to design an efficient RANSAC algorithm in this case. For the estimation of articulated motion subspaces the difficulty comes from the fact that both segmentation and subspace estimation are intertwined. In this case we show that a modified RANSAC can efficiently compute motion subspaces by making use of a prior that indicates how likely it is that two tracks are located on the same articulated part.

The remainder of the paper discusses these approaches in more detail. Section 5.2 presents the silhouette-based approach for camera network calibration. Section 5.3 discusses the segmentation and computation of articulated motions. Section 5.4 contains the conclusion and some discussion.

5.2   Silhouette-based camera network calibration

In surveillance camera networks, live video of a dynamic scene is often captured from multiple views. We aim to automatically recover the 3D reconstruction of the dynamic event, as well as the calibration and synchronization, using only the input videos. Our method simultaneously recovers the synchronization and epipolar geometry of such a camera pair. This method is particularly useful for shape-from-silhouette systems (Buehler *et al.*, 2001; Cheung *et al.*, 2003; Sand *et al.*, 2003) as visual hulls can now be reconstructed from uncalibrated and unsynchronized video of moving objects. Different aspects of this work have been published earlier (Sinha and Pollefeys, 2004a, b, c).

Different existing structure-from-motion approaches using silhouettes (Vijayakumar *et al.*, 1996; Wong and Cipolla, 2001; Yezzi and Soatto, 2003) either require good initialization or work only for certain camera configurations, and most of them require static scenes. Traditionally, calibration objects like checkerboard patterns or LEDs have been used for calibrating multi-camera systems (Zhang, 1999) but this requires physical access to the observed space. This is often impractical and costly for surveillance applications and could be impossible for remote camera networks or networks deployed in hazardous environments. Our method can calibrate or recalibrate such cameras remotely and also handle wide-baseline camera pairs, arbitrary camera configurations and a lack of photometric calibration.

Our algorithm exploits the constraints arising from the correspondence of frontier points and epipolar tangents (Astrom *et al.*, 1996; Porrill and Pollard, 1991; Wong and Cipolla, 2001). Frontier points on an object's surface are 3D points which project to points on the silhouette in the two views. In Figure 5.1a, X and Y are frontier points on the apparent contours C_1 and C_2, which project to points on the silhouettes S_1 and S_2 respectively. The projection of Π, the epipolar plane tangent to X gives

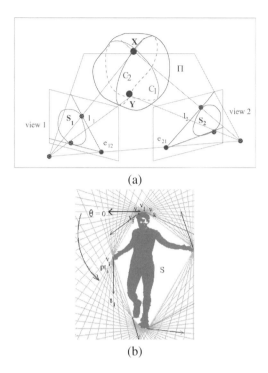

(a)

(b)

Figure 5.1. (a) Frontier points and epipolar tangents. (b) The tangent envelope. See the CD-ROM for a color version of this figure.

rise to corresponding epipolar lines l_1 and l_2 which are tangent to S_1 and S_2 at the images of X in the two images respectively. No other point on S_1 and S_2 other than the images of frontier points, X and Y correspond. Morever, the image of the frontier points corresponding to the outer-most epipolar tangents (Wong and Cipolla, 2001) must lie on the convex hull of the silhouette. The silhouettes are stored in a compact data structure called the tangent envelope (Sinha and Pollefeys, 2004a) (see Figure 5.1b). We only need of the order of 500 bytes per frame to store this representation.

Videos of dynamic objects contain many different silhouettes, yielding many constraints that are satisfied by the true epipolar geometry. Unlike other algorithms, (see Furukawa *et al.*, 2004) who search for all possible frontier points and epipolar tangents on a single silhouette, we search only for the outermost frontier points and epipolar tangents, but for many silhouettes. Using only the outermost epipolar tangents allows us to be far more efficient because the data structures are simpler and there are no issues of self-occlusion. Sufficient motion of the object within the 3D observed space gives rise to a good spatial distribution of frontier points and increases the accuracy of the fundamental matrix.

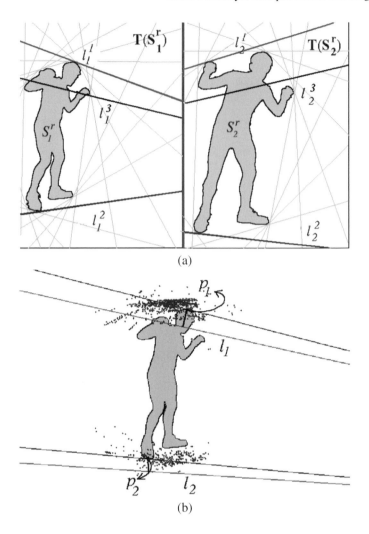

Figure 5.2. (a) The 4D hypothesis of the epipoles (not in picture). (b) All frontier points for a specific hypothesis and a pair of transferred epipolar lines l_1, l_2. See the CD-ROM for a color version of this figure.

5.2.1   Computing the epipolar geometry

Computing the epipolar geometry from silhouettes is not as simple as computing it from points. The reason is that having two corresponding silhouettes doesn't immediately yield usable equations. We first need to know where the frontier points are and this is dependent on the epipolar geometry. This is thus a typical "chicken and egg" problem. However, this is not as bad as it seems. We do not need the full epipolar geometry. The location of the epipoles (four out of seven parameters) is sufficient to determine the epipolar tangents and the frontier points. Our approach will thus consist of randomly generating epipole hypotheses and then verify that the bundle of epipolar tangents to all the silhouettes are consistent. One of the key elements to the success of our algorithm is to have a very efficient data representation and to generate a proper distribution of epipoles in our sampling process. This approach is explained more in detail in the remainder of this section.

RANSAC algorithm   The RANSAC-based algorithm takes two sequences as input, where the jth frame in sequence i is denoted by S_i^j and the corresponding tangent envelope by $T(S_i^j)$. We denote F_{ij} as the fundamental matrix between view i and view j (transfers points in view i to epipolar lines in view j) and e_{ij}, the epipole in view j of camera center i. While a fundamental matrix has seven degrees of freedom (dofs), we only randomly sample in a 4D space because if the epipoles are known, the frontier points can be determined, and the remaining degrees of freedom of the epipolar geometry can be derived from them. The pencil of epipolar lines in each view centered on the epipoles, is considered as a 1D projective space (Hartley and Zisserman, 2000). The epipolar line homography between two such 1D projective spaces can be represented by a 2D homography to be applied to the 2D representation of the lines. Knowing the epipoles e_{ij}, e_{ji} and the epipolar line homography fixes F_{ij}. Three pairs of corresponding epipolar lines are sufficient to determine the epipolar line homography $H_{ij}^{-\top}$ so that it uniquely determines the transfer of epipolar lines (note that $H_{ij}^{-\top}$ is only determined up to three remaining degrees of freedom, but those do not affect the transfer of epipolar lines). The fundamental matrix is then uniquely given by $F_{ij} = [e_{ij}]_\times H_{ij}$.

Hypothesis generation   At every iteration, we randomly choose the rth frames from each of the two sequences. As shown in Figure 5.2a, we then randomly sample independent directions l_1^1 from $T(S_1^r)$ and l_2^1 from $T(S_2^r)$ for the first pair of tangents in the two views. We choose a second pair of directions l_1^2 from $T(S_1^r)$ and l_2^2 from $T(S_2^r)$ such that $l_i^2 = l_i^1 - x$ for $i = 1, 2$ where x is drawn from the normal distribution, $N(180, \sigma)$.[1] The intersections of the two pair of tangents produces the epipole hypothesis (e_{12}, e_{21}). We next randomly pick another pair of frames q, and compute either the first pair of tangents or the second pair. Let us denote this third pair of lines by l_1^3 tangent to $CH(S_1^q)$ and l_2^3 tangent to $CH(S_2^q)$ (see Figure5.2a). Then H_{ij} is computed from $(l_i^k \leftrightarrow l_j^k; k = 1 \ldots 3)$.[2] The entities ($e_{ij}$, e_{ji}, H_{ij}) form the model hypothesis for an iteration of our algorithm.

Hypothesis verification   Once a model for the epipolar geometry is available, we verify its accuracy. We do this by computing tangents from the hypothesized epipoles to the whole sequence of silhouettes in each of the two views. For unclipped silhouettes we obtain two tangents per frame, whereas for clipped silhouettes there may be one or even zero tangents. Every tangent in the pencil of the first view is transferred through

---

[1] We use $\sigma = 60$ in our experiments. In case silhouettes are clipped in this frame, the second pair of directions is chosen from another frame.

[2] For simplicity we assume that the first epipolar tangent pair corresponds as well as the second pair of tangents. This limitations could be easily removed by verifying both hypotheses for every random sample.

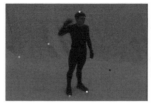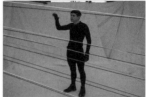

Figure 5.3. Example of computed epipolar geometry. Points in the left column are transferred to epipolar lines in the right column.

$H_{ij}^{-\top}$ to the second view (see Figure 5.2b) and the reprojection error of the transferred line from the point of tangency in that particular frame is computed. We count the outliers that exceed a reprojection error threshold (we choose this to be 5 pixels) and throw away our hypothesis if the outlier count exceeds a certain fraction of the total expected inlier count. This allows us to abort early whenever the model hypothesis is completely inaccurate. Thus tangents to all the silhouettes S_i^j, $j \in 1 \dots M$ in view i, $i = 1, 2$, would be computed only for a promising hypothesis. For all such promising hypotheses an inlier count is maintained using a lower threshold (we choose this to be 1.25 pixels).

Solution refinment   After a solution with a sufficiently high inlier fraction has been found, or a preset maximum number of iterations has been exhausted, we select the solution with the most inliers and improve our estimate of F for this hypothesis through an iterative process of nonlinear Levenberg–Marcquardt minimization while continuing to search for additional inliers. Thus, at every iteration of the minimization, we recompute the pencil of tangents for the whole silhouettes sequence S_i^j, $j \in 1 \dots M$ in view i, $i = 1, 2$ until the inlier count converges. The cost function minimized is the distance between the tangency point and the transferred epipolar line (see Figure 5.2b) in both images. At this stage we also recover the frontier point correspondences (the points of tangency) for the full sequence of silhouettes in the two views.

Results   This approach works well in practice and has been demonstrated on multiple datasets recorded by ourselves and by others (Sinha and Pollefeys, 2004a). Here we show some results obtained from a four-view dataset. In Figure 5.3 the computed epipolar geometry F_{14}, F_{24} and F_{34} is shown. The black epipolar lines correspond to the initial epipolar geometry computed as discussed in this section, the colored epipolar lines correspond to the epipolar geometry once it is made consistent over a triplet of cameras.[3] One can notice the significant improvement for pair 2–4 once three-view consistency is enforced. The result for pair 3–4 is less accurate. This is due to clipping of the silhouette at the feet in most of the frames, therefore only yielding a small number of extremal frontier points at the bottom of the image. The result is still sufficient to successfully initialize a bundle adjustment.

---

[3]Note that the final epipolar geometry is refined even further through bundle adjustment, see next section.

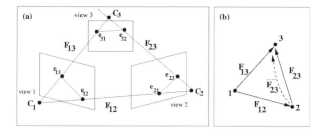

Figure 5.4. (a) Three non-degenerate views for which we estimate all F matrices. (b) The three-view case. $\overline{F}_{23}$ is the closest approximation of F_{23} we compute.

5.2.2 Camera network calibration from pairwise epipolar geometry

Typical approaches for computing projective structure and motion recovery require correspondences over at least three views. However, it is also possible to compute them based on only two-view correspondences. Levi and Werman (2003) have recently shown how this could be achieved given a subset of all possible fundamental matrices between N views with special emphasis on the solvability of various camera networks. Here we briefly describe our iterative approach which provides a projective reconstruction of the camera network.

The basic building block that we first resolve is a set of three cameras with non-colinear centers for which the three fundamental matrices F_{12}, F_{13} and F_{23} have been computed (Figure 5.4). Given those, we use linear methods to find a consistent set of projective cameras P_1, P_2 and P_3. Choose P_1 and P_2 as follows :

$$P_1 = [I|0] \quad P_2 = [[e_{21}]_\times F_{12}|e_{21}]. \tag{5.1}$$

It follows that P_3 is determined up to an unknown 4-vector v:

$$P_3(v) = [[e_{31}]_\times F_{13}|0] + e_{31}v^T. \tag{5.2}$$

Expressing F_{23} as a function of P_2 and P_3 we obtain:

$$\overline{F}_{23}(v) = [e_{32}]_\times P_3(v)P_2^+, \tag{5.3}$$

which is also linear in v, such that all possible solutions for F_{23} span a 4D subspace of P^8 (Levi and Werman, 2003). We solve for v which yields the closest appromixation to F_{23} within the subspace (in the Frobenius norm sense):

$$\overline{v} = \arg\min_v \|\overline{F}_{23}(v) - F_{23}\|_F. \tag{5.4}$$

The projection matrices $P_1, P_2, P_3(\overline{v})$ are fully consistent with F_{12}, F_{13} and $\overline{F}_{23}(\overline{v})$.

Using the camera triplet as a building block, we can handle an N-view camera network by induction. The projective reconstruction of a triplet (as described above) initializes the projective reconstruction of the whole network. At every step a new view

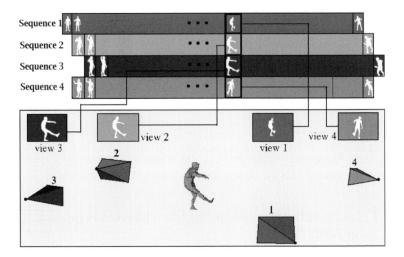

Figure 5.5. Recovered camera configuration and visual hull reconstruction of person.

that has edges to any two views within the set of cameras reconstructed so far forms a new triplet which is resolved in identical fashion. This process is repeated until all the cameras have been handled.

This projective calibration is first refined using a projective bundle adjustment which minimizes the reprojection error of the pairwise frontier point matches. Next, we use the linear self-calibration algorithm (Pollefeys *et al.*, 1999) to estimate the rectifying transform for each of the projective cameras. We rectify these projective cameras into metric cameras, and use them to initialize a Euclidean bundle adjustment (Triggs *et al.*, 2000). The Euclidean bundle adjustment step produces the final calibration of the full camera network.

Results   Here we present results from full calibration of the four-view video dataset which is 4 min long and captured at 30 fps (Sand *et al.*, 2003) (see Figure 5.5). We computed the projective cameras from the fundamental matrices $F_{12}, F_{13}, F_{23}, F_{14}, F_{24}$. On average, we obtained one correct solution, one which converged to the global minimum after nonlinear refinement for every 5 000 hypotheses.[4] This took approximately 15 s of computation time on a 3 GHz PC with 1 GB RAM. Assuming a Poisson distribution, 15 000 hypotheses would yield approximately 95% probability of finding the correct solution and 50 000 hypotheses would yield 99.99% probability.

Note that F_{23} and F_{24} were adjusted by the method described earlier, which actually improved our initial estimates.[5] The projective camera estimates were then refined through a projective bundle adjustment (reducing the reprojection error from 4.6 pixels to 0.44 pixels). The final reprojection error after self-calibration and metric bundle

---

[4]For all different camera pairs we get respectively one in 5 555, 4 412, 4 168, 3 409, 9 375 and 5 357. The frequency was computed over a total of 150 000 hypothesis for each viewpair.

[5]By projecting the least accurately computed fundamental matrices on the subspace compatible with other fundamental matrices the results can, in general, be improved.

adjustment was 0.73 pixels, which is comparable to the accuracy obtained by using an explicit calibration procedure.

In typical video, outermost frontier points and epipolar tangents often remain stationary over a long time. Such static frames are redundant and representative keyframes must be chosen to make the algorithm more efficient and avoid trivial consensus sets that could fool RANSAC. We do this by considering hypothetical epipoles (at the four image corners), pre-computing tangents to all the silhouettes in the whole video and binning them and picking representative keyframes such that at least one from each bin is selected. For the four-view dataset, we ended up with 600–700 keyframes selected out of the 7500 frames contained in the original videos.

For unsynchronized video sequences, this approach can easily be extended to also take a temporal offset into account. In stead of sampling over the four parameters of the epipoles, a fifth parameter is added to represent the temporal offset. In Sinha and Pollefeys (2004b), we proposed an efficient hierarchical approach and synchronized video sequences within $1/100$ s starting from an initial range of ± 500 frames. As we will see in the next section, the subframe temporal offset can be used to improve the visual hull reconstruction results.

5.2.3   Visual hull reconstruction from video streams

Once the calibration is available, it becomes possible to reconstruct the shape of the observed person by using visual hull techniques (Buehler *et al.*, 2001; Laurentini, 1994; Matusik *et al.*, 2000). However, one remaining difficulty when using unsynchronized video cameras is that the temporal offsets between the multiple video streams are in general not an integer number of frames. Given a specific frame from one video stream, the closest frame in other 30 Hz video streams could be as far of as $1/60$ s. While this might seems small at first, this can be significant for a moving person. This problem is illustrated in Figure 5.6 where the visual hull was reconstructed from the closest original frames in the sequence. The gray area represents what is inside the visual hull reconstruction and the white area corresponds to the reprojection error (points inside the silhouette carved away from another view). The motion of the arm and the leg that takes place during the small temporal offset between the different frames is sufficient to cause a significant error.

To deal with this problem, we propose to use temporal silhouette interpolation. Given two frames i and $i + 1$, we compute the distance $d_i(\mathbf{x})$ and $d_{i+1}(\mathbf{x})$ to the closest point on each silhouette for every pixel $\mathbf{x}$ (Mauch, 2003; Sethian, 1996). For the purpose of interpolation we can limit ourselves to the convex hull of both silhouettes. Then we compute an interpolated silhouette for subframe temporal offset $\Delta \in [0, 1]$ as the 0-level set of $S(\mathbf{x}) = (1 - \Delta)d_i(\mathbf{x}) - \Delta d_{i+1}(\mathbf{x})$. More details on this approach can be found in Sinha and Pollefeys (2004c).

Results   We use this approach in combination with the subframe temporal offsets. We choose some frames recorded from view three as a reference and generate interpolated silhouettes from the other viewpoints that correspond to the appropriate temporal offset. In Figure 5.7 the visual hull reprojection error is shown with and without subframe

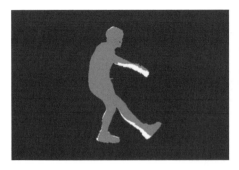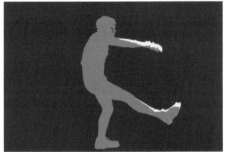

Figure 5.6. Visual hull reprojection error (white) induced by subframe temporal offset.

silhouette interpolation. We show an overal improvement by a factor of two or better of the reprojection error.

5.3   Articulated shape recovery from video

In this section we present our RANSAC-based approach to efficiently segment and recover articulated motion subspaces. First we discuss in detail the shape subspaces of articulated motions in comparison to those of independent motions. Then we present our algorithm which uses the concept of shape interaction to determine a prior that indicates if tracks are likely to belong to the same articulated part or not. A more detailed discussion of this approach can be found in (Yan and Pollefeys, 2005a). An alternative segmentation approach for articulated shapes which is based on spectral clustering is proposed in (Yan and Pollefeys, 2006).

5.3.1   Articulated shape subspaces vs. independent shape subspaces

The articulated motion subspace is a set of intersecting rigid motion subspaces (Yan and Pollefeys, 2005b). These are not orthogonal to each other as independent motions are. We will show this by using a canonical factorization form for both independent motions and articulated motions. The formulation is based on the Tomasi–Kanade factorization (Tomasi and Kanade, 1992) assuming orthographic projection.

Independent motions   For independent motions Costeira and Kanade (1998) proposed a motion segmentation algorithm that is based on the orthogonality property of

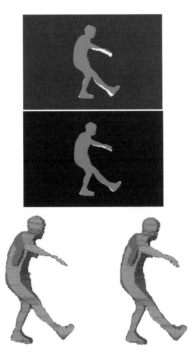

Figure 5.7. Reprojection error reduced from 10.5% to 3.4% of the pixels contained in the silhouette (2785 to 932 pixel). The overall improvement for the four corresponding silhouettes was from 5.2% to 2.2% reprojection error. The 3D visual hull reconstruction from silhouettes extracted from original video frames (bottom left) and from interpolated video frames (bottom right).

subspaces representing independent motions:

$$W = (R_1|T_1|R_2|T_2|...|R_N|T_N) \begin{pmatrix} S_1 \\ 1 \\ & S_2 \\ & 1 \\ & & \ddots \\ & & & S_m \\ & & & 1 \end{pmatrix}. \qquad (5.5)$$

Each motion has its own sequence of rotations and translations while the shape matrix consists of columns belonging to orthogonal shape subspaces.

Articulated motions For articulated motions it was shown by Yan and Pollefeys (2005b) (and independently by Tresadern and Reid (2005)) that the motion subspaces are intersecting. There are two cases for articulated motions.

- Articulation with two or three degree of freedom. In this case the motion subspaces for the two related parts have a one-dimensional intersection. This can easily be shown by assuming that the joint is located at the origin of both parts, as in this case the factorization equations can be written as follows:

$$W = [R_1\ R_2\ T] \begin{bmatrix} S_1 & 0 \\ 0 & S_2 \\ 1 & 1 \end{bmatrix}. \tag{5.6}$$

Hence the joining of the two 4D subspaces spans only a 7D subspace instead of 8D.

- Articulation with one degree of freedom. This represents the case where two parts are related by a rotation axis. In this case the motion subspaces for the two related parts have a two dimensional intersection. Here we show this by assuming that the rotation axis is aligned with the X-axis:

$$W = [r_1\ r_2\ r_3\ r_2'\ r_3'\ T] \begin{bmatrix} x_1 & x_2 \\ y_1 & 0 \\ z_1 & 0 \\ 0 & y_2 \\ 0 & z_2 \\ 1 & 1 \end{bmatrix}, \tag{5.7}$$

where $R_1 = [r_1\ r_2\ r_3]$ and $R_2 = [r_1\ r_2'\ r_3']$.

In this case the joining of the two 4D subspaces spans only a 6D subspace.

Shape interaction of articulated motions   Each trajectory has a corresponding column vector in the shape matrix which is the right-most matrix in Eqs. (5.5), (5.6) and (5.7). For independent motions (Eq. (5.5)), column vectors of different shape subspaces have zero inner products while column vectors of the same subspace generally do not. The shape interaction matrix (Costeira and Kanade, 1998) consists of these inner products of every pair of trajectories, so it can be used to group features of the same motion.

For articulated motions (Eqs. (5.6) and (5.7)), though the shape subspaces are not orthogonal, column vectors of the same shape subspace generally have larger inner products than those from different shape subspaces in magnitude. We will show that in the following. The first shape subspace in Eq. (5.6) can be represented by a base (e_1, e_2, e_3, e_7) where $e_i = [0, ..., 1, ...0]^T$ with i indicating the position of 1. Similarly, the second shape subspace can be represented by a base (e_4, e_5, e_6, e_7). It is easy to see that the inner product of column vectors from different shape subspaces has only one coefficient not canceled out while that of column vectors from the same shape subspace has four. This observation implies that the magnitude of the former is generally smaller than that of the latter. A similar analysis applies to Eq. (5.7).

So the inner products of column vectors may tell us how likely two trajectories are of the same motion. This key observation is what RANSAC with priors builds upon. In the following section we will describe how to estimate the priors with regard to how likely every pair of trajectories belong to the same motion and present our segmentation approach, RANSAC with priors.

5.3.2 RANSAC with priors

In this section, we will first describe how to build the priors to guide RANSAC. Then we will discuss RANSAC with priors.

The prior matrix   Though the magnitude of the entries in the shape interaction matrix (Costeria and Kanade, 1998) may be used directly for estimating how likely two trajectories are of the same motion. There is a better way.

The shape interaction matrix is actually an affinity matrix (Weiss, 1999). We adopt a spectral clustering algorithm (Ng *et al.*, 2002) to analyze the affinity matrix without carrying out the clustering part. Instead, we build an affinity matrix from the normalized spectral representations of each trajectory and use it to estimate the priors of how likely every pair of trajectories are of the same motion.

The procedure is described as followed.

- Build an affinity matrix M from the trajectory matrix W: $M = W^T W$.

- Normalize M into $N = D^{-1/2} M D^{-1/2}$ where $D_{ii} = \sum_j M_{ij}$

- Form a matrix $X_{p \times K}$ whose columns are the K dominant eigenvectors of N.

- Normalize each row vector of $X_{p \times K}$. This new matrix is $Y_{p \times K}$. Each row y_i of Y is the normalized spectral representation of trajectory i in R^K.

- Unlike spectral clustering which will cluster y_i into different groups at this step, we compute the affinity between each pair of y_i and y_j and use it to build the prior matrix P:

$$P_{ij} = \frac{2}{\sqrt{\pi}} \int_0^{y_i y_j^T} e^{-t^2} dt, \tag{5.8}$$

  where P_{ij} represents the probability of trajectory i belonging to the same motion as trajectory j.

A few remarks can now be made.

- The choice of the number of eigenvectors K. Ideally, K should be the rank of N. In practice, owing to noise, the rank of N can only be estimated. We may use a model selection algorithm inspired by a similar one in Vidal *et al.* (2004) to detect the rank:

$$r_n = \arg\min_r \frac{\lambda_{r+1}^2}{\sum_{K=1}^r \lambda_K^2} + \kappa\, r,$$

  with λ_i, the ith singular value of the matrix, and κ a parameter. If the sum of all λ_i^2 is below a certain threshold, the estimated rank is zero.

  Notice that because of outliers the estimated rank may be larger than the rank of the motion subspace. However, the spectral affinity turns out to be not very sensitive to a larger K.

- Any reasonable distribution function may substitute for Eq. (5.8). The point is to use the spectral affinity to build priors with regard to how likely two trajectories belong to the same motion.

RANSAC with priors   Here P_{ij} represents the probability of trajectory (or data) i belonging to the same motion (or model) as trajectory (or data) j.

We outline our segmentation approach, RANSAC with priors, as follows.

- Form a sample set of k data based on the priors P_{ij}.

  (1) Randomly choose the first data s_1 based on a probability distribution formed by the sums of each row of the prior matrix. A larger row sum indicates that the data is more likely to be part of the same motion as other data.

  (2) Randomly choose the subsequent data, s_i with $i = 2, \ldots, k$, based on a probability distribution formed by the priors related to data $s_1, \ldots, s_{i-1}$.

- Instantiate a model from this sample set.

- Determine the set of data S_i that are within a threshold t of the model.

- Repeat this N times. The largest consensus set is selected and the model is re-estimated using all the points in that consensus set. If the largest consensus set has a size less than some threshold T, terminate.

- Remove the data set S_i from the original data and repeat the above to find a new consensus set and its model until either the data are exhausted or no more models can be found from the remaining data.

A few remarks can be made here.

- The model that we use is the factorization model (Tomasi and Kanade, 1992) which states that the trajectories of a full rigid motion generally span a rank-4 subspace. So k is 4 in our experiments.

- Model selection can be naturally combined with RANSAC with priors to deal with degenerate shape and motion. This will be discussed in the next section.

Experiments   We present three experiments to show the effectiveness of our approach. The first experiment consists of a toy truck sequence with a moving shovel. Connected by an axis, the motion dependency is as high as it can get for articulated motions. To demonstrate the robustness of our approach, besides those erroneous trajectories due to tracking, outliers are created by adding large random noise (larger than 10%) to some existing trajectories. The prior matrix is shown in Figure 5.8. The actual rank of the articulated motion subspace is 6 while the detected rank is 13 because of outliers and noise. For illustration purposes, the trajectories have been grouped into the truck body, the shovel and random outliers. Notice the priors for random outliers have very small values which makes them unlikely to be selected into a sample set. And the erroneous trajectories are rejected when RANSAC with priors tries to find a largest possible consensus set. Each time, 50 samples are generated to find the largest possible consensus set from the current data. RANSAC with priors finds two motions and terminates when the largest possible consensus set that it can find has a size six which is less

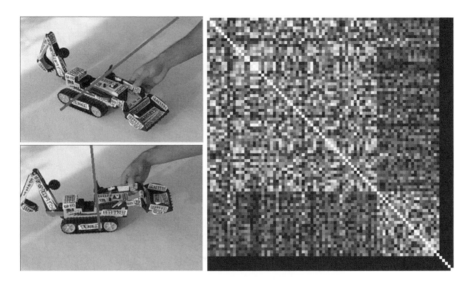

Figure 5.8. Two frames from the truck sequence with computed rotation axis overlaid (left) and prior matrix of the truck sequence with added outliers (right). Lighter color indicates higher probability.

than the threshold $T = 8$. Those six trajectories are some of the erroneous trajectories on the shovel and on the body. The remaining data consist of erroneous trajectories and the outliers that we add (Figure 5.9).

The second experiment is from a sequence of synthetic data of four linked parts. Each parts has 10 features to represent its 3D shape. Small random noise (less than 1%) is added to the trajectories. Four outliers are created by adding large random noise (larger than 10%) to some existing trajectories.

This experiment is challenging. First, each part has a small number of trajectories which provides too few constraints for GPCA (Vidal and Hartley, 2004) to work; secondly, RANSAC WITHOUT priors will require a large number of samples before it may obtain a valid sample set, i.e. a sample set consisting of trajectories from the same part. In this synthetic experiment only $1/4 \times 1/4 \times 1/4 = 1/64$ would be a sample set located on a single 4D subspace if priors are not taken into account. In practice, without knowing the number of motions beforehand, it is impossible to determine a sufficient number of random sets that have to be generated. With a large number of motions, generating random sets would be incredibly inefficient.

On the other hand, RANSAC with priors gets on average one valid sample set out of every three in this experiment and this rate does not depend on the total number of motions. It depends on the number of dependent motions. Parts that are further away generally have much less dependency which make the corresponding priors very small, thus their trajectories are unlikely to be chosen into a sample set. Each time 50 sample sets are generated to find the largest possible consensus set from the current data in this experiment. The actual rank of the articulated motion subspace is 13 but the detected rank is 17, owing to outliers. RANSAC with priors finds four motions

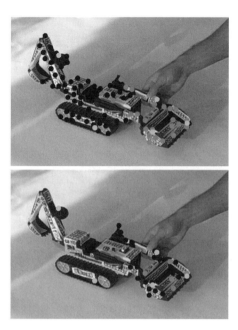

Figure 5.9. Top: RANSAC with priors finds the first consensus set indicated by the dark blue dots. The orange and light blue dots are the remaining data. The light blue dots are outliers. The orange dots on the truck body are erroneous trajectories. Bottom: the dark blue dots indicate the second consensus set found by RANSAC with priors. The orange and light blue dots are the remaining data. The light blue dots are the outliers. The orange dots are erroneous trajectories.

within the trajectories. The remaining data are four random outliers after RANSAC with priors can not find any consensus set of size more than $T = 8$. The result matches the ground truth.

Last but not the least, we test RANSAC with priors in a more complex scenario. For this experiment we combine the tracks from two video sequences as if they were seen simultaneously. Using our approach, independent motions are only a special case and can be treated the same way. The prior matrix for two independently moving articulated objects from a real sequence is shown in Figure 5.10. Each of these two articulated objects has two parts. Notice the priors between every pair of trajectories from different objects are very small. RANSAC with priors is able to segment four motions from these trajectories.

5.4   Conclusions and discussion

In this chapter we have presented a complete approach to determine the 3D visual hull of a dynamic object from silhouettes extracted from multiple videos recorded using an uncalibrated and unsynchronized network of cameras. The key element of our ap-

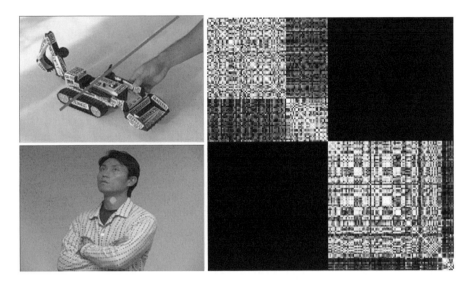

Figure 5.10. One frame from each of the two sequences for which the tracks were combined (left) and the prior matrix of two independently moving articulated objects (right). The truck has its two parts linked by a rotation axis while the person has body and head linked by a joint. Lighter color indicates higher probability.

proach is a robust algorithm that efficiently computes the temporal offset between two video sequences and the corresponding epipolar geometry. The proposed method is robust and accurate and allows calibration of camera networks without the need for acquiring specific calibration data. This can be very useful for applications where sending in technical personnel with calibration targets for calibration or recalibration is either unfeasible or impractical. We have shown that for visual hull reconstructions from unsynchronized video streams subframe silhouette interpolation allows us to significantly improve the quality of the results.

The second part of this chapter discussed an approach for efficiently performing motion segmentation for articulated objects based on RANSAC with priors. It can segment articulated motions as well as independent motions. It does not require prior knowledge of how many motions there are. It is both efficient and robust. The priors are derived from the spectral affinity between every pair of trajectories.

It is interesting to notice that at the core of both approaches presented in this chapter one can find a modified RANSAC algorithm. The standard RANSAC algorithm consists of selecting a minimal random subset of the data that allows us to compute a hypothesis which is then validated with respect to the remainder of the data. This procedure is repeated until a hypothesis with sufficient support from the data is obtained. The most important feature of this algorithm is the robustness to outliers.

The problem with applying RANSAC to silhouette-based epipolar geometry computation is that silhouettes do not provide constraints that can be solved directly. Our solution to this problem consisted of randomly generating hypotheses for the epipoles (four parameters) and then use three silhouettes to complete the epipolar geometry hypothesis. In this case many more samples have to be generated, but both the exploration of the parameter space and the robustness to outliers are addressed together by this modified RANSAC algorithm. It would be interesting to study how this approach can be used to deal with uncertainty on some of the parameters in other estimation problems.

The problem with applying RANSAC to the estimation of articulate motion subspaces is that the percentage of inliers for any single motion might be very small, and therefore a uniform sampling of feature tracks to generate hypotheses would be very inefficient. Our proposed solution consists of favoring tracks that are likely to be located on the same subspace. We show that this approach can be very effective in solving motion segmentation in the presence of dependent motions.

Acknowledgements

We would like to thank Peter Sand for providing us with the four-view dataset from MIT (Sand *et al.*, 2003). The partial support of the NSF Career award IIS 0237533, NSF ITR grant IIS-0313047 and a Packard Fellowship are gratefully acknowledged.

References

Astrom, K., Cipolla, R. and Giblin, P. (1996) Generalised epipolar constraints. *European Conf. on Computer Vision* II, pp. 97–108.

Buehler, C., Matusik, W. and Mcmillan, L. (2001). Polyhedral visual hulls for real-time rendering. *Eurographics Workshop on Rendering*.

Cheung, G., Baker, S. and Kanade, T. (2003). Visual hull alignment and refinement across time: a 3d reconstruction algorithm combining shape-from-silhouette with stereo. *IEEE Conf. on Computer Vision and Pattern Recognition*, II, pp. 375–382.

Costeira, J. and Kanade, T. (1998). A multibody factorization method for independently moving objects. *Int. J. Computer Vision*, **29**, 159–179.

Furukawa, Y., Sethi, A., Ponce, J., and Kriegman, D. (2004). Structure and motion from images of smooth textureless objects. *European Conf. on Computer Vision*, II, pp. 287–298.

Hartley, R. and Zisserman, A. (2000). *Multiple View Geometry in Computer Vision*. Cambridge University Press.

Laurentini, A. (1994). The visual hull concept for silhouette-based image understanding. *IEEE Trans. on Pattern Analysis and Machine Intelligence*, **16**, 150–162.

Levi, N. and Werman, M. (2003). The viewing graph. *IEEE Conf. on Computer Vision and Pattern Recognition*, I, pp. 518–522.

Matusik, W., Buehler, C., Raskar, R., Gortler, S. and McMillan, L. (2000). Image-based visual hulls. *SIGGRAPH*, pp. 369–374.

Mauch, S. (2003). *Efficient Algorithms for Solving Static Hamilton–Jacobi Equations*. PhD. thesis, California Institute of Technology.

Ng, A., Jordan, M. and Weiss, Y. (2002). On spectral clustering: analysis and an algorithm. *Advances in Neural Information Processing Systems 14*. MIT Press.

Pollefeys, M., Koch, R. and Van Gool, L. (1999). Self calibration and metric reconstruction inspite of varying and unknown intrinsic camera parameters. *Int. J. of Computer Vision*, **32**, 7–25.

Pollefeys, M., Van Gool, L., Vergauwen, M. *et al.* (2004). Visual modeling with a hand-held camera. *Int. J. of Computer Vision*, **59**, 207–232.

Porrill, J. and Pollard, S. (1991). Curve matching and stereo calibration. *Image and Vision Computing*, **9**, 45–50.

Sand, P., McMillan, L. and Popovic, J. (2003). Continuous capture of skin deformation. *SIGGRAPH*, pp. 578–586.

Sethian, J. (1996). A fast marching level set method for monotonically advancing fronts. *Proc. Nat. Acad. Sci.*, **94**, 1591–1595.

Sinha, S. and Pollefeys, M. (2004a). Camera network calibration from dynamic silhouettes. *IEEE Conf. on Computer Vision and Pattern Recognition*, pp. 195–202.

Sinha, S. and Pollefeys, M. (2004b). Synchronization and calibration of camera networks from silhouettes. *Int. Conf. on Pattern Recognition*, I, pp. 116–119.

Sinha, S. and Pollefeys, M. (2004c). Visual-hull reconstruction from uncalibrated and unsynchronized video streams. *2nd Int. Symp. on 3D Data Processing, Visualization & Transmission*.

Tomasi, C. and Kanade, T. (1992). Shape and motion from image streams under orthography: a factorization method. *Int. J. Computer Vision*, **9**, 137–154.

Tresadern, P. and Reid, I. (2005). Articulated structure from motion by factorization. *IEEE Conf. on Computer Vision and Pattern Recognition*, II, pp. 1110–1115.

Triggs, B., McLauchlan, P., Hartley, R. and Fitzgibbon, A. (2000). Bundle adjustment – A modern synthesis. *Vision Algorithms: Theory and Practice*. LNCS, Springer Verlag, pp. 298–375,

Vidal, R. and Hartley, R. (2004). Motion segmentation with missing data using power factorization and GPCA. *IEEE Conf. on Computer Vision and Pattern Recognition*, pp. 310–316.

Vidal, R., Ma, Y. and Piazzi, J. (2004). A new GPCA algorithm for clustering subspaces by fitting, differentiating and dividing polynomials. *IEEE Conf. on Computer Vision and Pattern Recognition*, p. 510.

Vijayakumar, B., Kriegman, D. and Ponce, J. (1996). Structure and motion of curved 3d objects from monocular silhouettes. *IEEE Conf. on Computer Vision and Pattern Recognition*, pp. 327–334.

Weiss, Y. (1999). Segmentation using eigenvectors: A unifying view. *Int. Conf. on Computer Vision*, pp. 975–982.

Wong, K. and Cipolla, R. (2001). Structure and motion from silhouettes. *Int. Conf. on Computer Vision*, II, pp. 217–222.

Yan, J. and Pollefeys, M. (2005a). Articulated motion segmentation using RANSAC with priors. *Workshop on Dynamic Vision*.

Yan, J. and Pollefeys, M. (2005b). A factorization-based approach to articulated motion recovery. *IEEE Conf. on Computer Vision and Pattern Recognition*, II, pp. 815–821.

Yan, J. and Pollefeys, M. (2006). A general framework for motion segmentation: Independent, articulated, rigid, non-rigid, degenerate and non-degenerate. *European Conf. on Computer Vision*.

Yezzi, A. and Soatto, S. (2003). Structure from motion for scenes without features. *IEEE Conf. on Computer Vision and Pattern Recogntion*, I, pp. 525–532.

Zhang, Z. (1999). Flexible camera calibration by viewing a plane from unknown orientations. *Int. Conf. on Computer Vision*, pp. 666–673.

6 Specular planar target surface recovery via coded target stereopsis

Arlene Ripsman, Piotr Jasiobedzki and Michael Jenkin

6.1 Introduction

Traditional computer vision algorithms are designed with non-specular surfaces in mind. Diffuse or Lambertian reflectance models are common. The basic premise of many stereopsis and optic flow algorithms is that the intensity of the surface remains constant or that the intensity changes in a slow predictable manner. Specularities are often ignored, and the intent in many approaches is to treat specularities as noise and to hope that the dramatic changes in intensity with illumination-viewing geometry can be detected and the region around the specularity can be rejected (see Bhat and Nayar, 1995; Li *et al.*, 2002). That being said, a number of recent stereo algorithms have begun to examine more complex surface–light interactions. Treuille *et al.* (2004) developed a multi-camera stereo system that support general BRDFs provided that appropriate reference objects are available. Recently, several groups of researchers have begun to use visual approaches to reconstruct highly specular surfaces. Kutulakos and Steger (2005) and Bonfort *et al.* (2006) use triangulation methods. Savarese *et al.* (2004) reconstruct mirror-like surfaces by looking at the distortion of a reflected target in an image.

Specularities occur naturally (e.g. at the surfaces of liquids) and many man-made structures are built to be highly specular. For example, much of the external surface of orbital equipment is designed to be highly specular in order to avoid unwanted heating due to the absorption of sunlight by non-specular surfaces. Space structures are notorious for their highly specular surfaces. Figure 6.1 shows an astronaut servicing the Hubble Space Telescope. The central body of the telescope is wrapped in a highly

Computational Vision in Neural and Machine Systems, ed. L. Harris and M. Jenkin. Published by Cambridge University Press. © Cambridge University Press 2007.

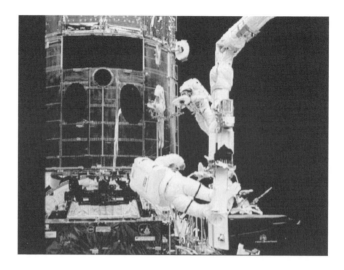

Figure 6.1. An astronaut servicing the Hubble Space Telescope.

specular surface (note the reflection of the astronaut in the telescope's surface). The highly specular nature of the surface poses a challenge to existing vision-based surface recovery algorithms.

Rather than attempting to patch existing algorithms that rely on a non-specular surface model, here we present a novel approach to the reconstruction of surfaces of highly specular objects. Instead of attempting to recover the surface structure of a specular object directly, we approach the problem by looking at the effects of specular surfaces on the appearance of other objects reflected within them. A commercial trinocular stereo vision system is coupled with an addressable video target to project controlled two-dimensional light patterns, and surface structure is inferred indirectly by the way in which the known light pattern is imaged after reflection in the surface. This method is intended to be used on a portable apparatus that can be moved around an object allowing reconstruction to proceed one portion at a time. Both highly specular and diffuse portions of the object are reconstructed simultaneously.

6.2   Exploiting properties of planar specular surfaces

Specular surfaces exhibit specular reflections. A perfectly specular surface is a mirror and reflects incident light in one direction – it reflects light such that the angle of incidence equals the angle of reflection. An object reflected in a planar mirror appears behind the surface of the mirror by exactly the same distance that the actual object is in front of the mirror (see Figure 6.2 and Halliday, Resnick and Walker, 1997). Suppose a known target point P is projected onto a unknown planar specular surface and then viewed as P' (P' is the reflection of P). Knowledge of P and P' can be used to infer structural information about the specular surface. Given P and P', the virtual planar mirror within which P is reflected can be computed as follows. Let $P_0 = (P + P')/2$.

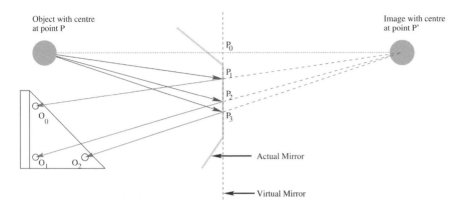

Figure 6.2. Recovery of points on a specular surface.

Then the virtual planar mirror in which P is reflected is given by the plane that is perpendicular to $\vec{PP'}$ that passes through P_0. If P' is viewed by an observer O_i, then the point P_i on the planar surface at which O_i observes P (and P') is given by the intersection of the line O_iP' with the virtual planar mirror. Note that if P' was originally located via a multi-camera system, then each camera of the multi-camera system defines its own O_i and hence provides its own point P_i on the specular surface (see Jenkin and Jasiobedzki, 1998; Ripsman, 2002; Ripsman and Jenkin, 2001a, b; and Figure 6.2 for details of this construction).

As illustrated in Figure 6.2, the point P_0 need not actually exist as a physical point on the mirror. The mirror need only exist and be planar in the region of the reflection of the rays joining the O_is and P_is.

6.3 Actively recovering 3D specular surface structure

Given that specular surface structure can be constructed given a 3D point P and its reflection in the surface P', all that remains is to establish some process to generate points P, acquire the 3D virtual points P', and to establish (as necessary) the correspondences between P and P'. Various approaches to each of these tasks are possible. For example, naturally occurring structure in the scene might be used along with its reflection. Here we take an alternative approach and actively generate potential real points P for which the true 3D position is known. We use an addressable two-dimensional illuminant to generate candidate real points P, and use a trinocular camera system to obtain the three-dimensional locations of the virtual points P'.

In brief, the algorithm is described in terms of the following six steps.

(1) The portion of the object that is to be reconstructed is illuminated in a systematic manner with an addressable illuminant. A purely specular surface will have no inherent texture of its own, and thus will be invisible unless some textured pattern is reflected within it.

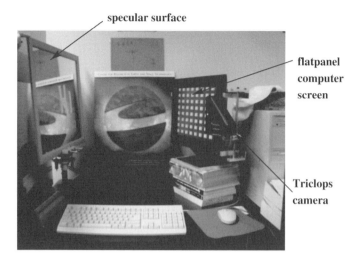

Figure 6.3. Experimental setup.

(2) Three-dimensional points are obtained from the illumination of the surface. The Triclops system is used to recover three-dimensional points (both specular and diffuse) within its field of view.

(3) The recovered three-dimensional points are divided into specular (virtual) and diffuse (real) points.

(4) For each specular point recovered, the true position of the illuminant that gave rise to the point is established.

(5) The points P and P' are used to transform the virtual specular points into real points on the object's surface.

(6) The diffuse and specular points are merged into a single representation of the object.

Each of these steps is described in some detail below, after details regarding the hardware setup and calibration are presented.

6.3.1   Experimental setup

A proof-of-concept system has been constructed consisting of a Triclops trinocular camera rigidly affixed to a flatpanel LCD display (see Figure 6.3). The LCD display serves as a controlled two-dimensional illuminate. The Triclops Stereo Vision system is a commercially available trinocular vision system. Triclops consists of three 1/3" CCD cameras that simultaneously capture three gray-scale images of the scene. The Triclops software uses a proprietary multi-baseline approach to stereo processing, based on the work of Kanade *et al.* (1995), and computes a disparity image from which the three-dimensional location of points in the scene can be determined. The Triclops hardware and software defines a global 3D coordinate frame for the system described here.

In order to use the LCD display it must be calibrated to the global coordinate frame. Recovering local surface structure from P and P' requires knowledge of the three-dimensional position of the illuminant. This is accomplished by establishing an affine mapping between pixel locations on the illuminate and three-dimensional points in space that define the plane of the illuminant. This calibration was accomplished through a two step calibration process. First, a planar mirror was covered with a diffuse target and imaged using the trinocular camera system. The resulting depth map was used to obtain the plane of the mirror in the camera coordinate frame via a robust linear least-squares procedure. Once this plane was identified, the diffuse target covering was removed, and points on the mirror were were illuminated using the controlled illuminant and corresponding virtual image points in the mirror determined. Using the known plane of the mirror, we determined the three-dimensional coordinate of each illuminant. Robust linear regression was used to determine an affine mapping between (u, v) coordinates on the illuminate and corresponding points (x, y, z) in camera space.

6.3.2 Obtaining virtual points P'

In order to solve the stereopsis correspondence problem there must exist visible features in each view that can be combined interocularly. Since many space-based objects involve surfaces that are large, relatively smooth and featureless, the surface may not contain sufficient texture or may not reflect sufficient naturally occurring texture. In order to overcome this problem, the required texture is provided using textured light patterns that are projected onto the object. We project n (where $n > 2$) different patterns onto the object and a disparity map is obtained for each pattern. Each of the patterns is chosen so that it is equiluminant *on average*.

Recovered disparities may correspond to either specular reflected points or diffuse surface points. In order to reconstruct highly specular planar surfaces with diffuse components, it is necessary to determine which image points correspond to specular reflections and which correspond to diffuse illumination. Once this has been accomplished, the three-dimensional location of diffuse points can be obtained directly from the disparity image produced by the Triclops system. The three-dimensional location of specular points can be determined by the passive target method.

In order to divide the recovered points into specular and diffuse, intensity images are captured along with disparity maps for each illumination condition. For each pixel, the grayscale intensity in each of Triclops' three images is recorded. The system assumes a point is diffuse when its intensity is relatively invariant to the light emitted by the projector over all of the images.

6.3.3 Using structured light to identify and locate the illuminant

Given a disparity image, it is necessary to identify which point on the illuminant gives rise to a particular disparity value. A controlled illuminant could be provided in a variety of different ways. Individual points on the illuminant could be controlled although this could result in a very time-intensive procedure. An alternative approach would be to project a range of different patterns designed to illuminate the scene in a controlled manner (Mouaddib *et al.*, 1997). Following this latter approach, a sequence of grid

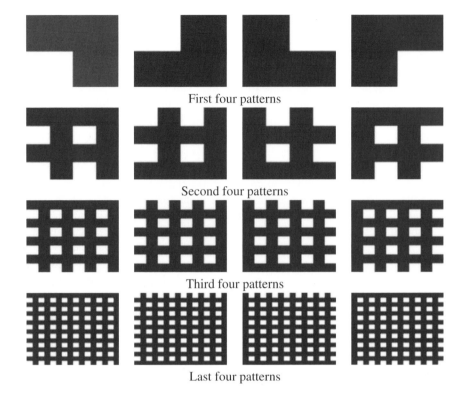

First four patterns

Second four patterns

Third four patterns

Last four patterns

Figure 6.4. Coded light patterns used to identify emitted light.

patterns is projected, and depth and intensity images are recovered for each illuminant. With each successive iteration the projection pattern is divided into finer grids. Each iteration consists of four frames. In each frame exactly one quarter of the screen is illuminated. After each iteration all parts of the screen have been illuminated exactly once. After an iteration each of the illuminated areas are again divided into four parts and each part is illuminated in a different frame in the next iteration. The process terminates when the resolution limit of the screen and the Triclops camera is reached. In our case, this occurs after four iterations, shown in Figure 6.4.

Based on the images obtained by the trinocular stereo rig, we are now able to determine, for each pixel in the image, the region on the computer screen which emitted the illuminant. After each iteration we can determine which frame illuminated each pixel by choosing the frame in which the pixel's intensity is brightest. Through this process the possible source of the illumination is reduced to one illuminant square in the final iteration (see Figure 6.5). The center of this surviving region is used as an approximation of a point illuminant. The error in this assumption depends on the size of the regions illuminated in the final iteration, as well as the distance of the reflected light from the emitted light. A derivation of the error in this approximation can be found in Ripsman (2002).

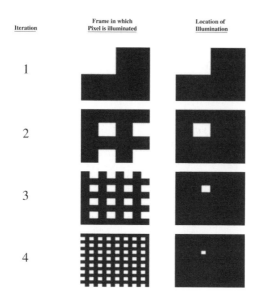

Figure 6.5. Identification of illuminant through coded patterns.

Providing a controlled illumination enables the establishment of the depth of true points corresponding to objects in the environment, as well as establishing virtual points that correspond to specular reflection.

6.3.4 Dealing with multiple planar surfaces

The passive target technique assumes that the target is a single, infinitely large, planar surface. In order to deal with objects with multiple planar surfaces, instead of assuming that all recovered surface points belong to a single plane, the points are divided into local regions and each region is assumed to be locally planar. Once the points are recovered, a set of overlapping regions are constructed and a plane is fit to each region.

Now consider surfaces with both specular and diffuse regions. Since we are modeling surfaces that may be composed of multiple planes, the region of interest is defined less clearly. For example, if the object has two planes at an angle to one another, the projected pattern could be reflected in each plane. In non-planar surfaces, diffuse points identified by the system can arise in several ways. We are interested only in modeling diffuse areas that lie on the surface of the object not those points that lie behind the projector or between the projector and the object.

In order to reconstruct a specular surface with diffuse components the method is applied in two passes. In the first pass only points initially identified as specular are used. As described above, these points are divided into regions and locally planar surfaces are determined. The algorithm is then run a second time. This time the points identified as diffuse by the system are included in solving for the surface. These diffuse points enable the system to refine the calculations of the local planar surfaces determined in the first pass. If a surface for the region was not calculated in pass one of the algorithm

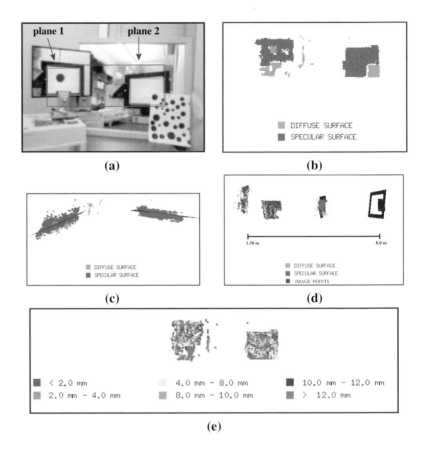

Figure 6.6. Reconstruction of two planar specular surfaces at an angle.

(this could be caused, for example, by the entire region being diffuse), then neighboring regions are used to guide the surface calculation. More details on this method are provided in Ripsman (2002).

6.3.5 Experimental results

In order to demonstrate that the system can effectively reconstruct multiple planar surfaces with diffuse components, an experiment was conducted. The system was placed in front of two planar surfaces at approximately a $30°$ angle to one another, each with diffuse components. The results of the experiment are shown in Figure 6.6 and Table 6.1.

Figure 6.6a shows the actual surfaces. The red rectangle outlines the area of interest as defined by the system. Figure 6.6b, c and d show front, top, and side views of the surface with the recovered specular surface shown in red and the recovered diffuse surface shown in green. The black plane seen in Figure 6.6c and d is the actual surface

	Plane 1	Plane 2	Total
Number of specular points	1687	2628	4315
Number of diffuse points	371	217	588
Number of points	2058	2845	4903
Mean distance from actual plane	0.0097 m	0.0058 m	0.0074 m
Standard deviation	0.0077 m	0.0045 m	0.0061 m

Table 6.1. *Statistics on recovered planar surfaces with diffuse components.*

and the blue points shown in Figure 6.6d are the points recovered by the Triclops system. Table 6.1 provides some statistics on the reconstruction broken down by the two planes labeled in Figure 6.6a.

6.4   Discussion

This chapter describes a novel approach to reconstructing the surface structure of large, smooth, planar objects with highly specular surfaces. The underlying concept is that by observing how a known point is reflected in the surface it is possible to infer local surface structure. A similar observation is used by Morris and Kutulakos (2005) to infer the surface structure of liquids by the refractive effect of the liquid medium. Here an addressable illuminant is used to generate illuminants in a controlled manner. This addresses the need to determine correspondences between illuminates and reflected image points. This is accomplished by using stereo (trinocular) vision in combination with a structured light technique. Results obtained demonstrate that the system can produce local reconstructions of simple, highly specular objects. The prototype system was able to produce range data for planar and multiple planar surfaces. The surfaces explored included those that were completely specular and those that had diffuse components. The points recovered were generally accurate to within an average of ±0.005 m of the actual surface.

Acknowledgments

The support of the Natural Sciences and Engineering Research Council of Canada (NSERC), The Canadian Space Agency, CRESTech and MDA is gratefully acknowledged.

References

Bhat, D. N. and Nayar, S. K. (1995). Stereo in the presence of specular reflection. *Proc. ICCV'95*, pp. 1086–1092.

Bonfort, T., Sturm, P. and Gargallo, P. (2006). General specular surface triangulation. *Proc. Asian Conference on Computer Vision*, Hyderabad, India, Volume II, pp.

872–881.

Halliday, D., Resnick, R. and Walker, J. (1997). *Fundamentals of Physics Extended Fifth Edition*. New York: John Wiley and Sons, Inc.

Jenkin, M. and Jasiobedzki, P. (1998). Computation of stereo disparity for space materials. *Proc. IEEE/RSJ IROS*, Victoria, Canada.

Kanade, T., Kato, H., Kimura, S., Yoshida, A. and Oda, K. (1995). Development of a video-rate stereo machine. *Proc. IEEE/RSJ IROS*, Pittsburgh, PA.

Kutulakos, K. N. and Steger, E. (2005). A theory of refractive and specular 3D shape by light-path triangulation. *Proc. ICCV'05*, pp. 1448–1455.

Li, Y., Lin, S., Lu, H., Kang, S. B. and Shum, H.-Y. (2002). Multibaseline stereo in the presence of specular reflections. *Proc. ICPR'02*.

Morris, N. and Kutulakos, K. (2005). Dynamic refraction stereo. *Proc. ICCV'05*, pp. 1573–1580.

Mouaddib, E., Salvi, J. and Batlle, J. (1997). An overview of the advantages and constraints of coded pattern projection techniques for autonomous navigation. *Proc. IEEE/RSJ IROS*, Grenoble, France.

Ripsman, A. (2002). *Local Surface Reconstruction of Orbital Objects*. M.Sc. Thesis, Department of Computer Science, York University.

Ripsman, A. and Jenkin, M. (2001a). Local surface reconstruction of orbital objects. *IEEE Int. Symp. on Computational Intelligence (CIRA-2001)*, Banff, Alberta.

Ripsman, A. and Jenkin, M. (2001b). Surface reconstruction of objects in space. *Proc. ISAIRAS 2001*, Montreal, Quebec.

Savarese, S., Chen, M. and Perona, P. (2004). Recovering local shape of a mirror surface from reflection of a regular grid. *Proc. of European Conference of Computer Vision*, Prague, Czech Republic.

Treuille, A., Herzmann, A. and Seitz, S. M. (2004). Example-based stereo with general BRDFs. *Proc. ECCV*, Prague, Czech Repulbic.

7 Neural construction of objects from parts

Charles E. Connor

From a subjective viewpoint, visual perception of objects is one of the richest and most ubiquitous aspects of human cognitive experience. From an objective viewpoint, the human abilities to recognize, comprehend, and remember objects are phenomenal. No machine-based visual systems have come close to duplicating those abilities. Human object perception depends on extensive neural processing through a series of stages in the ventral pathway of visual cortex. That processing is not yet understood in any deep, detailed, mechanistic way. This chapter summarizes our recent analyses of how information about objects is represented and transformed in higher-level ventral pathway cortex so as to produce our remarkable perceptual capacities and our vivid visual experiences of objects. The large-scale picture that emerges from these studies is one of active construction of object representations from neural signals for simple, standard object parts. We think it is this process that eventuates in a neural code compact, consistent, and explicit enough to support visual experience and perceptual performance.

In humans and non-human primates, the ventral visual pathway (Ungerleider and Mishkin, 1982), begins in primary visual cortex (V1) and continues through areas V2, V4, and multiple stages in ventral occipital/temporal cortex. In humans these more advanced areas include V8, lateral occipital (LO), and parts of the fusiform and parahippocampal regions (Epstein *et al.*, 1999; Kanwisher *et al.*, 1997a, b; Kourtzi and Kanwisher, 2000; Lerner *et al.*, 2001). Overall levels of neural activity in these human brain regions can be studied using functional magnetic resonance imaging (fMRI). However, the computational magic of human vision takes place at the level of neurons and neural networks. The study of visual information processing at this level requires invasive microelectrode recording of neural action potentials. This can be accomplished in humans under rare clinical circumstances (Quiroga *et al.*, 2005), but control over anatomical sampling and the amount of obtainable data is limited. Systematic study of visual computation in the brain thus depends mainly on non-human primates, especially macaque monkeys. Macaques have visual perceptual capacities comparable

Computational Vision in Neural and Machine Systems, ed. L. Harris and M. Jenkin. Published by Cambridge University Press. © Cambridge University Press 2007.

to those of humans, and the organization of visual cortex is strongly homologous between macaques and humans. Our studies focus on neural processing of object shape in higher-level stages of the macaque ventral pathway: area V4 (homologous to human area V4) and inferotemporal cortex (IT), which comprises a posterior-to-anterior series of processing stages with potential homology to human V8, LO, fusiform and parahippocampal cortex.

The step-wise transformation of visual information in the ventral visual pathway must culminate in representations that are (1) compact (sparse) enough to be stored in memory (Olshausen and Field, 1997; Vinje and Gallant, 2000), (2) consistent enough to support object recognition across multiple viewing circumstances, and (3) explicit enough to be easily accessed and interpreted by other parts of the brain. Presumably this widespread accessibility of explicit object information supports our vivid experience and extensive knowledge of objects. The original representation of objects at the retinal level is not compact but instead highly distributed, across approximately 10^6 retinal ganglion cells, which function like pixels on a display screen to signal brightness or color contrast in a local image region. This representation is anything but consistent – the activity pattern evoked on the retina by any given object changes completely with alterations of position, distance, orientation, and illumination. Finally, the retinal representation contains no explicit information about object identity or object characteristics. The information is all there, but in a hopelessly implicit form, no more readable than an endless list of pixel values on a display screen. The ventral visual pathway exists to translate this unwieldy mass of neural information into knowledge about objects in our world. Our results suggest this is achieved by initially deriving information about local object part geometry, representing a given object's constituent parts with a multi-peaked basis function code, and ultimately synthesizing part signals into representations of larger multi-part configurations. As described below, the neural coding dimensions in which parts and their relationships are represented, the synthetic process of integrating multiple parts, and the inherent general characteristics of parts-based representations all conspire toward compactness, consistency, and explicitness.

7.1   Basis function representation of object parts

Our empirical results tie together and substantiate two theoretical principles: basis function coding and representation by parts. Basis function coding is an efficient method for representing and processing multi-dimensional properties in populations of neurons with gradual tuning (Deneve *et al.*, 1999, 2001; Pouget *et al.*, 1998, 2000). We find that neurons in higher-level ventral pathway cortex represent object components with basis function coding on dimensions relating to local contour geometry: curvature, orientation, and relative position. Coding contour shape in terms of curvature and orientation takes advantage of statistical regularities in real-world contour structure to maximize compactness. Transformation from retinotopic to object-relative position coding helps achieve consistency across image changes.

Representation of objects in terms of their constituent parts (Biederman, 1987; Hoffman and Richards, 1984; Marr and Nishihara, 1978) also helps to achieve consistency, in the sense that the list of an object's parts remains constant across different views. Representation by parts has the combinatorial power to encode the virtual infinity of object shapes in this world in terms of a finite number of common components. Thus, the total number of neurons required to adequately represent real-world shapes is minimized. Our post hoc reconstructions of neural population activity indicate that the constituent parts of an object are represented by multiple local activity peaks along contour-related basis function dimensions. Previous examples of basis function coding analyses (Georgopoulos *et al.*, 1983) have focused on the representation of single values on one or two dimensions. The complexity and variety of object shape requires basis function representation of multiple values in a high-dimensional space.

Some sensitivity to contour curvature may exist in V1 and V2 (Dobbins *et al.*, 1987; Hegde and Van Essen, 2000; Heggelund and Hohmann, 1975), but explicit basis function-like tuning for contour curvature is first evident at the V4 level. Many individual V4 neurons recorded from awake macaque monkeys performing a fixation task show gradual, Gaussian-like tuning for both the curvature and orientation of luminance contours spanning their receptive fields (Pasupathy and Connor, 1999).[1] A given neuron, for example, might respond at 30 spikes (action potentials) per second to a sharply-curved convex contour oriented (pointing) downward, at 20 spikes/s to slightly different contours (e.g. broader convexities oriented downward, sharp convexities oriented toward lower left or lower right), and at progressively lower rates to more dissimilar contour stimuli (see Figure 7.1a). When more complex and complete shapes are present in the receptive field, V4 responses are still determined by local contour shape (Pasupathy and Connor, 2001). Thus, a neuron responsive to sharp convex curvature oriented to the right would respond to any variety of shapes containing such curvature (e.g. Figure 7.1b). This is a critical characteristic for parts-based coding. For combinatorial coding to work, it is essential that a given neuron consistently signal the same component shape values in all global shape contexts.

Curvature and orientation are derivatives useful for describing object shape in a more compact fashion. At the retinal level, shape information is widely distributed across large numbers of pixel-like retinal ganglion cells. In our world, the luminance patterns that define shape tend to contain many elongated contrast regions (contours), often representing the boundaries of objects. The brain takes advantage of this statistical characteristic, beginning in V1, by representing local contour regions not as large numbers of pixels but in terms of their orientation (Hubel and Wiesel, 1968). Orientation is the derivative of one spatial dimension with respect to the other on the 2D image plane. Orientation is often fairly constant on the scale of V1 receptive fields (fractions of a degree of visual angle), making it a useful dimension for compactly and accurately summarizing contour shape. At the larger scales that V4 neurons deal with (several degrees), orientation tends to change, but often at a roughly constant rate. Thus, larger contour regions can be described by additionally representing the second derivative, curvature (the rate of change in orientation along the contour), producing an even more compact description of shape. In addition, curvature representation provides an explicit signal for a significant aspect of object shape to which we are keenly sensitive

---

[1]Sensitivity to curvature is even more prominent at subsequent processing stages in IT (Brincat and Connor, 2004).

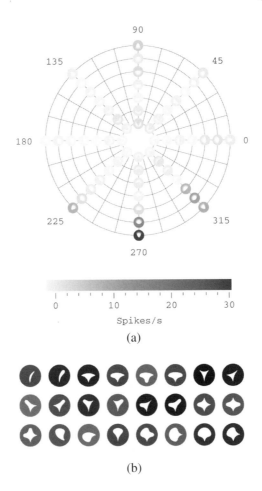

Figure 7.1. Basis function tuning for local boundary curvature in area V4. (a) Responses of a hypothetical V4 neuron exemplifying gradual tuning for orientation and curvature of boundary fragments. Average response rates in spikes per second are indicated by the gray level of the background circle (see scale). In this case, the tuning peak corresponds to sharp convex curvature oriented at 270° (pointing downward). (b) Responses of the same hypothetical V4 neuron to complex shapes, exemplifying how V4 neurons consistently respond to the same boundary feature (in this case, convex curvature at 270°) in different global shape contexts.

(Andrews *et al.*, 1973; Treisman and Gormican, 1988; Wilson *et al.*, 1997; Wolfe *et al.*, 1992).

In parallel to the emergence of curvature tuning in V4 and IT, there is a gradual transformation of position coding from retinotopic to object-relative coordinates. A given V1 neuron responds to stimuli only in a restricted region of retinotopic space. In V4, the retinotopic receptive fields are larger, and within those receptive fields, neurons are sensitive to object-relative position. For example, a neuron might respond strongly to sharp convex contour fragments near the bottom of an object but weakly to convexities near the right or left. In posterior IT, retinotopic receptive fields are even larger (on the order of $10°$) and tuning for object-relative position is stronger and more prevalent (Brincat and Connor, 2004). In anterior IT, retinotopic receptive fields can span most of the visual image.

The transformation from retinotopic to object-relative position coding produces increasing consistency of the neural representation across changes in object position across the retina. If the object-relative coordinate system scales with object size, consistency across changes in object size is also achieved. The remarkable consistency of shape tuning across multiple octaves of size difference argues that this is the case (Brincat and Connor, 2004), although it has not been investigated systematically. The transformation into an bject-relative reference frame is also a key element of any parts-based representation. For an adequate description of a given object, it is essential not only to represent part identities but also to represent how those parts are spatially related to each other. Finally, the appearance of basis function representation of object-relative position provides explicit spatial information of the kind we perceive and operate on. We do not naturally describe the positions of objects and object parts in exact Cartesian coordinates (even though that is the nature of spatial information in the original retinal image). Instead, we describe relative positions in local reference frames defined by objects (e.g. "Fred is standing behind Mary", "The handle is on the side of the teacup").

At the population level, parts-based representation requires that multiple values (corresponding to different parts) be represented in the same shape space. This stands in contrast to most neural basis function coding situations, where only a single value must be represented (e.g. reach direction; see Georgopoulos *et al.*, 1983). In single value cases, under standard conditions, there is a single hill of activity in the neural population. Those neurons with basis function tuning peaks closest to the true value are most active (i.e. they are at the top of the hill). Neurons with tuning peaks slightly offset from the true value are moderately active (forming the shoulders of the hill). K. O. Johnson suggested that if each neuron is considered to be a vector pointing to its tuning peak, and its activity level is considered to be the length of that vector, the true value can be derived from the total population by averaging all the vectors (Mountcastle, 1995). This can also be thought of as fitting a function to the distribution of activity levels (Deneve *et al.*, 1999). The brain appears to interpret basis function representations using some comparable operation, drawing on the entire pattern of response rates for greater accuracy and robustness, except under exceptional circumstances (Groh *et al.*, 1997).

In experiments on macaque area V4, we found that the contour fragments making up an object's boundary are represented by multiple hills of activity across the neural basis function space (Pasupathy and Connor, 2002). Our analysis was based on the responses of 109 neurons to a set of 366 parametrically varying silhouette shapes. To estimate the population response to a given shape, we treated each neuron as a vector pointing toward its tuning peak in curvature-angular position space, (the stimulus set was simple enough to characterize on this 2D domain). In particular, angular position and orientation were always identical – e.g. projections at the top always pointed upward – so the angular position dimension can also be thought of as the orientation dimension.) We treated the activity of the neuron (in response to the shape in question) as the magnitude or vector length. We then convolved the vectors with a 2D Gaussian to produce a smooth surface estimate of V4 population activity. The convolution is roughly equivalent to fitting a multi-peaked function to the neural vectors.

For each shape, the estimated population response surface contained local peaks corresponding to its constituent boundary components. For the valentine-heart-like shape in Figure 7.2, the sharp projection at the bottom was represented by an activity peak near 1.0 (infinitely sharp convex curvature) and 270° (pointing downward, near the bottom) on the curvature-angular position domain. The shallow indentation at the top was represented by an activity peak near −0.3 (moderate concave curvature) and 90° (pointing upward, near the top). Other peaks in the population activity pattern corresponded to the other boundary fragments making up the rest of the shape. The veridical representation of the shape in this domain is of course a continuous line (see Figure 7.2), but we suggest that the V4 activity pattern reflects a perceptual parsing of boundary shape into components with singular curvature/orientation/position values. This distills the large number of pixel values making up the boundary down to an explicit representation of a small number of contour components of the type we tend to perceive and describe. If asked to describe a valentine heart, we would mention the indentation at the top, the two broad shoulders on the upper right and upper left, the sharp corner at the bottom. Thus, our cognitive access to parts-level structure of visually perceived objects is reflected by (and presumably owing to) explicit representation of object parts in ventral pathway cortex.

This compact representation could be efficiently stored in memory, and the small number of peaks could be readily interpreted by the rest of the brain using a local version of vector averaging or other peak estimation method. We modeled this by applying a local peak detection algorithm to the fitted population surface, and used the results to reconstruct the stimulus shapes. In all cases, the multiple peaks in the neural population activity surface contained sufficient information to generate a reasonable approximation to the original stimulus (Pasupathy and Connor, 2002). Thus, the basis function representation of simple object parts (specifically single-curvature contour fragments) we observed in area V4 efficiently encodes boundary shapes of at least moderate complexity.

7.2   Synthesis of part signals into representations of multi-part configurations

Object representation at the V4 level is complete, relatively compact, and includes explicit signals for simple contour fragments. It does not, however, reflect our experience and knowledge of more complex objects and object parts common in our world. That is, it does not include explicit signals for the combinations of contour fragments that define more complex structures. Such signals begin to appear in the next ventral pathway processing stage, in posterior IT.

As described in the previous section, up to the V4 level, and up to the level of

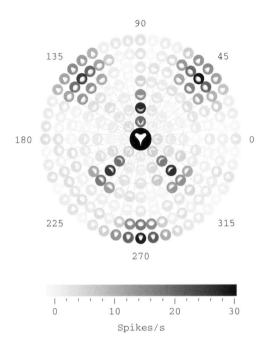

Figure 7.2. Population representation of shape in area V4. In this idealized plot, each circular element corresponds to V4 neurons responding to the boundary fragment appearing in that circle. Responses rates across the population are indicated by background gray level (see scale). The V4 population representation contains local peaks corresponding to the major boundary features of the shape in question (the heart-like shape at the center): the concavity at the top, the broad convexities at the upper right and upper left, the shallow concavities at the lower right and lower left, and the sharp convexity at the bottom.

medium-sized contour fragments, compact coding is achieved by extracting derivatives of contour shape. Beyond this level, however, larger object parts cannot be summarized simply with further mathematical transformations. Except in specific cases, the elements constituting larger shape constructs are not assembled according to any single, standard rule. Thus, to represent those higher-order constructs, it is necessary to integrate lower-level inputs not just in a single way (e.g. to extract a derivative) but in a variety of ways, to capture the full range of larger-scale shape structure. This is what we have observed in posterior IT.

The responses of posterior IT neurons can be characterized in the same dimensions – curvature, orientation, relative position, absolute position – we used to characterize V4 responses. But whereas most V4 neurons are best described by a single Gaussian tuning function in those dimensions, posterior IT neurons are best described by models based on 2–4 Gaussian tuning regions. (Most tuning regions correspond to excitatory driving, but many neurons have one or more inhibitory tuning regions.) This

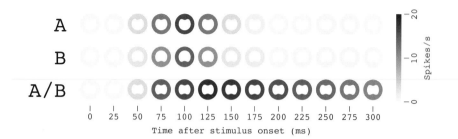

Figure 7.3. Synthesis of parts information in IT cortex. This hypothetical neural response exemplifies the transition from early signals for individual parts to specific representation of multi-part configurations. This neuron is sensitive to concavities at top and bottom. At early time points following stimulus onset (75–125 ms) the cell responds to shapes containing only the top concavity (A), only the bottom concavity (B), or both (A/B). At later time points (near 200 ms) the cell responds only shapes containing both features. Thus, the initially ambiguous signal for individual parts resolves into an explicit signal for the multi-part configuration.

presumably reflects IT neurons integrating information from multiple types of V4 input, in order to represent higher-order combinations of contour fragments with diverse curvatures, orientations and positions.

For some IT neurons, this integration process is clearly linear. Imagine a neuron sensitive to two regions in contour space, A and B, corresponding respectively to concavity opening upward near the top of the object and concavity opening downward near the bottom. A linear neuron might respond at 10 spikes/s to shapes containing A, 15 spikes/s to shapes containing B, and 25 spikes/s to shapes containing both A and B. This is a straightforward summation of inputs corresponding to two types of contour fragments. This type of integration, by itself, does not yield clear and explicit signals for multi-part configurations. A given response rate could represent something in the A tuning region, something in the B tuning region, or a combination of A and B. Information about A, B, and A/B combinations would be at least as distributed and laborious to decipher as at the V4 level.

Other IT neurons integrate contour signals in a highly nonlinear way. A nonlinear neuron might respond very weakly (e.g. 5 spikes/s) to shapes containing either part A or part B alone, but strongly (e.g. 30 spikes/s) to shapes containing both A and B, at say 30 spikes/s. Such a neuron would convey an unambiguous, easily deciphered signal for the A/B combination, making the representation of A/B more explicit, and the representation of shapes containing A/B more compact. Many neurons in posterior IT show some mixture of linear and nonlinear integration of contour signals. Such a neuron might respond at 10 spikes/s to shapes containing part A, 15 spikes/s to shapes containing part B, and 40 spikes/s to shapes containing A and B. This would correspond to a 15 spikes/s nonlinear A/B response component on top of the 10 and 15 spikes/s linear responses to A and B individually.

The above discussion has treated response rates as unitary values, averaged over some stimulus presentation period, but in fact we found that parts integration evolves over time following stimulus onset (Brincat and Connor, 2006). Specifically, neurons with primarily linear integration tend to begin responding earlier and peak at earlier time points, around 120 ms after stimulus onset. Highly nonlinear neurons tended to begin responding earlier and to peak at much later time points, around 180 ms after stimulus onset (Figure 7.3). Neurons with mixed linear/nonlinear response properties tended to be more linear at early time points and more nonlinear at later time points. This is exemplified by the mixed neuron in Figure 7.3, which has an early phasic response to A, B, or A/B. At later time points, responses to indvidual parts drop out, and the tonic response is associated only with the A/B combination. The response of such a cell is ambiguous at early time points, but resolves into an unambiguous, explicit signal for the multi-part configuration.

These trends at the level of individual neurons determine how information at the population level about parts (specifically single-curvature contour fragments) and multi-part configurations evolves through time. Immediately after the appearance of a new object, the initial representation is dominated by linear signals for separate parts. This preliminary sketch peaks in power at about 120 ms following object onset. Then, over the course of the next 60 ms, linear signals decline, while explicit nonlinear signals for multi-part configurations emerge, peaking at 180 ms post onset. This changeover is partly the result of a shift in the active population (from linear to nonlinear cells) and partly because of transitions in tuning within the mixed linear/nonlinear cell population. The result is a refined object representation containing more compact, explicit signals for multi-part configurations.

This temporal pattern suggests that the first feedforward pass through ventral pathway neural networks carries information mainly about disparate parts. This could be sufficient to accomplish the rough categorization tasks that require processing times on the order of only 100 ms (Thorpe *et al.*, 1996). Finer shape discrimination involving configural processing requires 30–50 ms longer (Arguin and Saumier, 2000; Wolfe and Bennett, 1997). This implies a need for recurrent network processing of shape configurations at the neural level, consistent with the gradual emergence of configurational information we observed. To analyze the role of recurrent processing, we simulated a neural network with an architecture based on previous models in which units varied continuously in their ratio of feedforward to recurrent inputs (Chance *et al.*, 1999; Salinas and Abbott, 1996). Recurrent connectivity had a difference of Gaussians pattern; units with similar tuning had mutual excitatory connections, units with dissimilar tuning had inhibitory connections. Neurons with primarily feedforward inputs behaved like the linear cells we observed neurophysiologically, responding rapidly in an ambiguous fashion to individual parts and their combinations. Neurons with primarily recurrent inputs behaved like nonlinear cells, encoding delayed signals for specific multi-part configurations. The continuum of feedforward/recurrent connectivity produced a range of mixed linear/nonlinear response patterns, as observed neurophysiologically. A few simple assumptions (like a 15 ms membrane time constant) yielded temporal patterns comparable to those observed in monkeys, with a delay between linear and nonlinear signal peaks in the range of 50 ms. This number, consistent in our neurophysiological and modeling analyses, is also strikingly similar to the time required in the dorsal pathway for motion signals to evolve from components to whole moving patterns (Pack *et al.*, 2001; Smith *et al.*, 2005). Thus, recurrent network processing of initially ambiguous combined component signals may be a general brain mechanism for inferring specific higher-order combinations.

At yet higher stages in the ventral pathway, further integration of this type may yield explicit signals for larger, more complex configurations and even entire objects. The limit on this progression is the combinatorial explosion of shape complexity. It is numerically impossible to have a separate neuron dedicated to signaling each object in our world (the "grandmother cell" argument; Connor, 2005). However, it is possible to have an extremely sparse representation of at least certain objects of learned behavioral importance. Thus, there is evidence for highly specific neural tuning for behaviorally relevant combinations of complex object halves (Baker *et al.*, 2002) and for multiple views of very familiar objects (Booth and Rolls, 1998). Extremely compact and explicit signals for important objects, derived from further stages of parts integration, would be especially amenable to memory storage, formation of memory associations, and accessibility by other parts of the brain. Thus, shape part synthesis up to the level of holistic object recognition could underlie our sense of familiarity, keen discrimination, and expert interactions with important and common objects in our lives.

References

Andrews, D. P., Butcher, A. K. and Buckley, B. R. (1973). Acuities for spatial arrangement in line figures: human and ideal observers compared. *Vis. Res.*, **13**, 599–620.

Arguin, M. and Saumier, D. (2000). Conjunction and linear non-separability effects in visual shape encoding. *Vis. Res.*, **40**, 3099–3115.

Baker, C. I., Behrmann, M. and Olson, C. R. (2002). Impact of learning on representation of parts and wholes in monkey inferotemporal cortex. *Nat. Neurosci.*, **5**, 1210–1216.

Biederman, I. (1987). Recognition-by-components: a theory of human image understanding. *Psychol. Rev.*, **94**, 115–147.

Booth, M. C. and Rolls, E. T. (1998). View-invariant representations of familiar objects by neurons in the inferior temporal visual cortex. *Cereb. Cortex*, **8**, 510–523.

Brincat, S. L. and Connor, C. E. (2004). Underlying principles of visual shape selectivity in posterior inferotemporal cortex. *Nat. Neurosci.*, **7**, 880–886.

Brincat, S. L. and Connor, C. E. (2006). Dynamic shape synthesis in posterior inferotemporal cortex. *Neuron*, **49**, 17–24.

Chance, F. S., Nelson, S. B. and Abbott, L. F. (1999). Complex cells as cortically amplified simple cells. *Nat. Neurosci.*, **2**, 277–282.

Connor, C. E. (2005). Neuroscience: friends and grandmothers. *Nature*, **435**, 1036–1037.

Deneve, S., Latham, P. E. and Pouget, A. (1999). Reading population codes: a neural implementation of ideal observers. *Nat. Neurosci.*, **2**, 740–745.

Deneve, S., Latham, P. E. and Pouget, A. (2001). Efficient computation and cue integration with noisy population codes. *Nat. Neurosci.*, **4**, 826–831.

Dobbins, A., Zucker, S. W. and Cynader, M. S. (1987). Endstopped neurons in the visual cortex as a substrate for calculating curvature. *Nature*, **329**, 438–441.

Epstein, R., Harris, A., Stanley, D. and Kanwisher, N. (1999). The parahippocampal place area: recognition, navigation, or encoding? *Neuron*, **23**, 115–125.

Georgopoulos, A. P., Caminiti, R., Kalaska, J. F. and Massey, J. T. (1983). Spatial coding of movement: A hypothesis concerning the coding of movement direction by motor cortical populations. *Exp. Brain Res. Supp.*, **7**, 327–336.

Groh, J. M., Born, R. T. and Newsome, W. T. (1997). How is a sensory map read Out? Effects of microstimulation in visual area MT on saccades and smooth pursuit eye movements. *J. Neurosci.*, **17**, 4312–4330.

Hegde, J. and Van Essen, D. C. (2000). Selectivity for complex shapes in primate visual area V2. *J. Neurosci.*, **20**, RC61.

Heggelund, P. and Hohmann, A. (1975). Responses of striate cortical cells to moving edges of different curvatures. *Exp. Brain Res.*, **23**, 211–216.

Hoffman, D. D. and Richards, W. A. (1984). Parts of recognition. *Cognition*, **18**, 65–96.

Hubel, D. H. and Wiesel, T. N. (1968). Receptive fields and functional architecture of monkey striate cortex. *J. Physiol. (Lond.)*, **195**, 215–243.

Kanwisher, N., McDermott, J. and Chun, M. M. (1997a). The fusiform face area: a module in human extrastriate cortex specialized for face perception. *J. Neurosci.*, **17**, 4302–4311.

Kanwisher, N., Woods, R., Iacoboni, M. and Mazziotta, J. (1997b). A locus in human extrastriate cortex for visual shape analysis. *J. Cog. Neurosci.*, **9**, 133–142.

Kourtzi, Z. and Kanwisher, N. (2000). Cortical regions involved in perceiving object shape. *J. Neurosci.*, **20**, 3310–3318.

Lerner, Y., Hendler, T., Ben Bashat, D., Harel, M. and Malach, R. (2001). A hierarchical axis of object processing stages in the human visual cortex. *Cereb. Cortex*, **11**, 287–297.

Marr, D. and Nishihara, H. K. (1978). Representation and recognition of the spatial organization of three-dimensional shapes. *Proc. R. Soc. Lond.*, **B200**, 269–294.

Mountcastle, V. B. (1995). The parietal system and some higher brain functions. *Cereb. Cortex*, **5**, 377–390.

Olshausen, B. A. and Field, D. J. (1997). Sparse coding with an overcomplete basis set: a strategy employed by V1. *Vis. Res.*, **37**, 3311–3325.

Pack, C. C., Berezovskii, V. K. and Born, R. T. (2001). Dynamic properties of neurons in cortical area MT in alert and anaesthetized macaque monkeys. *Nature*, **414**, 905–908.

Pasupathy, A. and Connor, C. E. (1999). Responses to contour features in macaque area V4. *J. Neurophysiol.*, **82**, 2490–2502.

Pasupathy, A. and Connor, C. E. (2001). Shape representation in area V4: position-specific tuning for boundary conformation. *J. Neurophysiol.*, **86**, 2505–2519.

Pasupathy, A. and Connor, C. E. (2002). Population coding of shape in area V4. *Nat. Neurosci.*, **5**, 1332–1338.

Pouget, A., Zhang, K., Deneve, S. and Latham, P. E. (1998). Statistically efficient estimation using population coding. *Neural Comput.*, **10**, 373–401.

Pouget, A., Dayan, P. and Zemel, R. (2000). Information processing with population codes. *Nat. Rev. Neurosci.*, **1**, 125–132.

Quiroga, R. Q., Reddy, L., Kreiman, G., Koch, C. and Fried, I. (2005). Invariant visual representation by single neurons in the human brain. *Nature*, **435**, 1102-1107.

Salinas, E. and Abbott, L. F. (1996). A model of multiplicative neural responses in parietal cortex IV. *Proc. Natl. Acad. Sci USA*, **93**, 11 956–11 961.

Smith, M. A., Majaj, N. J. and Movshon, J. A. (2005). Dynamics of motion signaling by neurons in macaque area MT. *Nat. Neurosci.*, **8**, 220–228.

Thorpe, S., Fize, D. and Marlot, C. (1996). Speed of processing in the human visual system. *Nature*, **381**, 520–522.

Treisman, A. and Gormican, S. (1988). Feature analysis in early vision: evidence from search asymmetries. *Psychol. Rev.*, **95**, 15–48.

Ungerleider, L. G. and Mishkin, M. (1982). Two cortical visual systems. In D. G. Ingle, M. A. Goodale and R. J. Q. Mansfield, eds.,, *Analysis of Visual Behavior*, Cambridge, MA: MIT Press, pp. 549–586.

Vinje, W. E. and Gallant, J. L. (2000). Sparse coding and decorrelation in primary visual cortex during natural vision. *Science*, **287**, 1273–1276.

Wilson, H. R., Wilkinson, F. and Asaad, W. (1997). Concentric orientation summation in human form vision. *Vis. Res.*, **37**, 2325–2330.

Wolfe, J. M. and Bennett, S. C. (1997). Preattentive object files: shapeless bundles of basic features. *Vis. Res.*, **37**, 25–43.

Wolfe, J. M., Yee, A. and Friedman-Hill, S. R. (1992). Curvature is a basic feature for visual search tasks. *Percept.*, **21**, 465–480.

Part II

Attention, motion, and eye movements

8 Attention and action

James J. Clark, Ziad M. Hafed and Li Jie

8.1 Introduction

This article provides a historical overview of the work carried out by the first author and his co-workers in the area of visual attention and its connection to active vision. It is written, in parts, in the first person, from the perspective of the first author. This is not intended, however, to in any way minimize the contributions of the second and third authors, which are significant and extensive, particularly in the latter sections.

Attention has been studied in great detail by researchers since the beginnings of the scientific approach to cognitive psychology and the founding works of Hermann von Helmholtz (1896) and William James (James, 1890). To this day, however, there is no universally agreed-upon theory of how attention functions in humans, and there is even still controversy as to what attention actually is. Attention remains, therefore, a very active area of research. Most would agree that attention is a *selective* process, which acts to focus sparse computational resources onto relevant aspects of the sensory input. My particular interest originated in the application of attention processes to machine vision. In particular, I was interested in so-called *active* vision systems, which deal with the problems and opportunities that arise when various aspects of the sensing process, such as the position and orientation of cameras, can be actively controlled. My interest in machine vision systems has since been extended to biological vision systems. This paper recounts the line of research that has grown out of this interest.

8.2 Active vision and attention in robots

The line of research outlined in this article began when I was a neophyte professor working in the Harvard Robotics Lab, under the direction of Roger Brockett. Along with my Ph.D. student, Nicola Ferrier (now a professor at the University of Wiscon-

Computational Vision in Neural and Machine Systems, ed. L. Harris and M. Jenkin. Published by Cambridge University Press. © Cambridge University Press 2007.

sin), I was interested in building an artificial active vision system, capable of moving a pair of video cameras under computer servo control so as to orient their gaze to a desired location in space. The resulting piece of hardware, one of the first such to be built, was the so-called Harvard Head (Ferrier and Clark, 1993). Nowadays the Harvard Head seems primitive and ungraceful, but it did produce at least one interesting piece of research, namely the demonstration of how selective attention could be linked to the generation of saccadic camera movements. We implemented the Koch and Ullman (1985) saliency-map model of attention on a combination Datacube/Sun-3 image processing platform (details can be found in (Clark and Ferrier, 1992)) and used the peak of the saliency map to define the saccade target (Clark and Ferrier, 1988, 1989). This saccade target was input as a command to a modal-control system developed by Brockett (1988), which controlled the position and velocity of the camera pan, tilt, and vergence motors. The Harvard Head project was one of many in the field of active vision. The late 1980s and early 1990s was a productive era in the development of active vision hardware. From the Canadian perspective, one of the most important contemporary active vision hardware systems was the University of Toronto "Trish" system (Milios *et al.*, 1990). This system makes use of attentional mechanisms, and served as the development platform for much of John Tsotsos' influential work on attention modeling. An excellent overview of the state-of-the-art in the early 1990s in active vision is the report produced by an NSF panel of experts (Swain and Stricker, 1991). This report also has a good presentation of what was considered to be the important research issues in the area, and these issues are still relevant today.

In the mid 1990s I left Harvard University and joined the fledgling Nissan Cambridge Basic Research Laboratory. This lab was located near MIT in Cambridge, Massachusetts, and was under the scientific direction of Whitman Richards, Ken Nakayama, and Warren Seering. It was focused on understanding human cognition while driving, for the purposes of making driving safer and more enjoyable. Nissan was interested in using eye movement measurements as a way of tapping into the driver's attentive state. Perhaps the most significant piece of research to come out of the CBR was the work on change-blindness due to disruption of attention (Rensink *et al.*, 1995, 1997; O'Regan *et al.*, 1999). Attentional change blindness refers to the phenomenon of extreme difficulty in noticing image changes if these changes are masked by global transients in image salience. Normally, one would think of change-blindness as a bad thing, but the phenomenon reflects the active nature of information acquisition in biological systems. The basic idea follows O'Regan's (1992) view of the "world as an outside memory," where detailed internal representations of the world are not needed, since the world can form the representation itself. Information need only be acquired by the visual system when changes in the world are detected. In this view, attention serves to localize the location of scene change, which is then followed by detailed analysis of the nature of the change. If nothing changes, then there is no need to re-acquire the information.

After two years working at Nissan, I joined the Centre for Intelligent Machines at McGill University in Montreal. At McGill, my lab has continued applying attentional processes to the construction of active vision systems. In Clark (1998b), I describe how an attentive active vision system can exhibit change-blindness.

8.3 Attention and saccade generation in biological systems

While at the Nissan CBR, I learned a great deal about biological attention mechanisms and, in particular, the link between attention and eye movements. Along the way, I learned something about doing psychophysical experiments. My subsequent work at McGill has focused more on modeling of biological vision systems than on implementing machine vision systems. The remainder of this article will therefore concentrate on my work related to modeling and studying the characteristics of biological attention mechanisms, and their link to the generation of eye movements.

8.3.1 Models of saccade targeting and triggering

In my view, the first step in understanding the link between attention and eye movements is to have a working model of how eye movements are generated, and then to fuse this with a model of how attention is controlled. Modeling of the processes and neural circuitry underlying the generation of saccadic eye movements has occupied many researchers since the time of Helmholtz and James. Attention is to be found in these models with varying degrees of involvement. The oldest form of model considers the processes of saccadic eye movement generation and attention control to be completely independent. Examples of this type of model can be found in the works of Becker and Jurgens (1979), Reulen (1984a, b), and Deubel *et al.*, (1984). Posner (1980) accepted the notion that there is an apparent link between the activity of covert attention and the generation of saccades, but argued that this link was coincidental. He held that the two systems are only functionally related and suggested that covert attention and eye movements are both drawn to exogenous stimuli, but not to endogenous stimuli, and that the mechanism controlling these shifts are completely independent.

Some models do propose a connection between the generation of saccades and visual attention, but only require that attention be disengaged from the current locus for a saccade to occur. A representative of such a model is that of Fischer (1993). In Fischer's model, the target of a saccadic eye movement is computed during the disengaged-attention phase by a localization system.

Finally, there are many models that infer a very strong coupling between attention and saccade generation. One common form of such models require that attention be engaged at a target location before a saccade can be made to that location. An early theory along this line was proposed by Wurtz and Mohler (1976). They suggested that attention shifts were *programs* for saccadic eye movements, to be subsequently executed by the oculomotor system. Klein's (1980) *oculomotor readiness theory* provides what is perhaps the most influential of the early attention/saccade models. This theory links attention and saccade generation by supposing that an attention shift to a particular spatial location results from a preparation of, or an oculomotor readiness to generate, a saccade to that location. This oculomotor readiness has the effect of enhancing information processing at the target location. Klein *et al.* (1992) qualified this theory to restrict the linkage between attention and saccade generation to situations where the saccade target is defined by an exogenous (image-based) stimulus, and not to situations involving *endogenous* (internally defined) saccade targets.

Henderson (1992) introduced a *sequential attention* model that invoked a *saccadic programming* process. In this model, the saccadic programming process is executed after attention shifts to the peripheral stimulus only after processing of the foveal visual input has been completed. The amount of foveal processing (or foveal load) affects the latency of the eye movement (the time from the appearance of a peripheral stimulus to the start of the saccade). For light foveal loads, the latency is modeled as 80 ms beyond the time taken for the attention shift. A modified version of his theory allowed for the saccadic program to start before the attention shift, which will reduce the latency, but still keeps the principle that saccades are ultimately directed to the locus of attention.

A rather extreme, but influential, conception of the link between attention and saccades is the *premotor theory* of Rizzolati (1983). The main tenet of this theory is that the system that controls action is the same as that which controls spatial attention. One module performs both functions, leading to an economical architecture. One implication is that there can be many forms of attention, each associated with a different motor system (Rizzolati *et al.*, 1994). Each motor modality employs its own neural representation of space, referred to as a *pragmatic map*. One such pragmatic map is the superior colliculus motor map (Wurtz, 1996). Saccade targeting activity involving the superior colliculus motor map would then affect the allocation of spatial attention.

The models mentioned above that invoke a strong link between attention and saccades were motivated primarily by the results of psychophysical studies. Support for the idea of a strong link between attention and saccades has also been provided by a number of neuro-physiological studies. Desimone (1990) made the general observation that the oculomotor system and the covert attention system both involve the targeting of stimuli and could usefully share some common neural hardware. Desimone *et al.* (1989) observed an impairment of an animal's ability to attend to a target in the presence of a distractor when small areas of the superior colliculus were rendered non-functional. Conversely, Kustov and Robinson (1996) forced saccades to be generated in monkeys by injecting electrical current into various areas of the superior colliculus and observed that the trajectories of these induced saccades were altered by both exogenous and endogenous attentional shifts.

8.3.2   Saccadic latency phenomena

What are the implications of the premise that saccadic eye movements are linked to attention shifts? One is that manipulation of the attention process should result in measurable changes in eye movement characteristics, such as the amplitude, direction, or timing. In fact, each of these characteristics are indeed subject to measurable changes. In my work, I have concentrated mainly on looking at temporal modulation effects, as these are often quite strong as compared with spatial effects.

Saccadic eye movements to suddenly appearing peripheral targets are never instantaneous. There is always some time delay, referred to as the *saccadic latency*, before the saccade begins. This is not surprising, as clearly there must be some chain of processing that takes place between the arrival of the photons on the retina and the activation of the eye muscles. If one looks, however, at the shortest neural pathways from retina to eye muscle, the path propagation time is rather short, on the order of

50 ms (see Fischer 1993). Observed saccadic latencies, on the other hand, can be quite long, typically ranging from about 150 to 300 ms. So what is the additional delay due to? There are many theories as to the source of this delay, but most posit some time-consuming mechanism for preparing, or programming, the saccade in response to the onset of a visual target.

To judge the merits of the various proposals for saccade generation models, we can look at a number of well-known phenomena associated with conditions that can modulate the saccadic latency. Some of these phenomena are described in the following sections.

The gap effect   The *gap effect* was first reported by Saslow (1967), who observed that saccadic latencies were reduced when the temporal gap between the offset of the fixation stimulus and the onset of the target stimulus was increased. The latencies were seen to increase when there was a temporal overlap between the disappearance of the fixation mark and the appearance of the peripheral target. Reulen (1984a) performed a detailed study of the gap effect, and measured latencies as a function of the asynchrony between fixation offset and target onset in seven subjects. He found that the data could be fit by a simple piecewise linear model, consisting of three sections: a constant latency for negative asynchronies (overlap), a (lower) constant latency for large positive asynchronies (gap), and a linear transition region between these two constant regions, located at small positive asynchronies. Kingstone and Klein (1993) and Walker *et al.* (1995) observed that giving instructions to direct attention to a target location did not lead to any decrease in the magnitude of the gap effect although there was an overall reduction in latency. A similar result was observed experimentally by Reuter-Lorenz *et al.* (1991), who found that the gap effect is unaffected by the luminance of the target.

The global effect   When a saccade target is embedded in a field of distracting objects, the actual saccade often does not land right on the target, but instead tends to land on the "center-of-gravity" of the target and distractor group (Coren and Hoenig, 1972). Findlay (1982) called this phenomenon the *global effect*. It was later shown by Coëffé and O'Regan (1987) that the global effect is strongest when the saccadic latency is short. In their experiments, subjects made saccadic eye movements to a cued letter in a string of ten letters presented in the periphery of the visual field. When subjects made saccades with very short latencies, the landing position of the eye was seen to overshoot the cued location for targets on the end of the string nearest to the fixation point and undershoot the cued location for targets on the end of the string furthest from the fixation point. As latencies were increased, the amount of over- or under-shoot was decreased. No target location under- or over-shoot was observed when only single letters were present, indicating that it was the presence of the other, non-cued, letters in the string that were giving rise to the under- and over-shoots.

Retinal eccentricity effects   Wyman and Steinman (1973) observed that saccadic latency increases rapidly as the target gets very close to the fovea. Kalesnykas and Hallett (1994) examined in detail saccadic latency for a wide range of retinal eccentricities and several different stimulus conditions. They found that latencies increase sharply for very small eccentricities and increase slowly at high eccentricities. The peak at small eccentricities is broader for less salient stimuli. For example, for target stimuli near detection threshold, the peak is about $4°$ wide, while for target stimuli 1000 times foveal detection threshold the peak is only about $1.5°$ wide. Target color did not seem to affect the peak, ruling out effects due to wavelength dependent absorption of light by macular pigments. They also found that the presence of the central latency peak did not depend on head or eye position, and the peak appeared even when latency was plotted against saccadic amplitude rather than eccentricity.

8.3.3 Saccadic programming or attention shifting?

So, how can these various saccadic latency phenomena be accounted for? Perhaps the most frequently proposed explanation is in terms of a *saccadic programming* process (see, for example, Abrams, 1992; Abrams and Jonides, 1988; Findlay, 1992; He and Kowler, 1988; Sereno, 1992). The saccadic programming process is usually decomposed into two components – amplitude programming and direction programming. These components are usually thought of as computational processes, each running in their own architecturally distinct modules, that are initiated, run for a while, and then provide a result. In the saccadic programming view, saccadic latencies reflect the time taken by these processes to produce the required amplitude and direction parameters for the saccade.

The saccadic programming view is quite natural for an engineer, and a modular approach to camera movement control is frequently seen in active machine vision systems. But I would argue that the saccadic programming approach is unnecessarily complicated. Instead, I suggest that the premotor approach, in which attention and eye movement control mechanisms are shared, is a better way to go. My view of the saccade generation process makes three basic assumptions. (1) The target of a saccade is given by the current locus of attention, which itself is determined by a saliency map. (2) A command to make a saccade is generated every time attention shifts. (3) The execution of saccade commands can be suppressed.

In this premotor view, saccades are programmed, if they can be said to be programmed at all, by the attention mechanisms. Conversely, one could just as rightly say that attention shifts are programmed by the saccade generation mechanisms. In the premotor view, it is meaningless to separate these as the mechanisms are the same. No saccadic "programming" need take place as the amplitude and direction of saccades are implicit in the attentionally defined target locations, and are always available. There is no programming process that needs to be initiated or that needs to be reset, modified, or restarted in response to a change in target position (Clark, 1999).

In Clark (1998a), I showed that all of the saccadic latency effects described above can be explained by a premotor theory. The basic idea is that the main variable component of saccadic latency is the time needed for spatial attention to shift to the location of the target for the saccade. To motivate my conclusions, I developed a simple dynamical model of the attention shift process and its link to saccade generation, and the various latency phenomena were replicated in computer simulations of the simple attentional model.

There are a number of computational models that describe the dynamical mechanisms underlying attention shifts (see Koch and Ullman, 1985; Tsotsos, 1990). These differ greatly in their details, but generally use or exhibit a type of behavior known as "Winner-Take-All" (or WTA). A WTA system is one in which elements compete against each other using mutual inhibition. The positive feedback inherent in such a system results in a stable state wherein one of the elements (the "winner") is maximally enhanced and all the other elements are maximally inhibited. I used an uncomplicated version of these WTA models using a simple saliency map, which weights various visual features (as in Koch and Ullman, 1985). Following models of the human visual cortex, I posited two types of feature detectors in the model, transient and sustained. The transient feature detectors are fast responding but have relatively low spatial resolution. The sustained feature detectors are slower to respond but have higher spatial resolution. A number of researchers (Breitmeyer and Ganz, 1976; Lennie, 1980; Yantis and Jonides, 1984) have suggested that the transient effects observed in tasks requiring visual attention (e.g., those reported by Nakayama and Mackeben, 1989 and Posner *et al.*, 1982) may be caused by the transient responses of low level feature detectors. The dynamics of the feature detectors arise from the temporal properties of their constituent neurons.

As for the generation of the saccadic eye movements, following the proposal of Lee *et al.* (1988), my model assumes that the command for the saccadic eye movement is coded in a distributed fashion by a population of neurons, whose activity is attentionally modulated, such as in the superior colliculus (Wurtz, 1996). Thus the target will be specified by the centre of mass of this pattern of activity, and is continually available. It should be noted that in taking this approach, the saccade target is *always* defined. There is no distinct *saccadic programming* module which computes the saccade target in response to some trigger stimulus. The target is always defined, and the saccade target is that which is defined at the moment of triggering.

8.3.4   Explanation of the saccadic latency phenomena

In my view, the explanation of the phenomena described above lies in the dynamics of the WTA process. One of the principal features of a WTA process is that it is multistable. The output of a WTA system is stable until the input is perturbed sufficiently, at which time it can switch rapidly to another stable stage. Based on this aspect of WTA function, the saccadic latency, in our model, depends on the time taken for the WTA attention process to *switch* from one location to another when the visual input changes (for example, because of the appearance of a salient target).

Gap effect   In short, the explanation of the gap effect is that the time taken for a WTA system to switch from one location to another depends on the relative salience of the two locations. In the overlap condition, the feature detector activity at the target location and that at the fixation location compete against each other in the Winner-Take-All competition. If the fixation point and the target have similar salience, this competition may take a long time to resolve, resulting in a long latency. In the gap condition, the target location is unopposed in this competition and thus wins it quickly, with a speed dependent on the target salience.

Global effect   The explanation of the global effect is linked to two factors in my model. The first is the assumption of both transient and sustained features. For short latencies, the feature detector response is dominated by the transient component, which has a low spatial frequency cutoff, effectively blurring the target and distractors together. At longer latencies the sustained component dominates, which has a higher spatial frequency cutoff, and hence creates less blurring of the target and distractors. The second factor contributing to the dependence of feature centroid on latency is the action of the Winner-Take-All network. Increasing the latency allows more time for the ultimate winning feature location to suppress its neighboring distractors, thus reducing the effect of the spatial blurring.

Retinal eccentricity effects   The attentional model also provides an explanation for the increase in saccadic latency for targets with small retinal eccentricities. Once again, the explanation lies partly in the assumption that saccadic latencies reflect the time taken for the WTA network to shift from one stable state to another. This time is a function of the difference between the target saliency and the value of the local maximum function times some weight less than one. The other important piece of the puzzle comes from an assumption that the influence of a salient location in the WTA is not limited to its immediate neighborhood, nor is it constant spatially, but falls off rather slowly with distance. This implies a *local* implementation of the WTA, which is more plausible to be implemented under the constraints of biological architectures.

If we assume a local WTA, when the target is far from the fixation feature, the target will have little competition in the WTA process and latencies should be relatively short. If the target is near to the fixation, and if the salience at the fixation location is greater than the target salience, then the local maximum value may be larger than the target value, hence the Winner-Take-All transition time will be longer than when the target is far from fixation. As the target salience increases, the distance at which the local maximum value becomes equal to the target salience becomes smaller. Thus, the eccentricity at which the saccadic latency begins to increase should decrease as the target saliency increases. Conversely, it is seen in the simulations of the model that the drop-off in latency with eccentricity is slower for low saliency targets than for highly salient targets, in accordance with the results of the experiments of Kalesnykas and Hallett (1994).

8.4   Covert attention tracking and microsaccades

So far, we have seen that there is an apparent link between the processes of selective visual attention and the generation of saccades. Various characteristics of saccadic eye movements can be influenced by attentional manipulations. This implies that observations and measurements of the saccade characteristics can provide information on the attention process, beyond what is provided by the position of the eye alone. This being said, the eye position remains the most-widely used direction measure of attentional allocation. But what about the situations in which the eye is held fixed, with saccades volitionally suppressed? In such a case, there can be a significant disconnect between the position of the eye and the locus of spatial attention. This led me to consider more closely what information could be acquired regarding the allocation of attention during ocular fixation.

In 1995, while working at the Nissan CBR, I had a lunch-time discussion with co-workers Ron Rensink and Kevin O'Regan, where Ron pondered whether it would be possible to track the locus of covert attention, in much the same way that an eye-tracker can track the locus of overt attention. Ron Rensink thought that it would be difficult to do so, if only because covert attention has many non-spatial aspects (such as featural selection), and may have multiple spatial loci. Kevin O'Regan, playing the role of contrarian as usual, claimed (in jest?) that he did not believe in covert attention at all and stated that all observed effects attributed to attention could be explained by changes in acuity induced by small eye movements, or microsaccades. While I did not really give this idea much credence, I turned it backwards in my mind and thought that maybe microsaccades could be explained by attention processes. In particular, I had the thought that microsaccades could be residual motions resulting from imperfectly suppressed normal saccades linked to attention shifts. In this view, the only difference between covert and overt saccades, is the presence of a suppression in the former case, perhaps mediated by the fixation cells in the superior colliculus (Munoz and Wurtz, 1993). If microsaccades are simply suppressed targeting saccades, then they should be associated with a covert attention shift just as regular targeting saccades. If this is true, then microsaccades could provide a potentially useful probe into the state of covert attention.

When I came to McGill University, I presented my thinking to Ziad Hafed and suggested it as the basis of a Ph.D. thesis topic. Ziad had previously done a Master thesis developing a neural network model of the superior colliculus (Hafed and Clark, 2000), and he thought that the idea of microsaccades as suppressed regular saccades was at least conceivable given the current understanding of colliculus function. So, Ziad and I looked into the microsaccade literature, such as it is, and planned out an investigation of the hypothesis. The study of microsaccades has never been a glamorous affair, and the the history of microsaccade thinking has been quite spotty, with the occasional theory put forward now and then. In perhaps the most influential of the early works, Cornsweet (1956) theorized that microsaccades provide the function of correcting the intersaccadic drifts of the eye. It was subsequently proposed that microsaccades (also) serve to prevent vision from fading during fixation due to a static retinal image (Carpenter, 1988). Other researchers go so far as to say that there is no function associated with microsaccades, or that they just reflect noise in the oculomotor plant (Kowler and Steinman, 1980). Recently, however, microsaccades have drawn closer scrutiny and some other views of microsaccades have been proposed. For example, neurophysiological evidence has suggested that microsaccades might help maintain perception by modulating neural responses in the visual cortex (Martinez-Conde *et al.*, 2000; Leopold and Logothetis, 1998). Nobody had suggested a direct causal link between covert attention shifts and the generation of microsaccades, however, so Ziad set out to test this idea.

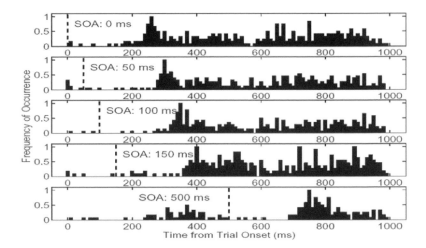

Figure 8.1. The frequency histogram of microsaccade occurrence aligned with the start of the trial. The dashed line indicates the onset of the peripheral stimulus, which occurs a variable length of time (the SOA) after the start of the trial.

8.4.1 Microsaccades during fixation

The experiments carried out by Ziad basically involved requiring the subject to maintain fixation and presenting the subject with attention-grabbing peripheral stimuli. The subjects were given a (color) discrimination task which required them to attend to both the fixation target and the peripheral stimulus. We recorded eye movement information (using an ISCAN head-mounted eye-tracker) while the subjects carried out the task and did an off-line analysis of the eye track data. The analysis detected the occurrence of microsaccades (defined as movements with a velocity above a set threshold, and with amplitudes less than $1°$). Details on the experiments can be found in Hafed (2003), and Hafed and Clark (2001, 2002, 2003).

The key to unlocking the secrets of the microsaccade data lay in looking at the *time course* of the microsaccade occurrences, relative to the onset of the peripheral visual stimulus. When we do this, as shown in Figure 8.1, a clearly visible peak in the microsaccade frequency is evident with a latency of around 250 ms. These latencies are very similar to those observed for regular saccades, suggesting that these microsaccades are directly related to the peripheral stimulus onsets. Furthermore, the horizontal *direction* of the microsaccades are biased in the horizontal direction of the peripheral stimuli, as shown in Figure 8.2. From the data depicted in this figure we can see that the majority of microsaccades were first directed towards the peripheral stimulus, at a latency of about 200 ms. At a later time, around 400 ms after stimulus onset, another peak in microsaccade frequency appears, in which the majority of the microsaccades were made in the other direction, suggesting an attention shift back to fixation. Keep in mind that the subjects were instructed to maintain fixation, and that

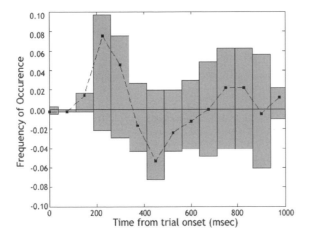

Figure 8.2. Microsaccades exhibited patterns of shifts towards the peripheral stimulus and back. The figure shows latency histograms of microsaccades as a function of peripheral stimulus location: positive bars indicate movements in its direction and negative bars indicate movements in the opposite direction. Bars are normalized by the total number of microsaccades shown in the figure. The thin line plots the difference between positive and negative bars for each latency bin.

information about the objects at fixation was needed to accomplish the task. Therefore the fixation area was highly salient to the subject, and hence it should not be surprising that attention would shift back to the fixation area. In Figure 8.1 many peaks are visible in the microsaccade time course plots, suggesting many shifts of attention during the performance of a task.

About the same time that we were carrying out our experiments, a group in Postdam, Germany, were working along a similar track, and published their work very soon after we did (Engbert and Kliegl, 2003). They also looked at the time course of microsaccade occurrence relative to a visual stimulus onset. Their results show a significant modulation of microsaccade activity related to the peripheral visual stimulus. As in our experiments, the direction of the microsaccades in the Engbert and Kliegl study appear to be biased in the direction of the stimulus. The work of Engbert and Kliegl (2003) provided, if not independent confirmation of, then at least additional independent evidence for, the link between covert attention and microsaccade occurrence.

8.4.2 Microsaccades related to non-visual events

A closer examination of Figure 8.1 shows significant tails of long latency microsaccades occurring well after the stimulus onsets (and, indeed, even before the stimulus onset). What do these long latency microsaccades correspond to? One might argue, as

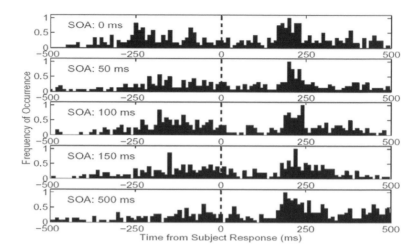

Figure 8.3. The frequency histogram of microsaccade occurrence aligned with the subjects' manual responses.

did Engbert and Kliegl (2003), that these long tail microsaccades simply correspond to a baseline, or steady state, population, the rate of which is merely *modulated* for a short while by attention shifts (revealing the low latency peaks). If this is in fact the case, then microsaccades may not be as useful a tool for indexing covert attention shifts as we are suggesting in the present work. This is so because with such a baseline rate, the observation of a microsaccadic occurrence at a particular time would only reflect an attention shift in some cases close to visual onsets but not others.

In neurobiology and psychophysics, baseline rates are often viewed with suspicion, and the suspicion is usually that a spread out population of events is a sign that the data is not aligned correctly. So, Ziad decided to try aligning the microsaccade data to various significant task times. In doing so, we hit pay-dirt and found a rather remarkable result. If we align the microsaccade data with the time of the subject's response, the so-called baseline population resolves into a well-defined peak of microsaccade activity. This is shown in Figure 8.3. The microsaccades that occurred after subject responses were concentrated around a fairly constant latency of 200 ms regardless of SOA. These microsaccades formed the diffuse long latency baseline population observed in Figure 8.1. The implication is that these microsaccades that they were elicited by an event occurring around subject response time. This suggests that there is really no baseline rate for microsaccades but, more importantly, it implies that there are detectable attention shifts that are time-locked to response execution in psychophysical tasks. In particular, if one considers the 250 ms lag of microsaccades that we observed here as an estimate for the time difference between an attention shift and a microsaccade, then the data in Figure 8.3 suggest that the response-related attention shifts in our task may have occurred approximately 50 ms before the execution of responses. The response-related microsaccades also show a significant modulation of microsaccade direction by peripheral stimulus location, generally in the direction of the peripheral stimulus. We hypothesize, based on this direction and on the relatively short time before the actual response, that the implied attention shift is to perhaps aid in a final check on the subject's decision before responding.

8.4.3   Microsaccades during pursuit

The initial studies done on the link between microsaccades and attention, those by our group, and those of Engbert and Kliegl, only looked at situations in which the eye is fixed. But humans are not always fixating. In most natural viewing conditions, in addition to fixation and normal saccades, large human eye movements consist of smooth pursuit of moving targets, vestibular-ocular reflex motions in response to head motion, vergence motions shifting the plane of gaze in depth, and optokinetic-nystagmus in response to large-scale rapid image flow. Thus, if the use of microsaccades as a probe of attentional state is to have wide applicability, it is important that the characteristics of microsaccades be studied in the non-fixational viewing situations. Recently, our lab has been investigating (Jie and Clark, 2005) the issue of whether microsaccades occur during pursuit and, if so, whether, and in what way, these microsaccades are related to covert attention shifts.

To determine whether humans engaged in pursuit generate microsaccades, current Ph.D. student Li Jie created a simple psychophysical task in which subjects pursued a moving object, and measured their eye movements. To study possible links to covert attention shifts, such shifts were induced while the subjects maintained pursuit by the abrupt onset of a peripheral square, something that is known to exogenously capture attention (Yantis and Jonides, 1984). The subjects were instructed to maintain pursuit, so the resulting attention shifts should be entirely covert. The details of the experiments are as follows. At the onset of every trial, a square cue appeared either on the left or right side edge of the display and remained visible for a variable period between 700 and 1100 ms in duration. The pursuit target, consisting of a cross shape appeared at the location of the cue and began to move horizontally as soon as the cue disappeared. The color of the cross shape changed periodically during the trial. The total duration for each trial after the cue's onset was 3.5 s. At some random time during the trial, a square object briefly appeared at a distance of $11°$ either to the left or to the right of the pursuit target. Subjects were instructed to maintain pursuit at all times on the moving cross and report as soon as possible after the onset of the distractor whether the pursuit target had the same color as the initial cue square.

The results of these experiments showed that microsaccades do indeed occur during ocular pursuit and that they have similar characteristics to those occurring during fixation. We observed that microsaccades appear either singly or in pairs of opposing movements during pursuit, similar to the patterns of microsaccadic motion discovered in fixation. After detecting all of the microsaccades that occurred during pursuit, we aligned all microsaccades to the onset time of the square object.

Following the same reasoning that we used in interpreting the microsaccade data during fixation, we associate the first peak in the microsaccade time histogram with the covert attention shift related to the onset of the flashed square. Microsaccades with longer latencies from the square onset are presumably, in this view, associated with

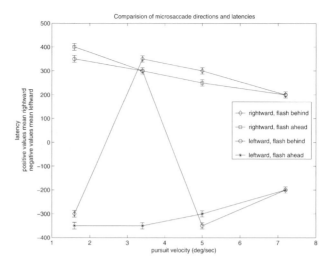

Figure 8.4. Comparison of the latencies and directions corresponding to the peak of the first population of microsaccades after stimulus onset, as a function of the pursuit velocity.

other covert attention shifts, perhaps back to the pursuit target.

In repeating the experiment at faster pursuit target velocities up to 7°/s, we found that the microsaccades contributing to the short latency peak tend to be biased in the direction of pursuit, and that this bias increases with the pursuit velocity. This phenomenon suggests that attention tends to shift more readily in the direction of pursuit with higher velocities. We also noted that the response time decreases as the pursuit velocity increases. Figure 8.4 shows the microsaccade directions and latencies as a function of the velocity of the pursuit target. Positive values on the vertical axis correspond to rightward microsaccades, while negative values correspond to leftward microsaccades. Actual latencies are the absolute value of the vertical dimension. It is clear that the directions and latencies of microsaccades are correlated with both the flash directions and the pursuit velocities. Microsaccade directions are biased in the direction of pursuit, and this bias increases with increases in pursuit velocities and microsaccade latencies decrease with increases of pursuit velocities. A similar result has been found for regular saccades during pursuit (Tanaka *et al.*, 1998). In that work, it was shown that that saccades in the same direction as the pursuit direction had shorter latencies than those in the opposite direction. This similarity supports the argument that saccades and microsaccades have the same dynamics and that they are generated by the same system responsible for saccade generation (Zuber *et al.*, 1965).

Our findings regarding attentional allocation (as indicated by the characteristics of microsaccades) during pursuit are supported by the studies reported by van Donkelaar (1999) and van Donkelaar and Drew (2002). They found that covert attention leads pursuit targets, with a lead amount that increases with the pursuit velocity. We can use the van Donkelaar and Drew result to construct a hypothesis regarding what is going on in our pursuit experiments. We assume that when a microsaccade occurs, it reflects a covert attention shift to one of three locations – the moving object itself, the location required to effectively pursue the moving object, or the distracting object. Van Donkelaar's research suggests that when pursuing a fast-moving object, attention is normally allocated to a location ahead of the moving object, with a distance that increases with pursuit velocity. As pursuit velocity increases, the salience of the location ahead of the pursuit object increases, owing to the increased difficulty of maintaining pursuit (i.e. the pursuit control system gain becomes higher). If attention is actually at this location when the distractor appears, then most of the time no attention shift will be generated, and a few times an attention shift will be made to the distractor. If attention is located on the moving object when the distractor appears, then most of the time there will be a covert attention shift to the optimal pursuit lead location, and a few times to the distractor. In both situations, the percentage of shifts to the distractor will drop as the pursuit velocity increases. This, then, would predict the type of bias towards the pursuit directions that we observe in our experiments.

8.5 What is next?

The research described in this article makes the case for a strong link between attention and the generation of eye movements. We think that we can make use of this link both to further our understanding of the human visual system, and to construct intelligent man–machine interfaces. Knowledge of where people are attending is invaluable in presenting information to them. For example, in automotive or aviation applications, information should be presented in ways that are at once non-intrusive or distracting, yet quickly assimilated. If we know when, and where, people are attending to a display, we can present information at that location. Presumably, if someone is attending to a location then they can access information at that location more quickly and accurately. Conversely, if we wish to make changes to a display that are not distracting, we could use the change blindness phenomenon to our advantage and make the changes at locations deemed to have low probability of being attended to currently. Such information would then have to be accessed by a slow search strategy, but in some applications, such as demanding search-and-rescue helicopter piloting, this may be a reasonable price to pay for the lack of distraction.

Currently in our lab, we are developing statistical covert attention tracking models, which fuse many sources of information regarding the allocation of covert attention. These sources include macro- and micro-eye movement measurements to keep track of gaze, and to detect microsaccades, as well as image information. The image data is used to compute image based salience measures. Pursuit eye movements are also detected, in which case attention leading of the pursued object is modeled. One of our goals is to apply the covert attention tracking system to real-time modification of visual displays in a video game. We are also looking into applying our ideas to automotive displays.

Finally, attention processes in the brain are not restricted to the visual modality. They operate in all sensory modalities. We are planning to extend our work to multimodal (visual, audio, tactile) attention control and tracking, and apply the resulting models to practical user-interface design for products such as cellular telephones. Stay tuned for future reports from our lab!

Acknowledgements

Portions of the research described in this article were carried out in the Harvard Robotics Laboratory (HRL), Nissan Cambridge Basic Research (CBR), and in the Centre for Intelligent Machines (CIM) at McGill University. We would like to acknowledge the contributions of Roger Brockett and Nicola Ferrier (now at the University of Wisconsin) from the HRL, and Ron Rensink (now at the University of British Columbia) and Kevin O'Regan (now at the Université de Paris V) at Nissan CBR.

All psychophysical studies performed by our group at McGill have received the approval of the Ethics Review Committee of the Faculty of Education at McGill University.

References

Abrams, R. A. (1992). Planning and producing saccadic eye movements. In K. Rayner, ed., *Eye Movements and Visual Cognition*. Springer-Verlag, pp. 66-88.

Abrams, R. A. and Jonides, J. (1988). Programming saccadic eye movements, *J. Exp. Psych.: Hum. Percept. Perf.*, **14**, 428–443.

Becker, W. and Jurgens, R. (1979). An analysis of the saccadic system by means of double step stimuli. *Vis. Res.*, **19**, 967–983.

Breitmeyer, B. and Ganz, L. (1976). Implications of sustained and transient channel for theories of visual pattern masking, saccadic suppression and information processing. *Psych. Rev.*, **83**, 1–36.

Brockett, R. (1988). On the computer control of movement. Proc. IEEE ICRA, Philadelphia, pp. 534–540.

Carpenter, R. (1988). *Movements of the Eyes*. London: Pion.

Clark, J. J. (1998a). Spatial attention and latencies of saccadic eye movements, *Vis. Res.*, **39**, 583–600.

Clark, J. J. (1998b). Spatial attention and saccadic camera motion. *Proc. IEEE CVPR*, Leuven, Belgium, pp. 3247–3252.

Clark, J. J. (1999). Linking covert and overt attention. *Behavioural and Brain Sci.*, **22**, 676.

Clark, J. J. and Ferrier, N. J. (1988). Modal control of an attentive vision system, *Proc. ICCV*, Tarpon Springs, Florida, pp. 514–523.

Clark, J. J. and Ferrier, N. J. (1989). Control of visual attention in mobile robots, *Proc. IEEE ICRA*, pp. 826-831.

Clark, J. J. and Ferrier, N. J. (1992). Attentive visual servoing. In A. Blake and A. L. Yuille, eds., *An Introduction to Active Vision*, Cambridge, MA: MIT Press, pp. 137–154.

Coeffe, C. and O'Regan, J. K. (1987). Reducing the influence of non-target stimuli on saccade accuracy: predictability and latency effects, *Vis. Res.*, **27**, 227–240.

Coren, S. and Hoenig, P. (1972). Effect of non-target stimuli upon length of voluntary saccades. *Percept. Motor Skills*, **34**, 499–508.

Cornsweet, T. N. (1956). Determination of the stimuli for involuntary drifts and saccadic eye movements. *J. Opt. Soc. Am.*, **46**, 987–993.

Desimone, R. (1990). Complexity at the neuronal level (commentary on *Vision and complexity*, by J. K. Tsotsos), *Behav. Brain Sci.*, **13**, 446.

Desimone, R., Wessinger, M., Thomas, L. and Schneider, W. (1989). Effects of deactivation of lateral pulvinar or superior colliculus on the ability to selectively attend to a visual stimulus. *Soc. Neurosci. Abst.*, **15**, 162.

Deubel, H., Wolf, W. and Hauske, G. (1984). The evaluation of the oculomotor error signal. In A. G. Gale and F. Johnson, eds., *Theoretical and Applied Aspects of Eye Movement Research*, Elsevier Science Publishers, pp. 55–62.

Engbert, R. and Kliegl, R. (2003). Microsaccades uncover the orientation of covert attention. *Vis. Res.*, **43**, 1035–1045.

Ferrier, N. J. and Clark, J. J. (1993). The Harvard Binocular Head. *Int. J. Patt. Recog. Artif. Intell.*, **7**, 9–32.

Findlay, J. M. (1982). Global visual processing for saccadic eye movements, *Vis. Res.*, **22**, 1033–1045.

Findlay, J. M. (1992). Programming of stimulus-elicited saccadic eye movements. In K. Rayner, ed., *Eye Movements and Visual Cognition*, New York: Springer-Verlag, pp. 31–45.

Fischer, B. (1993). Express saccades and visual attention. *Behav. Brain Sci.*, **16**, 553–610.

Hafed, Z. M. (2003). Motor theories of attention: how action serves perception in the visual system. Ph.D. Thesis, McGill University.

Hafed, Z. M. and Clark, J. J. (2000). Neural network model of saccade generation and control. *Invest. Ophthalmol. Vis. Sci.*, **41**(Suppl.), 315.

Hafed, Z. M. and Clark, J. J. (2001). Microsaccades reflect covert attention shifts. *European Conference on Visual Perception*, Turkey.

Hafed, Z. M. and Clark, J. J. (2002). Microsaccades as an overt measure of covert attention shifts. *Vis. Res.*, **42**, 2533–2545.

Hafed, Z. M. and Clark, J. J. (2003). Detecting patterns of covert attention shifts in psychophysical tasks using microsaccades. *Vision Sciences Society Annual Meeting*, Sarasota, Florida.

He, P. and Kowler, E. (1989). The role of location probability in the programming of saccades: Implications for Center-of-Gravity tendencies. *Vis. Res.*, **29**, 1165–1181.

Helmholtz, H. von (1896). *Handbuch der Physiologischen Optik*, 2nd edition. Leipzig and Hamburg: Leopold Voss.

Henderson, J. M. (1992). Visual attention and eye movement control during reading and scene perception. In K. Rayner, ed., *Eye Movements and Visual Cognition*, Springer-Verlag, pp. 260–283.

Hikosaka, O., Takikawa, Y. and Kawagoe, R. (2000), Role of the basal ganglia in the control of purposive saccadic eye movements. *Physiol. Rev.* **80**, 953–978.

James, W. (1890). *The Principles of Psychology*, Volume 1, chapter 11. New York: Dover Publications (reprint).

Jie, L. and Clark, J. J. (2005). Microsaccadic eye movements during ocular pursuit. *Vision Sciences Society Annual Meeting*, Sarasota, Florida.

Kalesnykas, R. P. and Hallett, P. E. (1994). Retinal eccentricity and the latency of eye saccades. *Vis. Res.*, **34**, 517–531.

Kingstone, A. and Klein, R. M. (1993). Visual offsets facilitate saccadic latency: does predisengagement of visuospatial attention mediate this gap effect? *J. Exp. Psych., Hum. Percept. Perf.*, **19**, 1251–1265.

Klein, R. M. (1980). Does oculomotor readiness mediate cognitive control of visual attention? In Nickerson, ed., *Attention and Performance VIII*, Hillsdale, NJ, Erlbaum.

Klein, R., Kingstone, A. and Pontefract, A. (1992). Orienting of visual attention. In K. Rayner, ed., *Eye Movements and Visual Cognition*. New York: Springer-Verlag, pp. 46–65.

Koch, C. and Ullman, S. (1985). Shifts in selective visual attention: Towards the underlying neural circuitry. *Hum. Neurobiol.*, **4**, 219–227.

Kowler, E. and Steinman, R. M. (1980). Small saccades serve no useful purpose. *Vis. Res.*, **20**, 273–276.

Kustov, A. A. and Robinson, D. L. (1996). Shared neural control attentional shifts and eye movements. *Nature*, **384**, 74–77.

Lee, C., Rohrer, W. H. and Sparks, D. L. (1988). Population coding of saccadic eye movements by the superior colliculus. *Nature*, **332**, 357–359.

Lennie, P. (1980). Parallel visual pathways: A review. *Vis. Res.*, **20**, 561–594.

Leopold, D. A. and Logothetis, N. K. (1998). Microsaccades differentially modulate neural activity in the striate and extrastriate visual cortex. *Exp. Brain Res.*, **123**, 341–345.

Martinez-Conde, S., Macknik, S. L. and Hubel, D. H. (2000). Microsaccadic eye movements and firing of single cells in the striate cortex of macaque monkeys. *Nature Neurosci.*, **3**, 251–258.

Milios, E., Jenkin, M. and Tsotsos, J. K. (1990). Design and performance of TRISH, a binocular robot head with torsional eye movements. *Int. J. Pat. Recog. Artif. Intell.*, **7**, 51–68.

Munoz, D. P. and Wurtz, R. H. (1993). Fixation cells in monkey superior colliculus. I. Characteristics of cell discharge. *J. Neurophysiol.*, **70**, 559–575.

Nakayama, K. and Mackeben, M. (1989). Sustained and transient components of focal visual attention. *Vis. Res.*, **29**, 1631–1647.

O'Regan, J. K. (1992). Solving the 'real' mysteries of visual perception: The world as an outside memory. *Can. J. Psychol.*, **46**, 461–488.

O'Regan, J. K., Rensink, R. A. and Clark, J. J. (1999). Change blindness as a result of mudsplashes. *Nature*, **398**, 34.

Posner, M. I. (1980). Orienting of attention. *Quart. J. Exp. Psych.*, **32**, 3–25.

Posner, M. I., Cohen, Y. and Rafal, R. D. (1982). Neural systems control of spatial orienting, *Phil. Trans. Roy. Soc. Lond.*, B **298**, 187–198.

Rensink, R. A., O'Regan, J. K. and Clark, J. J. (1995). Image flicker is as good as saccades in making large scene changes invisible. *European Conference on Visual Perception*, Tubingen, Germany. *Percept.*, **24** (suppl.), 26–28.

Rensink, R. A., O'Regan, J. K. and Clark, J. J. (1997). To see or not to see: the need for attention to perceive changes in scenes. *Psychol. Sci.*, **8**, 368–373.

Reulen, J. P. H. (1984a). Latency of visually evoked saccadic eye movements. I. Saccadic latency and the facilitation model. *Biol. Cybern.*, **50**, 251–262.

Reulen, J. P. H. (1984b). Latency of visually evoked saccadic eye movements. II. Temporal properties of the facilitation mechanism. *Biol. Cybern.*, **50**, 263–271.

Reuter-Lorenz, P., Hughes, H. C. and Fendrich, R. (1991). The reduction of saccadic latency by prior offset of the fixation point: An analysis of the gap effect. *Percept. Psychophys.*, **49**, 167–175.

Rizzolati, G. (1983). Mechanisms of selective attention in mammals. In J. P. Ewart, R. R. Capranica and D. J. Ingle, eds., *Advances in Vertebrate Neuroethology*. New York: Plenum, pp. 261–297,

Rizzolati, G., Riggio, L. and Sheliga, B. M. (1994). Space and selective attention. In C. Umilta and M. Moscovitch, eds., *Attention and Performance XV*. Cambridge, MA: MIT Press, pp. 231–265.

Saslow, M. G. (1967). Effects of components of displacement-step stimuli upon latency for saccadic eye movement. *J. Opt. Soc. Am.*, **57**, 1024–1029.

Sereno, A. B. (1992). Programming saccades: The role of attention. In K. Rayner, (ed.), *Eye Movements and Visual Cognition*. Springer-Verlag, pp. 89–107.

Swain, M. J. and Stricker, M. (eds.) (1991). Promising directions in active vision. *University of Chicago Technical Report*, CS-91-27.

Tanaka, M., Yoshida, T. and Fukushima, K. (1998). Latency of saccades during smooth-pursuit eye movement in man. *Exp. Brain Res.*, **121**, 92–98.

Tsotsos, J. K. (1990). Analyzing vision at the complexity level. *Behav. Brain Sci.*, **13**, 423–469.

van Donkelaar, P. (1999). Spatiotemporal modulation of attention during smooth pursuit eye movements. *Neuroreport*, **10**, 2523–2526.

van Donkelaar, P. and Drew, A. (2002). The allocation of attention during smooth pursuit eye movements. *Prog. Brain Res.*, **140**, 267–277.

Walker, R, Kentridge, R. W. and Findlay, J. M. (1995). Independent contributions of the orienting of attention, fixation offset and bilateral stimulation on human saccadic latencies. *Exp. Brain Res.*, **103**, 294–310.

Wurtz, R. H. (1996). Vision for the control of movement. *Invest. Ophthalmol. Vis. Sci.*, **11**, 2130–2145.

Wurtz, R. H. and Mohler, C. W. (1976). Organization of monkey superior colliculus: Enhanced visual response of superficial layer cells. *J. Neurophysiol.*, **39**, 745–765.

Wyman, D. and Steinman, R. M. (1973). Latency characteristics of small saccades. *Vis. Res.*, **13**, 2173–2175.

Yantis, S. and Jonides, J. (1984). Abrupt visual onsets and selective attention: evidence from visual search. *J. Exp. Psychol.: Hum. Percept. Perf.*, **10**, 601–621.

Zuber, B. L., Stark, L. and Cook, G. (1965). Microsaccades and the velocity-amplitude relationship for saccadic eye movements. *Science*, **150**, 1459–1460.

9 Cueing visual search in clutter

Preeti Verghese

9.1 Background

How do we find something in a cluttered scene? In the classic children's book, *Where's Waldo?* (Handford, 1997), children are asked to find Waldo, a boy, dressed in a red striped shirt, blue pants and a beanie hat, amidst dense crowd scenes containing a random assortment of oddly dressed people and other diverse objects. The search is difficult because there are so many possible locations for Waldo, so many competitors with similar clothing, and so much stuff in the way. If the picture had only eight boys presented at discrete locations, a well-trained observer could judge that one of them was wearing a shirt with wider stripes than the others without scrutinizing each of the eight boys. Indeed, in the past decade, this type of simple visual search has been encompassed within traditional signal detection theory (Green and Swets, 1966; Palmer *et al.*, 1993; Verghese and Stone, 1995; Eckstein, 1998; Morgan *et al.*, 1998; Palmer *et al.*, 2000; Baldassi and Burr, 2000; Verghese, 2001).

The displays used in studies of simple visual search bear little resemblance to natural scenes because they are arranged to examine judgments made without focused attention on individual elements. They typically use isolated features that vary along a single dimension and are presented in a ring at the same eccentricity, thereby eliminating the complexities of natural scenes, such as masking by adjacent or superimposed features, variable eccentricity and multiple dimensions. While these simplifications permit straightforward modeling, they raise questions about the generality of the conclusions reached in these studies. A more challenging question is how target selection occurs in cluttered conditions and how factors such as external cues, prior knowledge and segmentation processes influence the selection of the target.

In recent work, I have examined the detection of targets in cluttered displays in the absence of any external cues. The novel aspect of this work is that it adds a biological front end to the signal detection theory (SDT) model. The front end was made up

Computational Vision in Neural and Machine Systems, ed. L. Harris and M. Jenkin. Published by Cambridge University Press. © Cambridge University Press 2007.

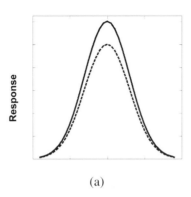 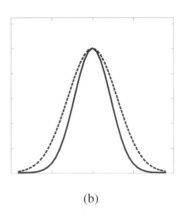

(a)   (b)

Figure 9.1. Effects of attention on the response of a hypothetical neuron as a function of an arbitrary feature value. (a) Attention can enhance the response across the entire tuning curve (solid line), effectively increasing the response at a given feature value by a multiplicative factor. The unattended tuning curve is depicted by a dashed line. (b) Attention can also increase the selectivity of the neuron by responding over a narrower region of feature space.

of local detectors that responded to both target and clutter. In two separate studies, one on motion detection and another on static orientation detection, I have shown that such a model does an excellent job of predicting the data if the target is a brief motion trajectory or a short oriented segment (Verghese *et al.*, 1999; Verghese and McKee, 2004). The targets in these studies occurred at unknown locations and had unknown directions/orientations. They were also embedded in dense noise that shared common aspects with the target. This work demonstrated that contemporary SDT models can, in principle, handle the clutter of natural scenes.

When searching natural environments, the observer typically has many cues to the target. How do external cues select a target, and how can these cueing effects be incorporated into the SDT models? It has been recognized for many decades that cueing enhances detection and discrimination by drawing attention to the cued location or feature (Posner 1980; Nakayama and Mackeben, 1989; Carrasco *et al.*, 2000). What exactly does attention do to the biological representation of the target? Attending to the cued attribute can aid target selection in three ways: (1) by reducing the uncertainty about the target, (2) by enhancing the gain of detectors tuned to the cued attribute and/or suppressing irrelevant detectors, and (3) by increasing the selectivity of detectors tuned to the cued attribute (by narrowing the tuning function of the detector); see Figure 9.1.

A cue can reduce uncertainty by specifying, for example, where the target will occur, or what its orientation will be. The observer then selects only those detectors that are tuned to the cued value of the target. Several studies have shown that cueing a subset of possible target locations makes location uncertainty equal to the number of cued locations (Palmer *et al.*, 1993; Foley and Schwartz, 1998; Palmer *et al.*, 2000; Burr *et al.*, 2003). For example, reducing uncertainty for location can be thought of as assigning a weight of 1 to the cued locations, and a weight of 0 to the uncued locations, without changing the properties of the individual detectors.

There is also evidence that the cue enhances the response of *individual detectors*. Physiological studies have shown that cueing a location or a feature has a profound effect on single neurons in awake, behaving monkeys. In fact, attending to a feature enhances the responses of a cell when the attended feature matches the cell's preference and suppresses the response when the feature is non-preferred (Moran and Desimone, 1985; Reynolds *et al.*, 1999; Treue and Martinez-Trujillo, 1999; Martinez-Trujillo and Treue, 2004). This modulation in response is evident over the entire tuning function as a change in the gain and is greatest when there are competing stimuli in the visual field (Motter, 1993; Treue and Martinez-Trujillo, 1999; McAdams and Maunsell, 1999). Psychophysical studies have shown enhanced gain at the cued location when the stimuli are clearly visible or embedded in low noise (Dosher and Lu, 2000a; Carrasco *et al.*, 2000).

The evidence that the *cue narrows the tuning of detectors* is mixed. In psychophysics, observers show a narrower spatial selectivity for the cued location only under conditions of clutter or high noise (Yeshurun and Carrasco, 1998; Dosher and Lu, 2000b). However, the classification image study of Eckstein *et al.* (2002) found little evidence for increased spatial selectivity in the presence of a location cue. In physiology, early studies suggested that attending to a stimulus resulted in both an increased gain and a narrower tuning of V4 neurons (Haenny and Schiller, 1988; Spitzer *et al.*, 1988). This is in contrast to later studies that carefully measured responses across the entire tuning function and only found evidence for increased gain (Treue and Maunsell, 1996; Reynolds *et al.*, 1999; Treue and Martinez-Trujillo, 1999; McAdams and Maunsell, 2000).

What implications do the different cueing effects have on signal detection theory models? The two critical variables in SDT are the number of detectors that respond to the signal relative to the total number of detectors responding (uncertainty) and the signal-to-noise ratio of each of these detectors. These two variables have different effects on the psychometric function that plots the observer's probability of a correct response versus signal strength. A decrease in uncertainty decreases the slope of the psychometric function (see Figure 9.3). Any change in signal-to-noise ratio is reflected in a horizontal shift of the psychometric function. The signal-to-noise ratio can by altered either by a greater sensitivity to the signal, or by a more selective filter. When the signal is presented in dense noise, it is not likely that increased gain across the entire bandwidth of the tuning function improves performance because gain would increase both the response to the signal and to the high level of external noise, and thus leave signal-to- noise ratio unchanged. In our experiments with cluttered backgrounds, it is more likely that performance is improved due to decreased uncertainty, or due to a more selective filter.

In daily life, we search for things, often without the aid of explicit cues. We have evidence from our own work that in such cases implicit cues may mimic the effect of explicit cues. The effect of implicit cues is likely built up from visual experience where the probability of one stimulus co-occurring with another is high. For example, given a contour segment of one orientation, it is highly likely that an adjacent segment will have a very similar orientation (Geisler *et al.*, 2001). In two separate studies, we have demonstrated that implicit cues enhance the visibility of contours and motion trajectories in noise. I have shown that the initial part of a motion trajectory acts a "cue" to subsequent segments, thus greatly enhancing the detection of an extended trajectory, in noise. I have also shown that a short oriented segment acts as a cue to nearby segments of similar orientation, thus bootstrapping the detection of a contour in noise. In these studies, a self-cue helps to select the target from the surrounding noise (clutter).

At what levels of visual processing do cues influence selection? There is now compelling evidence that attentive selection occurs at many levels of the visual hierarchy, including area V1 (Moran and Desimone, 1985; Motter, 1993; Treue and Maunsell, 1996; Gandhi *et al.*, 1999; Martinez *et al.*, 1999; Reynolds, *et al.*, 1999; Saenz *et al.*, 2002). This selection implicates a top-down modulation of the visual input. The self-cueing that we observe in the motion and orientation domains is consistent with a hierachical Bayesian framework that integrates the feedforward input with feedback from higher areas (Lee and Mumford, 2003; see also Thielscher and Neumann, 2005). The feedback provides the weights that modulate the incoming visual input. This top-down weighting might reflect priors learned through visual experience such as smoothness in contours and trajectories (see Geisler *et al.*, 2001, Elder and Goldberg, 2002), or might reflect explicit attention- or task-based weighting (Tsotsos *et al.*, 1995). Thus recurrent feedback/feedforward loops, along with interactions between neighboring units within a cortical area, allow the visual system to converge on an interpretation of the image. This is a rather general framework. Its greatest strength is its flexibility, which allows knowledge about target and context to shape processing at every level of the visual processing stream. This property is consistent with several studies that show how context influences the responses of neurons as early as V1 (Lamme, 1995; Lee *et al.*, 1998, 2002).

I will consider in detail two examples of attention acting through implicit cues to enhance the visibility of targets in clutter. The first study deals with detecting a signal dot moving along a smooth path among noise dots in Brownian motion, a task first used by Watamaniuk *et al.* (1995). The second task deals with linking roughly collinear contour segments embedded among noise patches of random orientation (as in Field *et al.*, 1993). I use a contrast probe on both the motion trajectory and contour segment to understand what mechanisms make these signals detectable in noise.

9.2 Detecting smooth motion paths in noise

Watamaniuk *et al.* (1995) and Verghese *et al.* (1999) showed that a single dot moving along a consistent trajectory in Brownian noise was easily detected.[1] The signal trajectory was 200 ms long and was defined by a dot moving in a consistent direction. The noise was made up of dots in Brownian motion that had the same magnitude of displacement as the signal on every frame, but moved in a random direction. Can

---

[1] A movie of the stimulus Traj-In-Noise.mov is available on the accompanying CD-ROM. For purposes of demonstration the movie is 500 ms long, whereas the stimulus display was only 200 ms long. The movie shows a single trial composed of two temporal intervals. The signal trajectory is present in the second interval and is moving down and to the left.

these results be explained by summation of stimulus energy within individual motion detectors? Or, do they require an interaction between motion detectors lying along the stimulus path?

To answer these questions, we compared human sensitivity to the predictions of a local motion energy model (details of the model are available in Verghese *et al.*, 1999). The model based its decision on the largest response of an array of local detectors that tiled the stimulus area. Local detectors were chosen to be of the optimal size given the speed of the signal. We also assumed that the local detectors had an integration time of 100 ms, consistent with estimates of temporal integration times from monkey MT and human psychophysics (Mikami *et al.*, 1986; Watson, 1979). One could postulate circular detectors large enough to see the entire signal trajectory that integrate motion signals over the length of the trajectory. However, such units have very poor signal-to-noise ratio, because they integrate more noise than signal with increasing area (Verghese *et al.*, 1999). Alternatively, it is possible that a unit elongated in the direction of motion can explain the detectability of trajectories, as suggested by van Doorn and Koenderink (1984) and Fredericksen *et al.* (1994). Additional simulations with detectors with aspect ratios as large as 10:1 (ratio of length along the motion axis to length along the orthogonal axis) show that this modified geometry is also inadequate to explain human performance.

The predictions of our local model show that when the trajectory duration is brief (100 ms), the model does an excellent job of predicting human performance. This is also true when there is more than a single 100 ms trajectory. Figure 9.2 compares predictions of the local model to human performance. When there were two independent 100 ms trajectory segments, both human and model performance improved by a factor of $\sqrt{2}$, consistent with probability summation of independent detectors. But when a single trajectory was extended (200 ms), human performance far exceeded the predictions of the model. Note that the model prediction for the single 200 ms trajectory are identical to those for two separate 100 ms segments, because the model assumes that the two responses are independent.

What makes an extended trajectory so much more detectable than the sum of its parts? A hint comes from a study in which we manipulated the spatial and temporal arrangements of two 100 ms trajectory segments. In this experiment, observers were asked to detect which of two intervals contained a trajectory. Our results show that a trajectory was most detectable when the second segment continued where the first one ended. Interestingly, detectability was only slightly impaired if the second component appeared in the vicinity of the first. This was true whether the second component deviated by $45°$ with respect to the first, or if it moved in the same direction, but within $2°$ of the first (Verghese and McKee, 2002). When the two segments were separated by more than $2°$, detectability was severely impaired. These results suggest that the first segment of the trajectory, i.e., the first 70–100 ms, acts as a cue that alerts the visual system to subsequent motion segments, thereby increasing their visibility.

As outlined in Section 9.1, a cue can improve performance by increasing the sensitivity of the cued detector, or by reducing uncertainty about which detector contains the signal, or by some mixture of both operations (Shiu and Pashler, 1994; Lu and Dosher, 1998; Dosher and Lu, 200a, b; Carrasco *et al.*, 2000; Verghese, 2001). In physiological terms, the change in sensitivity might be achieved by increasing the gain

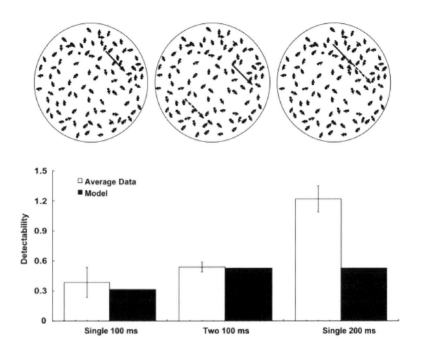

Figure 9.2. Comparison of human sensitivity to the predictions of a model composed of local motion energy units. The comparisons are shown for three conditions; a single 100 ms trajectory in noise (left), two 100 ms trajectories in noise (middle) and a single 200 ms trajectory (right). The long solid and dashed arrows depict 100 ms trajectories. The dashed arrow represents a trajectory that comes on in the latter 200 ms of the display. Model and observer performance was converted to a d' measure.

of the signal neurons (Treue and Maunsell, 1996) or by an increase in selectivity, and the reduction in uncertainty could be accomplished by a competitive interaction that results in the weaker neuronal responses being suppressed (Reynolds *et al.*, 1999). To determine how this cue enhances trajectory visibility, we measured the visibility of a contrast probe on the trajectory. The probe was a contrast increment that occurred either at the beginning (first 70 ms) or the end (last 70 ms) of a 200 ms trajectory in separate experimental blocks (movies demonstrating the stimulus are available on the accompanying CD-ROM.)[2] In this task, both intervals of the trial had trajectories, but observers were asked to choose the interval with the contrast increment. To prevent the observer from basing his or her decision on the interval with the brightest dot, each

---

[2]The movies of the contrast increment experiment show examples of the trajectory with the increment at the beginning, by itself and in the presence of noise (Inc_Beg.mov and Ing_Beg_Noise.mov, respectively). Again the movie is 500 ms long, whereas the actual stimulus lasted 200 ms. Also for ease of detection, the trajectory is always shown moving down and to the left, while it moved in one of eight directions in the experiment. (Movies that show the trajectory with the increment at the end, by itself and in noise are Inc_End.mov and Inc_End_Noise.mov, respectively.)

noise dot was randomly assigned one of five contrast values that straddled the contrast of the signal dot. The highest of these contrast values was greater than or equal to the largest value of contrast increment on the signal dot.

We reasoned that if the first part of a trajectory in noise were cueing the second part, then contrast increments would be more visible at the end of the trajectory. We also hypothesized that because we blocked the two conditions (increments at the beginning and at the end), observers should know exactly where the increment would appear if the trajectory were presented in a fixed location and direction without noise. Our results show that indeed for the trajectory-known condition, thresholds at the beginning and at the end of the trajectory were almost identical (not shown). When the trajectory was presented in noise and its location and direction were randomized, thresholds for the beginning of the trajectory were significantly higher. Furthermore the slope of the psychometric function for the beginning of the trajectory was much steeper than that for the end of the trajectory (Figure 9.3c). This is the classic uncertainty effect; observers appear much more uncertain about the beginning of the trajectory, rather than the end (Verghese and McKee, 2002).

The differential effect of noise on increment thresholds at the beginning and end of the trajectory supports the role of self-cueing. Because the trajectory appears at a random location, and moves in a random direction among dynamic noise dots, detecting the contrast increment is akin to a search task in which the location and direction of the target are unknown. Without prior information about the location and direction of the trajectory, the observer's attention is distributed and the observer potentially monitors multiple locations and directions. The first part of the trajectory generates a slightly larger response in local motion detectors than the surrounding noise and acts as a cue, thereby reducing the potential locations and directions of subsequent parts of the signal trajectory. A signal detection theory analysis (Green and Swets, 1966; Shaw, 1982,1984; Pelli, 1985) of our data shows that the improvement for increments at the end of the trajectory is largely due to a reduction in uncertainty (a reduction in the number of detectors that the observer monitors). The reduction in uncertainty suggests that the visual system uses consistent motion, by itself, as a cue to the most likely direction and future location of a moving feature.

Signal detection theory predicts that increasing the gain k and/or reducing the number of detectors M that the observer monitors can improve contrast discrimination. These two parameters have different effects on the psychometric function. Increasing the gain shifts the psychometric function leftwards to lower values (and lower thresholds), without changing its shape (Figure 9.3a). On the other hand, a reduction in uncertainty changes the slope of the psychometric function (Figure 9.3b). The curve is shallow when the observer monitors the single detector that contains the signal, and the curve is steep when the observer monitors many (32) detectors, only one of which contains the signal. Note that if contrast thresholds are specified as a criterion percentage correct, e.g. 75%, they will be lower when the observer is monitoring fewer detectors, even if there is no accompanying change in gain. These predictions are based on the uncertainty model outlined by Shaw (1982, 1984) and by Pelli (1985), that has been used extensively to model visual search performance (Eckstein, 1998; Palmer *et al.*, 1993; Verghese and Stone, 1995). Our intent was to fit the measured psychometric functions with the uncertainty model to determine how much of the improvement in

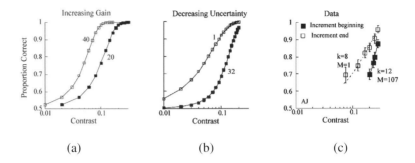

(a)   (b)   (c)

Figure 9.3. Predicted psychometric functions for two values of gain (a), and uncertainty (b). An increase in gain shifts the psychometric function leftward, and a decrease in uncertainty makes the function shallower. The filled and open symbols in (c) show data for detecting a contrast increment at the beginning and at the end of a motion trajectory in noise. The k and M values alongside each curve represent the best-fitting gain and uncertainty estimates. For this observer, the improved ability to detect contrast increments at the end of the trajectory is due to a 100-fold reduction in uncertainty.

contrast discrimination at the end of the trajectory is due to changes in gain and/or uncertainty (see Appendix for uncertainty model).

We used an iterative procedure to find the best-fitting values of k and M for psychometric functions at the beginning and end of a trajectory presented in noise (Figure 9.3c). This observer detected the increment at the end of the trajectory far more easily than the increment at the beginning of the trajectory. The calculated fits indicate that there are small changes in the gain parameter k, perhaps amounting to about a factor of 1.5 for end-increments relative to beginning-increments. However, there is a huge change, by more than a factor of 100, in the uncertainty parameter M. Three other observers also found detection of contrast increments to be easier at the end of the trajectory than at the beginning. Two of these observers showed the same large change in uncertainty with little change in gain, but the other observer showed a large change in gain (factor of three) with little change in the uncertainty parameter. Thus both gain and/or uncertainty can work to enhance increment detection.

The large decrease in uncertainty at the end of the trajectory suggests that the first part of the trajectory cues subsequent parts. This is consistent with our typical experience with motion in the real world. Objects often continue to move along a smooth trajectory and rarely change direction or speed abruptly. This suggests that we have a prior for smoothness that favors locations and directions that are close to the initial estimate. To examine the effect of this prior we measured contrast increments on a 200 ms trajectory where the second 100 ms segment changed direction with respect to the first. This direction change was always $45°$ clockwise, so the uncertainty of the stimulus configuration was identical to the case of the straight trajectory, where the second segment continued in the same direction as the first. When we measured sensitivity to the contrast probe for the bending trajectory, all three observers were much more sensitive

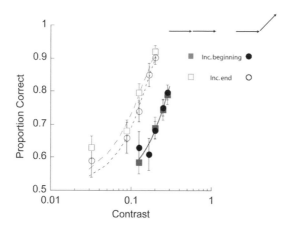

Figure 9.4. Comparison of straight and bent trajectories. The arrows in the upper right represent 100 ms trajectory fragments. Circle and square symbols show data for the straight and bent trajectories respectively. The two conditions were run in separate blocks and observers knew whether the contrast increment appeared at the beginning (solid symbols) or at the end (open symbols). The contrast increment at the beginning was equally detectable for both the straight and bent trajectories, whereas the improvement for increments at the end is consistently less for the bent trajectory than for the straight trajectory.

to increments at the end of the trajectory than to increments in the beginning, but the improvement was significantly smaller than for the straight trajectory (data for one observer are shown in Figure 9.4). Note that this result is consistent with our finding that a trajectory that bends by 45° is also slightly less detectable than a straight trajectory. Both findings support a role for a Bayesian prior for smoothness.

9.3 Self-cueing in contour formation

Amidst the clutter of the natural visual world, human observers effortlessly identify the bounding contours of discrete objects. The edges of natural objects tend to be smooth and not change orientation abruptly. Several studies have shown that contours in randomly oriented noise are most detectable when adjacent elements of the contour change orientation slowly (Field *et al.*, 1993, Kovacs and Julesz, 1993; Geisler *et al.*, 2001; Elder and Goldberg, 2002). Does self-cueing play a role in determining the visibility of contours in noise? To determine whether the implicit cueing effect in the motion domain extends to static contours, I measured sensitivity to contrast increments on a test patch that was cued by a contour (Verghese, 2003). The contour + test occurred at an unknown location, in the presence of randomly oriented noise. The contour cue was at various orientations with respect to the test patch, but the identity of the test patch was

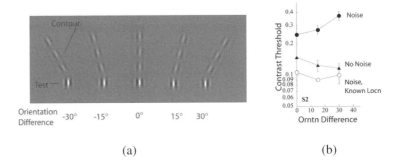

Figure 9.5. Detecting contrast increments at the end of a contour. (a) shows the five stimulus configurations. The test patch was always at the end of cueing string made up of three collinear Gabor patches. The angle between the string and test was varied in separate blocks of trials. Human observers detected a contrast increment on the test patch in the absence of noise (shown) or in a display with randomly oriented Gabor patches. (b) shows contrast increment thresholds for one observer as a function of the orientation difference between cueing string and test. Data are shown for three conditions, no noise, noise and noise with the test in a known location.

unambiguous; it was either at the right end or at the bottom of the contour (Figure 9.5). The orientation difference between the test and contour was also blocked, so that the test had a known relationship to the cue.

Figure 9.5 plots increment thresholds as a function of orientation difference for one of our three observers. Thresholds for clockwise and counterclockwise deviations were similar, so thresholds are combined and plotted as a function of absolute deviation. There are three points to note.

(1) In the absence of noise, thresholds were highest when the contour was collinear with the test and decreased as the angle between contour and test increased (solid triangles). These results are similar to Chen and Tyler (2001), who showed that collinear flanking patches elevated contrast increment thresholds compared to flankers of other orientations.

(2) In the presence of randomly oriented noise, thresholds (filled circles) showed the opposite pattern. Thresholds were lowest for the collinear case and increased with orientation difference.

(3) When the test (and contour) were presented in noise but at a known location and orientation, collinearity had no effect on thresholds. Thresholds in this condition (open circles) were independent of contour orientation, indicating that the contour cue was superfluous when test location was known.

What class of contour integration model accounts for these effects? One class of model predicts an overall increase in the activity of detectors coding for roughly collinear elements. These include models that implement long-range facilitatory interactions (see Li, 1998; Grossberg *et al.*, 1997) and those that maximize smoothness in contour grouping (Pettet *et al.*, 1998). The increased activation on the contour explains the increased detectability of contours in noise. Because of the increased activation and the higher variability associated with higher response levels, these models also predict higher increments thresholds on the contour, consistent with our no-noise results. Another class of model is based on contrast gain control that preferentially weights collinear signals in the normalization pool (Schwartz and Simoncelli, 2001). Gain control does not predict an increase in overall activity but rather increased contrast sensitivity. This latter model explains the higher sensitivity to increments in noise, when the cue is collinear with the test, but does not explain why contours are easily detected in noise. Neither class of model by itself explains both the visibility of contours in noise and the increased sensitivity for increments on a contour in the presence of noise.

It is possible that some combination of summation through long-range interactions and suppression through contrast-gain control can explain both (Gilbert, 1992; Kapadia *et al.*, 1995; Schwartz and Simoncelli, 2001). Alternately, I propose that a short contour segment acts as a cue to the rest of the contour. Cueing is thought to increase the sensitivity of the underlying detector and to reduce the number of competing responses. The increase in sensitivity can be achieved through a process akin to gain control and the increase in the visibility of the contour can be achieved through a reduction in the number of competitors (a decrease in uncertainty).

How can contour segments act as cues? At high contrast levels, any pair of roughly aligned Gabor patches may increase the response of an elongated orientation detector (Jones and Palmer, 1987; Solomon *et al.*, 1998) above that generated by the randomly oriented noise. However, a single pair is barely detected in dense noise, and even multiple pairs scattered throughout the noise are not as detectable as an extended contour formed of a comparable number of patches. I am proposing that each pair acts as a selective cue for adjacent patches of similar orientation. Competitive interaction between the cue and noise also suppresses the activity generated by patches of dissimilar orientation (Reynolds *et al.*, 1999). In short, the visual system uses a bootstrapping operation to connect the oriented segments. Identifying a contour is difficult in noisy, cluttered environments where there is considerable uncertainty about which oriented segments belong together. By removing competitors, self-cueing greatly enhances the signal-to-noise ratio of the responses generated by the real meandering contour. In fact Elder and Goldberg (2002), using an entropy measure, show that contour grouping cues such as proximity and good continuation significantly reduce the uncertainty about which oriented segments are to be grouped together.

Our result showing that a collinear contour improves contrast discrimination only when the test is presented at an unknown location in noisy conditions, indicates that the collinear contour implicitly cues the test and reduces uncertainty about its location. These results suggest that local collinearity is an important cue to contour formation, particularly under conditions of poor visibility (noise).

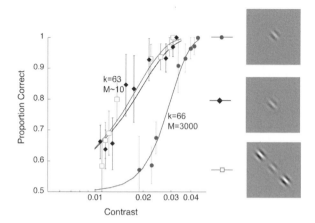

Figure 9.6. Uncertainty effects in a contrast detection paradigm. The graph plots proportion correct as a function of test contrast. The test was presented on its own (red circles), or surrounded by a low contrast circle (black diamonds), or flanked by high contrast collinear Gabor patches as in Polat and Sagi (1993) (green squares). The smooth lines are the fits of the uncertainty model to the data. It is interesting to note that for this observer a reduction in uncertainty accounts for all of the threshold improvement obtained in the presence of a circle or of flanking collinear patches. (A color version of this figure is available on the CD-ROM.)

9.4   Uncertainty and collinear facilitation at detection threshold

What about the ultimate low-visibility condition – detection threshold? Previous studies have shown that the detection of a Gabor patch is improved considerably in the presence of high contrast flanking patches that are collinear with the test (Polat and Sagi, 1993, 1994). This result has been interpreted as evidence for collinear facilitation. However, as collinear facilitation is observed only for low-contrast targets, and not at suprathreshold contrasts where the test is clearly visible (Chen and Tyler, 2002), the effect of the flankers may well be to reduce the uncertainty of the targets location and orientation. If this is true, then other cues to location and orientation should give rise to a similar decrease in thresholds. Moreover, SDT predicts that the slope of the psychometric function should decrease in the presence of cues that reduce uncertainty. To test this hypothesis, we measured contrast detection threshold for a Gabor target under three conditions: (1) target alone, (2) target surrounded by a low-contrast circle that served as a location cue and (3) target flanked by two collinear Gabor patches (Petrov *et al.*, 2006).

Figure 9.6 plots the psychometric functions obtained as a function of the test contrast for one observer. We replicate the findings of Polat and Sagi (1993) showing that the presence of collinear flankers (green squares) improved detection considerably compared to the case when the patch is presented by itself (red circles). The faint circular outline caused an intermediate improvement for three of our five observers (black diamonds), indicating that these observers used the additional orientation information provided by the collinear Gabors. Most interestingly, the remaining two observers show almost identical improvement with the circle as with the collinear flankers (only one observer's data are shown). An uncertainty analysis shows that the improvement in performance is largely due to a decrease in uncertainty, rather than a change in sensitivity as implied by Polat and Sagi (1993, 1994).

There have been hints in the literature that other factors beside collinear facilitation impact detection thresholds. In a modificiation of the original Polat and Sagi (1993) paradigm, Tanaka and Sagi (1998) showed that high-contrast collinear flankers improve the detectability of a test patch even if they are flashed up to 16 seconds before the test patch. The largest benefit was for simultaneous flankers, but at longer delays the facilitation was at least half the magnitude of the facilitation observed with a simultaneous flanker. The test and flanker paradigm pioneered by Polat and Sagi (1993, 1994) has elements of both an explicit cue and a contour cue. The flankers serve as an explicit cue because they specify the orientation and location of the test patch. At the same time the three-patch configuration can be thought of as a contour segment. The enhanced detection of the test patch in the three-patch configuration has been attributed to long-range connections among neurons of similar orientation preference that selectively enhance the processing of collinear contours. The suppression observed at high flanker contrasts is thought to be the result of a contrast normalization pool that preferentially weights signals from neurons along the preferred orientation of the cell (Cavanaugh *et al.*, Movshon, 2002; Chen and Tyler, 2001; Schwartz and Simoncelli, 2001). Such specific neural interactions probably have an effective duration on the order of hundreds of milliseconds rather than seconds. It is therefore likely that the benefit from flankers that appear long before the test is a cueing effect that reduces uncertainty. Several studies support a role for attention in contrast detection – they show that contrast detection of the test patch improves only when the observers attend to the collinear flankers (Giorgi *et al.*, 2004; Freeman *et al.*, 2001; Shani and Sagi, 2005).

9.5 Conclusions

The contrast detection results, along with the motion and contour cueing studies, suggest that implicit cues such as smooth segments in the motion and orientation domain can help to select a weak target. These implicit cues show the same benefits as explicit cues, with their largest effect being a reduction in uncertainty. There are two points to note: (1) the benefits of implicit cueing are most evident under conditions of poor visibility (clutter, noise, low contrast), and (2) implicit cues seem to enforce a prior for smoothness, which may be learnt from visual experience.

Acknowledgements

This work was supported by NSF grant 0347051 and by Smith Kettlewell.

Appendix

Model   The uncertainty model assumes that the observer monitors multiple detectors M in each interval. The detectors have a gain k, and each detector produces a noisy response from a Gaussian distribution. The observer finds the largest of these responses in each interval and then chooses the interval with the larger response. Errors arise when the interval without the increment produces a larger response and the probability of error increases with the number of detectors that the observer monitors. This formulation is based on Pelli's (1985) uncertainty model. For our two-interval forced choice task, the probability of a correct response is given by the probability that the interval with the increment produces the larger response. Alternately, the probability of a correct response is 1-probability that the non-increment interval produces the larger response.

$$
\begin{aligned}
P_{\text{correct}}(\Delta c) &= P_{\text{increment interval larger}} \\
&= 1 - P_{\text{non-increment interval larger}} \\
P_{\text{correct}}(\Delta c) &= \int_{\infty}^{+\infty} M.f(x - kc)F(x - kc)^{2M-2}F(x - k(c + \Delta c))\mathrm{d}x
\end{aligned}
$$
$$(9.1)$$

where c is the contrast of the trajectory, Δc is the contrast increment, $f(x)$ is the Gaussian probability density function and $F(x)$ is the cumulative Gaussian $\int_{-\infty}^{x} f(x')\mathrm{d}x'$.

The non-increment interval produces the largest response when one of the M detectors in the non-increment interval has a value x and all the other detectors have a value less than x. These other detectors includes a total of $2M - 2$ detectors that see the pedestal contrast c ($M - 1$ from the interval with the increment, and $M - 1$ from the non-increment interval), and one detector that sees the increment contrast $c + \delta c$. The probability that a detector in the non-increment interval produces a response x is given by the Gaussian density $f(x - kc)$ where k is the sensitivity parameter and c is the pedestal contrast. The probability that all the other detectors will produce a contrast less than x is the product of all their cumulative distributions, i.e. $F(x - kc)^{2M-2}F(x - k(c + \delta c))$, where the first term is from the $2M - 2$ detectors that see the pedestal contrast and the second term is from the one detector in the increment interval that sees the increment. The expression is multiplied by M because any one of the M detectors in the non-increment interval can produce the largest response. The integral calculates the probability of an incorrect response over all values of x.

References

Baldassi, S. and Burr, D. C. (2000). Feature-based integration of orientation signals in visual search. *Vis. Res.*, **40**, 293–300.

Burr, D. C., Morrone, M. C., Baldassi, S. and Verghese, P. (2003). Visual search for motion direction: pop-out and set-size dependencies explained by stimulus and intrinsic uncertainty. *Vis. Sci. Soc.*, http://www.journalofvision.org/3/9/41/

Carrasco, M., Penpeci-Talgar, C. and Eckstein, M. (2000). Spatial covert attention increases contrast sensitivity across the CSF: support for signal enhancement. *Vis. Res.*, **40**, 1203–1215.

Cavanaugh, J. R., Bair, W. and Movshon, J. A. (2002). Nature and interaction of signals from the receptive field center and surround in macaque V1 neurons. *J. Neurophysiol.*, **88**, 2530–2546.

Chen, C. C. and Tyler, C. W. (2001). Lateral sensitivity modulation explains the flanker effect in contrast discrimination. *Proc. R. Soc. Lond.*, B **268**, 509–516

Chen, C. C. and Tyler, C. W. (2002). Lateral modulation of contrast discrimination: flanker orientation effects. *J. Vis.*, **2**, 520–530.

Dosher, B. A. and Lu, Z. (2000a). Mechanisms of perceptual attention in precuing of location. *Vis. Res.*, **40**, 1269–1292.

Dosher, B. A. and Lu, Z. (2000b). Noise exclusion in spatial attention. *Psychol. Sci.*, **11**, 139–146.

Eckstein, M. P. (1998). The lower efficiency for conjunctions is due to noise and not serial attentional processing. *Psychol. Sci.*, **2**, 111–118.

Eckstein, M. P., Shimozaki, S. S. and Abbey, C. K. (2002). The footprints of visual attention in the Posner cueing paradigm revealed by classification images. *J. Vis.*, **2**, 25–45.

Elder, J. H. and Goldberg, R. M. (2002). Ecological statistics of Gestalt laws for the perceptual organization of contours. *J. Vis.*, **2**, 324–353.

Field, D. J., Hayes, A. and Hess, R. F. (1993). Contour integration by the human visual system: evidence for a local "association field". *Vis. Res.*, **33**, 173–193.

Fredericksen, R. E., Verstraten, F. A. J. and van de Grind, W. A. (1994). An analysis of the temporal integration mechanism in human motion perception. *Vis. Res.*, **34**, 3153–3170.

Freeman, E., Sagi, D. and Driver, J. (2001). Lateral interactions between targets and flankers in low-level vision depend on attention to the flankers. *Nature Neurosci.*, **4**, 1032–1036.

Foley, J. M. and Schwarz, W. (1998). Spatial atteniton: effect of position uncertainty and number of distractor patterns on the threshold-versus contrast function for contrast discrimination. *J. Opt. Soc. Am. A*, **15**, 1036–1047.

Gandhi, S. P., Heeger, D. J., and Boynton, G. M. (1999). Spatial attention affects brain activity in human primary visual cortex. *Proc. Natl. Acad. Sci. USA*, **96**, 3314–3319.

Geisler, W. S., Perry, J. S., Super, B. J. and Gallogly, D. P. (2001). Edge co-occurrence in natural images predicts contour grouping. *Vis. Res.*, **41**, 711–724.

Gilbert, C. D. (1992). Horizontal integration and cortical dynamics. *Neuron*, **9**, 1–13.

Giorgi, R. G., Soong, G. P., Woods, R. L. and Peli, E. (2004). Facilitation of contrast detection in near-peripheral vision. *Vis. Res.*, **44**, 3193–3202.

Green, D. M. and Swets, J. A. (1966). *Signal Detection Theory and Psychophysics*. New York: John Wiley and Sons.

Grossberg, S., Mingolla, E. and Ross, W. D. (1997). Visual brain and visual perception: how does the cortex do perceptual grouping? *Trends Neurosci.*, **20**, 106–111.

Handford, M. (1997). *Where's Waldo?* 2nd edition. Cambridge, MA: Candlewick Press.

Haenny, P. E. and Schiller, P. H. (1988). State dependent activity in monkey visual cortex. I. Single cell activity in V1 and V4 on visual tasks. *Exp. Brain Res.*, **69**, 225–244.

Jones, J. P. and Palmer, L. A. (1987). An evaluation of the two-dimensional Gabor filter model of simple receptive fields in cat striate cortex. *J. Neurophysiol.*, **58**, 1233–1258.

Kapadia, M. K., Ito, M., Gilbert, C. D. and Westheimer, G. (1995). Improvement in visual sensitivity by changes in local context: parallel studies in human observers and in V1 of alert monkeys. *Neuron*, **15**, 843–856.

Kovacs, I. and Julesz, B. (1993). A closed curve is much more than an incomplete one: Effect of closure in figure-ground segmentation. *Pro. Nat. Acad. Sci. USA*, **90**, 7495–7497.

Lamme, V. A. (1995). The neurophysiology of figure ground segregation in primary visual cortex *J. Neurosci.*, **15**, 1605–1615.

Lee, T. S. and Mumford, D. (2003). Hierarchical Bayesian inference in the visual cortex. *J. Opt. Soc. Am. A*, **20**, 1434–1448.

Lee, T. S., Mumford, D., Romero, R. and Lamme, V. A. (1998). The role of the primary visual cortex in higher level vision. *Vis. Res.*, **38**, 2429–2454.

Lee, T. S., Yang, C. F., Romero, R. D. and Mumford, D. (2002). Neural activity in early visual cortex reflects behavioral experience and higher-order perceptual saliency. *Nat. Neurosci.*, **5**, 589–597.

Li, Z. (1998). A neural model of contour integration in the primary visual cortex. *Neural Comput.*, **10**, 903–940.

Lu, Z. L. and Dosher, B. A. (1998). External noise distinguishes attention mechanisms. *Vis. Res.*, **38**, 1183–1198.

Martinez, A., Anllo-Vento, L., Sereno. M. I. *et al.* (1999). Involvement of striate and extrastriate visual cortical areas in spatial attention. *Nat. Neurosci.*, **2**, 364–369.

Martinez-Trujillo, J. C. and Treue, S. (2004). Feature-based attention increases the selectivity of population responses in primate visual cortex. *Cur. Biol.*, **14**, 744–751.

McAdams, C. J. and Maunsell, J. H. R. (1999). Effects of attention on orientation-tuning functions of single neurons in macaque cortical area V4. *J. Neurosci.*, **19**, 431–441.

McAdams, C. J. and Maunsell, J. H. (2000). Attention to both space and feature modulates neuronal responses in macaque area V4. *J. Neurophysiol.*, **83**, 1751–1755.

Mikami, A., Newsome, W. T. and Wurtz, R. H. (1986). Motion selectivity in macaque visual cortex. I. Mechanisms of directional and speed selectivity in extrastriate area MT. *J. Neurophysiol.*, **55**, 1308–1327.

Moran, J. and Desimone, R. (1985). Selective attention gates visual processing in the extrastriate cortex. *Science*, **229**, 782–784.

Morgan, M. J., Ward, R. M. and Castet E. (1998). Visual search for a tilted target:tests of spatial uncertainty models. *Quart. J. Exp. Psych.*, **51A**, 347–370

Motter, B. C. (1993). Focal attention produces spatially selective processing in visual cortical areas V1, V2, and V4 in the presence of competing stimuli. *J. Neurophysiol.*, **70**, 909–919.

Nakayama, K. and Mackeben, M. (1989) Sustained and transient components of focal visual attention. *Vis. Res.*, **29**, 1631–1647.

Palmer, J., Ames, C. T. and Lindsey, D. T. (1993). Measuring the effect of attention on simple visual search. *J. Exp. Psyc.: Hum. Percept. Perf.*, **19**, 108–130.

Palmer, J., Verghese, P. and Pavel, M. (2000). The psychophysics of visual search. *Vis. Res.*, **40**, 1227–1268.

Pelli, D. G. (1985). Uncertainty explains many aspects of visual contrast detection and discrimination. *J. Opt. Soc. Am. A*, **2**, 1508–1532.

Pettet, M. W., McKee, S. P. and Grzywacz. N. M. (1998). Constraints on long range connections mediating contour detection. *Vis. Res.*, **38**, 865–879.

Polat, U. and Sagi, D. (1993). Lateral interactions between spatial channels: Suppression and facilitation revealed by lateral masking experiments. *Vis. Res.*, **33**, 993–999.

Polat, U. and Sagi, D. (1994). The architecture of perceptual spatial interactions. *Vis. Res.*, **34**, 73–78.

Petrov, Y., Verghese, P. and McKee, S. P. (2006). Collinear facilitation is largely uncertainty reduction. *J. Vis.*, **6**, 170–178.

Posner, M. I. (1980). Orienting of Attention. *Quart. J. Exp. Psych.*, **32**, 3–25.

Reynolds, J. H., Chelazzi, L., and Desimone, R. (1999). Competitive mechanisms subserve attention in macaque areas V2 and V4. *J. Neurosci.*, **19**, 1736–1753.

Saenz, M., Buracas, G. T. and Boynton, G. M. (2002). Global effects of feature-based attention in human visual cortex. *Nat. Neurosci.*, **5**, 631–62.

Schwartz, O. and Simoncelli, E. P. (2001). Natural signal statistics and sensory gain control. *Nat. Neurosci.*, **4**, 819–825.

Shaw, M. L. (1982). Attending to multiple sources of information: I. The integration of information in decision making. *Cogn. Psych.*, **14**, 353–409.

Shaw, M. L. (1984). Division of attention among spatial locations: a fundamental difference between detection of letters and detection of luminance increments. In H. B. Bouma, ed., *Attention and Performance*, Vol. X, pp. 109–121.

Shani, R. and Sagi, D. (2005). Eccentricity effects on lateral interactions. *Vis. Res.*, **45**, 2009–2024.

Shiu, L.-P. and Pashler, H. (1994). Negligible effect of spatial precuing on identification of single digits. *J. Exp. Psych.: Hum. Percept. Perf.*, **20**, 1037–1054.

Solomon, J. A., Watson, A. B. and Morgan, M. J. (1999). Transducer model produces facilitation from opposite-sign flanks. *Vis. Res.*, **39**, 987–992.

Spitzer, H., Desimone, R., and Moran, J. (1988). Increased attention enhances both behavioral and neuronal performance. *Science*, **240**, 338–340.

Tanaka, Y. and Sagi, D. (1998). Long-lasting, long-range detection facilitation. *Vis. Res.*, **38**, 2591–2599.

Thielscher, A. and Neumann, H. (2005). Neural mechanisms of human texture processing: texture boundary detection and visual search. *Spat. Vis.*, **18**, 227–257.

Treue, S. and Maunsell, J. H. (1996). Attentional modulation of visual motion processing in cortical areas MT and MST. *Nature*, **382**, 539–541.

Treue, S. and Martinez-Trujillo, J. C. (1999). Feature-based attention influences motion processing gain in macaque visual cortex. *Nature*, **399**, 575–579.

Tsotsos, J. K., Culhane, S., Wai, W. *et al.* (1995). Modeling visual attention via selective tuning. *Artif. Intell.*, **78**, 507–547.

van Doorn, A. J. and Koenderink, J. J. (1984). Spatiotemporal integration in the detection of coherent motion. *Vis. Res.*, **24**, 47–53.

Verghese, P. (2001). Visual search and attention: a signal detection theory approach. *Neuron*, **31**, 523–535.

Verghese, P. (2003). The costs and benefits of grouping along a contour. *J. Vis.*, http://www.journalofvision.org/3/9/117/.

Verghese, P. and McKee, S. P. (2002). Predicting future motion. *J. Vis.*, **2**, 513–523.

Verghese, P. and McKee, S. P. (2004). Visual search in clutter. *Vis. Res.*, **44**, 1217–1225.

Verghese, P., and Stone, L. S. (1995). Combining speed information across space. *Vis. Res.*, **35**, 2811–2823.

Verghese, P., Watamaniuk, S. N. J., McKee, S. P. and Gryzwacz, N. M. (1999). Local motion detectors cannot account for the detectability of an extended trajectory in noise. *Vis. Res.*, **39**, 19–30.

Watamaniuk, S. N., McKee, S. P. and Grzywacz, N. M. (1995). Detecting a trajectory embedded in random-direction motion noise. *Vis. Res.*, **35**, 65–77.

Watson, A. B. (1979). Probability summation over time. *Vis. Res.*, **19**, 515–522.

Yeshurun, Y. and Carrasco, M. (1998). Attention improves or impairs visual performance by enhancing spatial resolution. *Nature*, **396**, 72–75.

10 Transsaccadic memory of visual features

Steven L. Prime, Matthias Niemeier and J. Douglas Crawford

10.1 Introduction

The visual world is rich with information distributed over a wide area. The fovea, however, only provides detailed information for a small portion of the visual world at one time. Consequently, to fully encode and process the surroundings humans make many fast, or "saccadic," eye movements (Yarbus, 1967; Stark and Ellis, 1981). Since vision is poor during a saccade (see Matin, 1974) the brain must somehow encode discrete "snapshots" of the visual scene during fixations between saccades if it is to integrate these into a perceptual whole. However, at this time it is not known how and to what extent the brain pieces together these spatially and temporally separated snapshots.

Intuitively, it might seem that the brain would retain a highly detailed representation of the visual world in a spatiotopic "integrative visual buffer" (McConkie and Rayner, 1976). However, several studies suggest that relatively little information is stored across saccades (Bridgeman *et al.*, 1975; Bridgeman and Mayer, 1983; Irwin *et al.*, 1983; O'Regan and Levy-Schoen, 1983; Rayner and Pollatsek, 1983; McConkie and Zola, 1979; Rayner *et al.*, 1980; Irwin *et al.*, 1988; Henderson *et al.*, 1987). Moreover, humans show "change blindness", an inability to detect even significant changes in the visual scene when these changes occur during saccades and other brief visual interruptions (Grimes, 1996; Simons, 1996; Simons and Levin, 1997; O'Regan *et al.*, 2000; Rensink *et al.*, 1997).

It may be erroneous to assume that transsaccadic change blindness is proof that we retain nothing across saccades. Change blindness may occur for different reasons besides limitations in visual short-term memory (Irwin, 1991, 1992; Irwin and Andrews,

Computational Vision in Neural and Machine Systems, ed. L. Harris and M. Jenkin. Published by Cambridge University Press. © Cambridge University Press 2007.

1996) or insufficient encoding of objects that are poorly attended (Scholl, 2000; Henderson and Hollingworth, 1999; Hollingworth *et al.*, 2001). In particular, a recent study shows that some forms of change blindness can be caused by a probabilistic process the brain employs to make optimal inferences about events such as sudden changes in the visual scene (Niemeier *et al.*, 2003). In brief, these authors argue that transsaccadic change blindness can occur because outside a vision lab sudden external events are unlikely to happen in perfect sync with a saccade, and thus, apparent changes in stimuli that coincide with a saccade are more likely to arise from unreliable sensorimotor signals. The brain is, therefore, inclined to ignore sensory information about visual changes that occur during saccades or to underestimate them.

These developments suggest that the question of what information is retained across saccades needs to be re-examined. Recently, most investigators have considered intermediate views between the extreme beliefs that visual information is either completely retained or not retained at all. So to understand how transsaccadic memory operates we first need to understand the basic "building blocks" of this process, like what and how much visual feature information is retained across saccades. For example, some models of transsaccadic integration assume that basic visual features are retained in transsaccadic memory (Irwin, 1992; Currie *et al.*, 2000; McConkie and Currie, 1996). In support of this, several studies have found evidence of transsaccadic retention of the visual features of shape (Pollatsek, Rayner, and Collins, 1984; Palmer and Ames, 1992; Schlingensiepen *et al.*, 1986; Carlson-Radvansky, 1999; Deubel *et al.*, 2002), colour (Hayhoe *et al.*, 1998; Irwin and Gordon, 1998; Irwin and Andrews, 1996), and orientation (Henderson and Hollingworth, 1999; Landman *et al.*, 2003; Verfaillie *et al.*, 1994; Henderson and Siefert, 1999; Moore *et al.*, 1998).

While the preceding studies suggest that features information is retained across saccades, they do not provide detailed psychometric functions for feature discrimination necessary to build a quantitative model of transsaccadic memory. The aim of the present study was to provide these building blocks by measuring to what degree subjects are able to retain visual features across saccades. Specifically, we studied our subjects performance in comparing probes both within and between fixations for changes in luminance, orientation, and shape in three experiments. To test the effect of spatial context on retention of these features, we had subjects make these comparisons in two separate spatial tasks. For the first task, same-retinal task, both probes shared the same retinal position. In contrast, the probes in the second task, same-spatial task, were presented at the same spatial position.

10.2   Methods

10.2.1   Subjects

A total of eight subjects (four males and four females; mean age 28.5 years) participated in this study, six subjects in each experiment. All subjects had normal or corrected-to-normal visual acuity. Informed consent was obtained from each subject. Two subjects were aware of the purpose of the experiments but followed the same trends as the naïve subjects.

10.2.2 General procedure and apparatus

We determined to what extent saccades affect transsaccadic memory for visual features in three experiments. Figure 10.1 illustrates the general experimental design for all three experiments. The four staggered rectangles of each panel illustrate the temporal order for presentation of ocular fixation targets (+) and the stimulus probes (•), and their relative spatial locations. Most studies on transsaccadic perception use some form of a *same-spatial task* (Figure 10.1c). This task involves subjects comparing stimuli that share one spatial location. So, typically the first stimulus appears in the retinal periphery, then the subject makes a saccade towards that location and after the saccade a second stimulus appears in the same spatial location. That is, this task looks at how we integrate visual information from a presaccadic peripheral preview and to a postsaccadic foveal view. Yet, transsaccadic perception may also serve to integrate the snapshots we obtain by discrete foveal views. Therefore, a second aim of this study was to examine how we integrate visual information that shares the same retinal location on the fovea by including a "*same-retinal task*" (Figure 10.1a). We were interested in seeing how transsaccadic memory may differ when stimuli at different fixation locations are compared, so when they share the same retinal positions rather than the same spatial position. As control conditions we simulated the same retinal stimulation patterns from these two saccade conditions but within a single fixation (Figure 10.1b, d).

The temporal sequence for an experimental trial was the same for all four conditions. Figure 10.2 shows horizontal eye position plotted as a function of time from one typical trial onto the respective stimulus events. Each trial began with a fixation cross, subtending $0.4°$ by $0.4°$ of visual angle, presented randomly at either $4°$ left or $4°$ right from subjects' head-center. Once fixation was detected the first probe was presented. Probe duration from onset to offset was 40 ms. In Experiments 2 and 3 this was followed immediately by a mask at the same spatial location to prevent confounds due to afterimages. Following the mask was the second fixation cross. Upon fixation on the second fixation cross the second probe was presented after a short delay. For saccade trials this delay would depend on the subject's saccade response latency. The delay during control trials was matched to the subject's saccade latency from saccade trials.

At the end of each trial subjects were required to compare the two probes by way of a two alternative forced-choice task. Subjects responded manually by pressing mouse buttons. Subjects were instructed to make their best guess if they were not sure. The second probe varied according to an adaptive test procedure that took the subjects' performance on a trial-by-trial basis into account (Kontsevich and Tyler, 1999).

Each experimental session began with a calibration and a block of 50 practice trials. The practice block consisted of trials from each condition. Each condition consisted of 100 trials for a total of 400 trials. A customized computer network system of three microprocessor personal computers was used for both stimulus presentation and data recording. A projector back-projected stimuli onto a 1.9 m by 1.4 m display screen spanning $100°$ of visual angle horizontally by $90°$ of visual angle vertically. The screen was unlit (black) with a luminance level of 0.015 cd/m^2. Eye position was monitored using the scleral search coil technique (Robinson, 1963) with a sampling rate of 1000 Hz. Saccades were detected using a velocity criterion of $36°$ per second

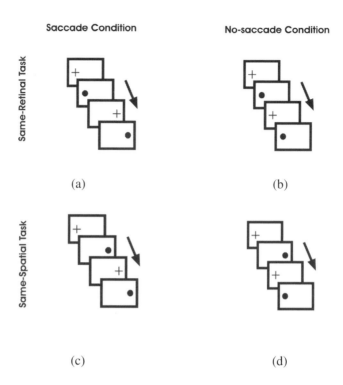

Figure 10.1. General experimental paradigm. Subjects were required to make two alternative forced choice comparisons between two probes (●). (a) Saccade condition of the same-retinal task. Subjects looked at a fixation cross (+), which was replaced with the first probe, and then, the second fixation cross on the opposite side of the display. Subjects made a saccadic eye movement to the second fixation cross and were presented with the second probe. (b) No-saccade condition of the same-retinal task. Subjects maintained eye fixation as the two probes were presented at the same, foveal location as in (a). (c) Saccade condition of the same-spatial task. The first probe was presented in the retinal periphery (position opposite to where the subject was fixating). After the subjects saccaded to the same location as the first probe, as shown by the second fixation cross, the second probe was presented. (d) No-saccade condition of the same-spatial task. This condition simulated the retinal stimulation of (c) as the subjects maintained eye fixation on the fixation cross.

and eye position criterion of 1.5° of visual angle from the fixation point. The subject's head was stabilized using a bite-plate made by dental compound.

10.2.3   Experiment 1: Luminance

For experiment 1 subjects were required to determine whether the second probe was brighter or darker than the first probe. The probes subtended 2° of visual angle in

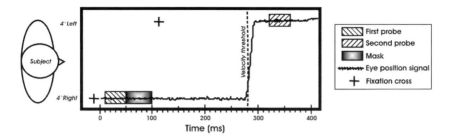

Figure 10.2. Time course for an experimental trial. The fixation cross is first presented to the right target location. Upon eye fixation the first probe (40 ms) and mask (50 ms) is presented. Following the mask is the presentation of the second fixation cross. After the subject saccades to the second fixation cross there is a short delay and the second probe (40 ms) is presented.

diameter. The first probe (standard) was always the same luminance value (13 cd/m^2). Luminance levels for the second probe ranged from a luminance of 32 cd/m^2 (white) to 3 cd/m^2 (dark gray). The order of presentation for all four conditions was randomized and the discrimination threshold was determined concurrently for all four conditions.

10.2.4 Experiment 2: Orientation

Subjects were required to discriminate whether the second probe was oriented clockwise or counter-clockwise relative to the first probe. The probes were circles 2° of visual angle in diameter and displayed as sinusoidal gratings of varying luminance. The gratings' mean luminance was 17 cd/m^2 and the spatial frequency was two cycles per degree of visual angle. The orientation of the first probe's (standard) grating was randomly selected from six possible orientations, 40°, 45°, or 50° clockwise or counter-clockwise relative to the straight-up direction. The second probes orientation varied by a step-size of 0.1° randomly presented on either side of the first probe. We deliberately did not test cardinal orientations as it has been shown that discrimination sensitivity for these angles are very high (Orban *et al.*, 1984; Regan and Price, 1986).

The mask was a white circle subtending 2° of visual angle in diameter, presented for 50 ms, and had a luminance of 33.61 cd/m^2. Conditions were blocked. Block A consisted of 50 trials from the same-retinal task with both the saccade and control conditions. Block B consisted of 50 trials from the same-spatial task with both the saccade and control conditions. Trials from each condition were randomized in both blocks. The order of blocks was either A-B-B-A or B-A-A-B and was counterbalanced between subjects.

10.2.5   Experiment 3: Shape

In this experiment, the probes were ellipses varying in size along the horizontal axis. Subjects discriminated whether the second probe was longer or shorter than the first probe. The first probe (standard) subtended $2°$ of visual angle vertically and $5.5°$, $5°$, or $4.5°$ of visual angle horizontally. The second probe changed by a step-size as small as $0.12°$ of visual angle either shorter or longer than the first probe. All ellipses were white (luminance: 33.61 cd/m^2). A mask was presented during the inter-probe interval. This mask was a white rectangle subtending $8°$ of visual angle horizontally and $2°$ of visual angle vertically, presented for 50 ms, and had a luminance of 33.61 cd/m^2. Again, conditions were blocked for the same-retinal task and the same-spatial task.

10.3   Results

Trials that contained errors in eye movements were removed from the data before analysis. Using Matlab's nlinfit procedure we fitted Weibull functions to the subjects' data to estimate the subjects' discrimination thresholds defined at 75% probability correct. Figure 10.3 provides the psychometric functions for each condition of experiment 1 for one typical subject. A two-way analysis of variance (ANOVA) for repeated measures was performed on the thresholds for each condition. The within-subject factors were Saccade (saccade condition versus control condition) and Task (same-retinal task versus same-spatial task). For these and all subsequent analyses, a p-value of 0.05 was adopted for significance. To examine transsaccadic memory directly we performed t-tests by comparing the saccade conditions with their respective control conditions within each task, that is, condition 1 (Figure 10.1a) with condition 2 (Figure 10.1b) and condition 3 (Figure 10.1c) with condition 4 (Figure 10.1d).

10.3.1   Experiment 1: Luminance

Figure 10.4 shows the average thresholds across all subjects for each condition derived from psychometric functions as in Figure 10.3. Subjects showed slightly lower thresholds when comparing probes within a single fixation rather than across saccades and lower thresholds for the same-spatial task than the same-retinal task. However, the ANOVA did not yield any significant effects. The main effect for the saccade factor was $F_{(1,5)} = 3.965$, $p = 0.103$ and the main effect for Task was $F_{(1,5)} = 2.120$, $p = 0.205$. Likewise, the interaction was not significant, $F_{(1,5)} = 0.020$, $p = 0.894$. Even without Bonferroni correction we found no significant difference for either of the two comparisons between the saccade conditions and control conditions for both tasks, $t_{(5)} = 1.338$, $p = 0.238$ and $t_{(5)} = 1.261$, $p = 0.263$, respectively. Based on these results we concluded that subjects were as accurate comparing the luminance levels between the two probes during the saccade conditions as they were during the control conditions. Moreover, we found no significant difference for accuracy in comparing probes between the two tasks.

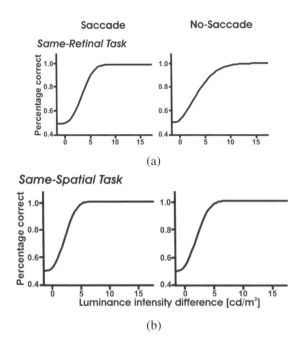

(a)

(b)

Figure 10.3. Psychometric functions of a typical subject for each condition in both the same-retinal task (a) and same-spatial task (b). Saccade conditions are shown in the left panels and no-saccade conditions are shown in the right panels. Absolute difference in stimulus intensity is plotted on the abscissa and percentage correct on the ordinate. Thresholds were determined at 75% correct.

10.3.2 Experiment 2: Orientation

Figure 10.5b shows the results of experiment 2 represented by the average thresholds for each condition derived from psychometric functions like those shown in Figure 10.5a from one typical subject. Subjects had significantly higher thresholds when performing the same-spatial task than the same-retinal task: $F_{(1,5)} = 11.502$, $p = 0.019$. Thus, it was more difficult to compare the probes when one of them was presented in the retinal periphery than when they both appeared on the fovea. However, the interaction and the main effect for saccade were non-significant: $F_{(1,5)} = 0.406$, $p = 0.552$ and $F_{(1,5)} = 0.103$, $p = 0.762$, respectively. No difference was found between saccade conditions and control conditions within both tasks; same-retinal task ($t_{(5)} = 0.742$, $p = 0.491$) and saccade-target task ($t_{(5)} = -0.317$, $p = 0.764$). These results suggest that subjects were able to compare the probes' orientation with the same accuracy during saccade conditions as non-saccade conditions. Moreover, these data are consistent with previous studies that show fine orientation discrimination in humans during fixation (Andrews *et al.*, 1973; Westheimer *et al.*, 1976).

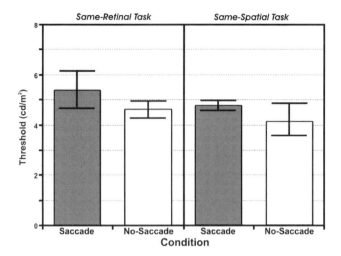

Figure 10.4. Results from experiment 1. The bars show the average thresholds across all subjects for each condition in both tasks. The results for the same-retinal task are shown in the left panel and the same-spatial task in the right panel. Within each task, the saccade condition (dark bar) was compared to the no-saccade condition (white bar). Subjects' discrimination thresholds were the same between saccade and no-saccade conditions in both tasks. Moreover, no significant difference of discrimination threshold was found between the two tasks.

10.3.3   Experiment 3: Shape

Figure 10.6a shows an example of one subject's psychometric functions for the same-retinal task and Figure 10.6b shows the average thresholds obtained for each condition of experiment 3. As with experiment 2 the same-spatial task yielded significantly higher thresholds than the same-retinal task: $F_{(1,5)} = 6.585$, $p = 0.05$. In contrast, again the main effect for saccade condition failed to be significant: $F_{(1,5)} = 0.038$, $p = 0.854$. And there was no evidence for a disrupting effect from saccades when we preformed individual t-tests (same-retinal task $t_{(5)} = -0.361$, $p = 0.733$; and same-spatial task $t_{(5)} = 0.31$; $p = 0.976$). Lastly, the interaction was non-significant: $F_{(1,5)} = 0.083$, $p = 0.785$. The relative low thresholds obtained by our subjects are consistent with previous studies that show that humans are very accurate at discriminating ellipses during fixation (see Laursen and Rasmussen, 1975). Our data show that subjects were able to compare probes for differences in shape across saccades with the same accuracy as within a single fixation. As found in experiment 2, the subjects' comparisons were more accurate when both probes were presented on the fovea rather comparing one probe presented on the periphery and the other on the fovea.

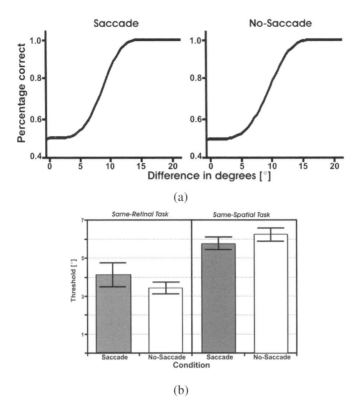

(a)

(b)

Figure 10.5. Experiment 2 results. (a) psychometric functions from a typical subject for both conditions in the *same-spatial task*. Absolute difference in stimulus intensity is plotted on the abscissa and percentage correct on the ordinate. Thresholds were determined at 75% correct. (b) The bars show the average thresholds across all subjects for each condition in both tasks. No difference was found between the saccade condition (dark bar) and the no-saccade condition (white bar) in either task. Subjects' comparisons were more accurate in the *same-retinal task* than in the *same-spatial task*.

10.4 Discussion

In this study, we investigated if the visual features of luminance, orientation, and shape are retained in transsaccadic memory and available for comparisons across saccades. We measured the extent to which subjects can retain these features across saccades by means of psychometric functions. For each of these three features tested in this study, we found that subjects were able to compare stimulus probes across saccades with statistically the same accuracy as when the probes appeared within a single fixation.

In addition, we used two tasks to study the effect of transsaccadic memory of these visual features at either same spatial or same retinal positions. For the *same-retinal task* both probes shared the same retinal position. In contrast, the probes in the second

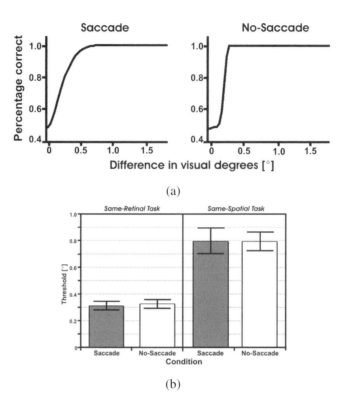

Figure 10.6. Experiment 3 results. (a) Psychometric functions from a typical subject for both conditions in the same-retinal task. Absolute difference in stimulus intensity is plotted on the abscissa and percentage correct on the ordinate. Thresholds were determined at 75% correct. (b) The bars show the average thresholds across all subjects for each condition in both tasks. No difference was found between the saccade condition (dark bar) and the no-saccade condition (white bar) in either task. Subjects' comparisons were more accurate in the *same-retinal task* than in the *same-spatial task*.

task, *same-spatial task*, were presented at the same spatial position. We found that for each experiment the discrimination thresholds were the same for the saccade and control conditions in both tasks. That is, our results suggest that transsaccadic memory works for both tasks and that visual information can be integrated regardless whether the stimuli were spatially or retinally fixed.

Our results from experiments 2 and 3 show that subjects had higher discrimination thresholds for the *same-spatial task* than the *same-retinal task*. One interpretation of this finding is that the visual system is better tuned for discriminating feature changes within local regions of the retina than it is for discriminating changes that occur within spatially, but not retinally, fixed regions. However, a simpler explanation could be that subjects were less accurate for orientation and shape comparisons when one probe was presented in the peripheral regions of the retina. These findings are consistent with previous studies that show that discrimination thresholds for orientation and shape are sensitive to retinal eccentricity (Paradiso and Carney, 1988; Whitaker *et al.*, 1993).

One possible solution to resolve this issue is to increase the size of the probes as a function of retinal eccentricity in the *same-spatial task*. Previous studies of orientation discrimination have found that discrimination thresholds are lowered (i.e. subjects are more sensitive) when stimulus-size is increased in scale as retinal eccentricity is increased (Makela *et al.*, 1993; Paradiso and Carney, 1988). If retinal eccentricity is the reason for the differences between the tasks in experiments 2 and 3, we should then expect lower discrimination thresholds in the *same-spatial task* by scaling the size of the probes. Theoretically thresholds of the *same-spatial task* may be able to equal thresholds of the *same-retinal task*.

Based on our findings we conclude that certain visual features are retained in transsaccadic memory and are available for comparisons across saccades. This is consistent with previous studies (Pollatsek *et al.*, 1984; Palmer and Ames, 1992; Schlingensiepen, *et al.*, 1986; Verfaillie, *et al.*, 1994; Henderson and Siefert, 1999; Moore *et al.*, 1998). Our study, however, provides quantitative data to show to what extent these visual features are retained transsaccadically.

Regarding more complex tasks, it has been suggested that transsaccadic memory is poor with limited capacities of storage (Irwin and Andrews, 1996) and of encoding of information across saccades (Scholl, 2000; Henderson and Hollingworth, 1999; Hollingworth *et al.*, 2001). This has been interpreted to mean that our subjective impression of perceiving a highly detailed representation of the visual world is an illusion. For example, O'Regan (1992) has proposed that there is no need to retain information across saccades because the world can be used as an "external memory store."

We agree in that it does make sense to use the physical visual scenery as a form of memory – at least to some extent. However, one limitation of a purely external storage of information is that the visual input has to be processed. This is a time and energy consuming procedure (Salthouse *et al.*, 1981; Henderson, 1992). It would be surprising if the brain discarded all processed information with each saccade. But it is rather likely that the brain's transsaccadic memory takes into account the costs and gains of storing visual information and integrating it with new information. Indeed, this is likely the reason why we scan the features of complex objects with multiple saccades (Yarbus, 1967; Stark and Ellis, 1981) rather than fixating some central point within the object.

Further evidence for transsaccadic memory comes from neurophysiological studies showing that the brain retains visual representations during eye movements. For instance, certain brain areas are involved in keeping track of spatial locations of objects in the world with corresponding changes in eye position. That is, spatial information is updated as the head or eyes move. This so called "remapping" has been found to take place on many levels of the primate's visual system including the lateral intraparietal area (Duhamel *et al.*, 1992), the frontal eye field (Umeno and Goldberg, 1997), the superior colliculuss intermediate layer (Walker *et al.*, 1995), and the striate and extrastriate cortex (Nakamura and Colby, 2000; 2002). Moreover, an object's orientation may be another form of visual information that is retained across saccades (Moore *et al.*, 1998). These researchers found that neurons from area V4 in the primate brain retain orientation information by a resurgent response in neurons selectively tuned to that orientation of a saccade target immediately prior to the saccade. Our current study suggests that similar studies should test the neural retention of luminance and shape information across saccades.

In conclusion, the mechanisms that govern transaccadic memory are only beginning to be understood. This study investigated the quantitative effect of saccades on the storage of visual features of luminance, orientation, and shape. We found that subjects were able to compare these visual features across saccades with the same accuracy as when comparing them within a single fixation. This is an essential condition for transsaccadic integration to occur. We suggest that further research is necessary to construct a quantitative model of transsaccadic memory. The data from the present study may serve as building blocks for such a model.

Acknowledgements

The authors thank Saihong Sun and Dr. Hongying Wang for technical assistance. This work was supported by grants from the Natural Sciences and Engineering Research Council of Canada and the Canadian Institutes of Health Research. J. D. Crawford holds a Canada Research Chair.

References

Andrews, D. P., Butcher, A. K. and Buckley, B. R. (1973). Acuities for spatial arrangement in line figures: human and ideal observers compared. *Vis. Res.*, **13**, 599–620.

Bridgeman, B. and Mayer, M. (1983). Failure to integrate visual information from successive fixations. *Bull. Psychonomic Soc.*, **21**, 285–286.

Bridgeman, B., Hendry, D. and Stark, L. (1975). Failure to detect displacement of the visual world during saccadic eye movements. *Vis. Res.*, **15**, 719–722.

Carlson-Radvansky, L. A. (1999). Memory for relational information across eye movements. *Percept. Psychophys.*, **61**, 919–934.

Currie, C. B., McConkie, G. W., Carlson-Radvansky, L. A. and Irwin, D. E. (2000). The role of the saccade target object in the perception of a visually stable world. *Percept. Psychophys.*, **62**, 673–683.

Deubel, H., Schneider, W. X. and Bridgeman, B. (2002). Transsaccadic memory of position and form. *Progress in Brain Res.*, **140**, 165–180.

Duhamel, J., Colby, C. L. and Goldberg, M. E. (1992). The updating of the representation of visual space in parietal cortex by intended eye movements. *Science*, **255**, 90–92.

Grimes, J. (1996). On the failure to detect changes in scenes across saccades. In K. Akins, ed., *Vancouver Studies in Cognitive Science: Vol. 2: Perception*, New York: Oxford University Press, , pp. 89-110.

Hayhoe, M., Bensinger, D. G. and Ballard, D. H. (1998). Task constraints in visual working memory. *Vis. Res.*, **38**, 125–137.

Henderson, J. M. (1992). Visual attention and eye movement control during reading and picture viewing. In K. Rayner, ed., *Eye Movements and Visual Cognition: Scene Perception and Reading*, New York: Springer, pp. 261–283.

Henderson, J. M. and Hollingworth, A. (1999). The role of fixation position in detecting scene changes across saccades. *Psychol. Sci.*, **10**, 438–443.

Henderson, J. M. and Siefert, A. B. C. (1999). The influence of enantiomorphic transformation on transsaccadic object integration. *J. Exp. Psych.: Human Percept. and Perf.*, **25**, 243–255.

Henderson, J. M., Pollatsek, A. and Rayner, K. (1987). Effects of foveal priming and extrafoveal preview on object identification. *J. Exp. Psych.: Human Percept. and Perf.*, **13**, 449–463.

Hollingworth, A., Schrock, G. and Henderson, J. M. (2001). Change detection in the flicker paradigm: The role of fixation position within the scene. *Memory and Cognition*, **29**, 296–304.

Irwin, D. E. (1991). Information integration across saccadic eye movements. *Cogn. Psych.*, **23**, 420–456.

Irwin, D. E. (1992). Memory for position and identity across eye movements. *J. Exp. Psych.: Learning, Memory, and Cognition*, **18**, 307–317.

Irwin, D. E. and Andrews, R. (1996). Integration and accumulation of information across saccadic eye movements. In T. Inui and J. L. McClelland, eds., *Attention and Performance XVI: Information Integration in Perception and Communication*, Cambridge: MIT Press, MA, pp. 125–155.

Irwin, D. E., Brown, J. and Sun, J. (1988). Visual masking and visual integration across saccadic eye movements. *J. Exp. Psych.: Gen.*, **117**, 276–287.

Irwin, D. E. and Gordon, R. D. (1998). Eye movements, attention, and trans-saccadic memory. *Vis. Cogn.*, **5**, 127–155.

Irwin, D. E., Yantis, S. and Jonides, J. (1983). Evidence against visual integration across saccadic eye movements. *Percept. Psychophys.*, **34**, 49–57.

Kontsevich, L. L. and Tyler, C. W. (1999). Bayesian adaptive estimation of psychometric slope and threshold. *Vis. Res.*, **39**, 2729–2737.

Landman, R., Spekreijse, H. and Lamme, V. A. F. (2003). Large capacity storage of integrated objects before change blindness. *Vis. Res.*, **43**, 149–164.

Laursen, A. M. and Rasmussen, J. B. (1975). Circle-ellipse discrimination in man and monkey. *Vis. Res.*, **15**, 173–174.

Makela, P., Whitaker, D. and Rovamo, J. (1993). Modelling of orientation discrimination across the visual field. *Vision Res.*, **33**, 723–730.

Matin, E. (1974). Saccadic suppression: A review and an analysis. *Psychol. Bull.*, **81**, 899–917.

McConkie, G. and Currie, C. (1996). Visual stability across saccades while viewing complex pictures. *J. Exp. Psych.: Human Percept. Perf.*, **22**, 563–581.

McConkie, G. W. and Rayner, K. (1976). Identifying the span of the effective stimulus in reading: literature review and theories in reading. In H. Singer and R. B. Ruddell, eds., *Theoretical Models and Processes of Reading*, Newark, NJ: International Reading Association, pp. 137–162.

McConkie, G. and Zola, D. (1979). Is visual information integrated across successive fixations in reading? *Percept. and Psychophys.*, **25**, 221–224.

Moore, T., Tolias, A. S. and Schiller, P. H. (1998). Visual representations during saccadic eye movements. *Proc. Nat. Acad. Sci. USA*, **95**, 8981–8984.

Nakamura, K. and Colby, C. L. (2000). Visual, saccade-related, and cognitive activation of single neurons in monkey extrastriate area V3A. *J. Neurophysiol.*, **84**, 677–692.

Nakamura, K. and Colby, C. L. (2002). Updating of the visual representation in monkey striate and extrastriate cortex during saccades. *Proc. Nat. Acad. Sci.*, **99**, 4026–4031.

Niemeier, M., Crawford, J. D. and Tweed, D. (2003). Optimal transsaccadic integration explains distorted spatial perception. *Nature*, **422**, 76–80.

O'Regan, J. K. (1992). Solving the "real" mysteries of visual perception: the world as an outside memory. *Can. J. Psych.*, **46**, 461–488.

O'Regan, J. K., Deubel, H., Clark, J. J. and Rensink, R. A. (2000). Picture changes during blinks: looking without seeing and seeing without looking. *Vis. Cogn.*, **7**, 191–211.

O'Regan, J. K. and Levy-Schoen, A. (1983). Integrating visual information from successive fixations: Does trans-saccadic fusion exist? *Vis. Res.*, **23**, 765–768.

Orban, G. A., van den Bussche, E. and Vogels, R. (1984). Human orientation discrimination tested with long stimuli. *Vis. Res.*, **24**, 121–128.

Palmer, J. and Ames, C. T. (1992). Measuring the effect of multiple eye fixations on memory for visual attributes. *Percept. Psychophys.*, **52**, 295–306.

Paradiso, M. A. and Carney, T. (1988). Orientation discrimination as a function of stimulus eccentricity and size: nasal/temporal retinal asymmetry. *Vis. Res.*, **28**, 867–874.

Pollatsek, A., Rayner, K. and Collins, W. (1984). Integrating pictorial information across eye movements. *J. Exp. Psych.: Gen.*, **113**, 426–442.

Rayner, K., McConkie, G. and Zola, D. (1980). Integrating information across eye movements. *Cogn. Psych.*, **12**, 206–226.

Rayner, K. and Pollatsek, A. (1983). Is visual information integrated across saccades? *Percept. Psychophys.*, **34**, 39–48.

Regan, D. and Price, P. (1986). Periodicity in orientation discrimination and the unconfounding of visual information. *Vis. Res.*, **26**, 1299–1302.

Rensink, R. A., O'Regan, J. K. and Clark, J. J. (1997). To see or not to see: the need for attention to perceive changes in scenes. *Psychol. Sci.*, **8**, 368–373.

Robinson, D. A. (1963). A method of measuring eye movement using a sclera search coil in a magnetic field. *IEEE Trans. Biomed. Eng.*, **10**, 137–145.

Salthouse, T. A., Ellis, C. L., Diener, D. C. and Somberg, B. L. (1981). Stimulus processing during eye fixations. *J. Exp. Psych.: Hum. Percept. and Perf.*, **7**, 611–623.

Schlingensiepen, K. H., Campell, F. W., Legge, G. E. and Walker, T. D. (1986). The . importance of eye movements in the analysis of simple patterns. *Vis. Res.*, **26**, 1111–1117.

Scholl, B. J. (2000). Attenuated change blindness for exogenously attended items in a flicker paradigm. *Vis. Cogn.*, **7**, 377–396.

Simons, D. J. (1996). In sight, out of mind: When object representations fail. *Psychol. Sci.*, **7**, 301–305.

Simons, D. and Levin, D. (1997). Change blindness. *Trends Cogn. Sci.*, **1**, 261–267.

Stark, L. W. and Ellis, S. R. (1981). Scanpaths revisited: Cognitive models, direct active looking. In D. F. Fisher, R. A. Monty, and J. W. Senders, eds., *Eye Movements: Cognition and Visual Perception*. Hillsdale, NJ: Lawrence Erlbaum, pp. 193–226.

Umeno, M. M. and Goldberg, M. E. (1997). Spatial processing in the monkey frontal eye field I. Predictive visual responses. *J. Neurophysiol.*, **78**, 1373–1383.

Verfaillie, K., De Troy, A. and van Rensbergen, J. (1994). Trans-saccadic integration of biological motion. *J. Exp. Psych.: Learning, Memory, and Cognition*, **20**, 649–670.

Walker, M. F., Fitzgibbon, E. J. and Goldberg, M. E. (1995). Neurons in the monkey superior colliculus predict the visual result of impending saccadic eye movements. *J. Neurophysiol.*, **73**, 1988–2003.

Westheimer, G., Shimamura, K. and McKee, S. P. (1976). Interference with line-orientation sensitivity. *J. Opt. Soc. Am.*, **66**, 332–338.

Whitaker, D., Latham, K., Makela, P. and Rovamo, J. (1993). Detection and discrimination of curvature in foveal and peripheral vision. *Vis. Res.*, **33**, 2215–2224.

Yarbus, A. L. (1967). *Eye Movements and Vision*. New York: Plenum Press.

11 Modeling what attracts human gaze over dynamic natural scenes

Laurent Itti and Pierre Baldi

11.1 Introduction and rationale

Visual attention is deployed based on a combination of bottom-up cues derived from visual stimuli, and of top-down cues derived from volition, expectations, previous observations, and internal goals of the observer (James, 1890). Through the interplay between bottom-up and top-down cues, attention rapidly prunes vast amounts of sensory information, to focus slower and more sophisticated analysis resources onto the most important subsets of the data (Itti and Koch, 2001). In real-life environments, rarely is there time for thoroughly analyzing all inputs: a savannah monkey must typically take action faster than it can fully recognize a rapidly approaching leopard. Consequently, evolving rapid and computationally efficient heuristics to important information is key to predation, escape, and mating. We show that a new mathematical definition of information surprise, – or simply surprise – predicts well where humans look while inspecting dynamic natural scenes, and represents an efficient shortcut to subjectively important information.

A productive approach to studying attentional selection and heuristics in complex scenes is to use eye-tracking devices to evaluate image statistics and neural responses at the locations that attract gaze (Vinje and Gallant, 2000). With static natural images, humans preferentially orient towards locations with higher contrast, entropy, and edge or corner density (Parkhurst *et al.*, 2002; Privitera and Stark, 2000; Reinagel and Zador, 1999; Tatler *et al.*, 2005); but how strongly these features attract attention, and why, remains poorly understood. With dynamic but synthetic stimuli, human attention is captured by flicker, onsets of novel stimuli, and abrupt luminance changes (Abrams and Christ, 2003; Theeuwes, 1995); but how these features would fare with natural

Computational Vision in Neural and Machine Systems, ed. L. Harris and M. Jenkin. Published by Cambridge University Press. © Cambridge University Press 2007.

scene stimuli, and what the tradeoff between static and dynamic attractors is, remains unknown. Moreover, single-unit recordings in the laboratory (Fecteau and Munoz, 2003; Müller *et al.*, 1999) show that neuronal responses are modulated by stimulus flicker and novelty, but how this eventually affects gaze shifts is also poorly understood. Finally, humans have been shown to specifically attend to objects in a scene which are more relevant to the task at hand (e.g. a jar of jelly while making a sandwich: see Hayhoe *et al.*, 2003), but these observations have thus far remained descriptive and no theory or computational model has yet been implemented which can reproduce such complex human behavior using only raw visual inputs.

Progress on these questions hinges on developing a unifying theory of attention that illuminates what has remained an heteroclitic collection of behavioral and neuronal observations, and on testing the theory against large amounts of data acquired in natural settings. To mathematically characterize important or subjectively valuable information, we have recently proposed that attention is attracted by features which are "surprising," and that surprise is a general, information-theoretic concept, which can be derived from first principles and formalized analytically across spatio-temporal scales and data types (Baldi, 2002, 2005; Baldi and Itti, 2005; Itti and Baldi, 2005, 2006). We briefly summarize the key highlights of Bayesian surprise in Section 11.2. In Section 11.3 we then describe how a computational model can be designed, which takes video streams as inputs and predicts in real-time how surprising each image location in the streams is. We finally validate the approach in Section 11.4 by comparing the model's outputs to human eye movements recorded while naïve observers watched the video clips. Compared with five other models which also attempt to predict regions of high human interest from raw video data, we find that the surprise model performs highly significantly better. Further discussion of the significance of this result is presented in Section 11.5.

11.2   Quantifying surprise

Although the concept of surprise is omnipresent in our everyday life – and certainly researchers are always on the lookout for surprising data or results – little theoretical and computational understanding has until now existed of the very essence of surprise. Indeed, while we know how to quantify information in bits, until now there has been no widely accepted quantitative unit of surprise. Qualities such as "wow factors" have remained vague and elusive to mathematical analysis. Within the Bayesian probabilistic framework, we have developed the first quantitative theory of surprise, outlined below.

11.2.1   Bayesian definition of surprise

Surprise is fundamentally a *relative* property of data with respect to observers and their expectations. As such, its definition must be independent of the specific nature or embodiment of the data or the observer. It must apply equally well across sensory modalities and datatypes, and to information processing observers that range from synapses to neuronal circuits, organisms, and computer devices. Surprise exists only in the presence of uncertain environments; therefore its essence must also be probabilistic. Consistently with the Bayesian approach to probabilistic data modeling and inference, the background information of observers is captured by their prior probability distribution $P(M)$ over the hypotheses or models M in a model space $\mathcal{M}$. The fundamental effect of a new data observation D on the observer is to change the prior distribution $P(M)$ into the posterior distribution $P(M|D)$ via Bayes theorem $P(M|D) = P(M)P(D|M)/P(D)$. Therefore we can formally measure surprise elicited by data as the distance between the posterior and prior distributions, which is best done using the relative entropy or Kullback–Leibler (KL) divergence (Kullback, 1959). Thus, surprise is defined by the average of the log-odd ratio

$$S(D, \mathcal{M}) = KL(P(M|D), P(M)) = \int_{\mathcal{M}} P(M|D) \log \frac{P(M|D)}{P(M)} dM \qquad (11.1)$$

taken with respect to the posterior distribution over the model space $\mathcal{M}$. While the term surprise has sometimes been used in reference to Shannon information, by our definition it is a fundamentally different quantity. Shannon's theory of communication focuses on "reproducing at one point either exactly or approximately a message selected at another point" (Shannon, 1948). As such it has been eminently successful for the development of modern computer and telecommunication technologies, because it allowed for the first time to objectively quantify the previously elusive concept of information. But this came at the price that subjective and semantic attributes of information, like value or importance to an observer, had to be ignored. Shannon's entropy

$$H(\mathcal{D}, M) = -\int_{\mathcal{D}} P(D|M) \log P(D|M) dD \qquad (11.2)$$

requires integration over the space of data $\mathcal{D}$ and quantifies information objectively under the assumption of a single, implicit observer (e.g. the Bell Labs communication engineer) and model M that define the distribution $\{P(D|M)\}_{D \in \mathcal{D}}$. Thus, a file on your computer occupies the same number of bits whether you subjectively consider it an important file or not, leading to the white snow paradox described below. In contrast, surprise requires integration over $\mathcal{M}$ and quantifies how data affects the distribution $\{P(M)\}_{M \in \mathcal{M}}$ of subjective beliefs an observer may have over the entire space of models. Thus, viewing a file on your computer may elicit different amounts of surprise for different viewers, or for a same viewer in different states.

11.2.2 Surprise, Shannon information, and the white snow paradox

The disconnect between Shannon information and surprise is evident from the paradox that random snow, the most boring of all television programs, carries the largest amount of Shannon information. Indeed, because pixel values in random snow are unpredictable and uncorrelated, transmitting a frame of snow requires that some information about every pixel be transmitted; in contrast, transmitting typical television frames requires less information because spatiotemporal correlations can be exploited. At onset, snow carries both surprise and information; indeed, snow may signal storm, earthquake, toddler's curiosity, or military putsch. This initial surprise is experienced as the viewer's beliefs shift towards more strongly favoring a random pixel model M_{snow}, correspondingly decreasing beliefs in models of other programs, like M_{CNN}, M_{BBC}, and M_{MTV}. After a moment, however, M_{snow} becomes the single most probable model, prior and posterior become identical, and additional snow frames carry very little surprise albeit megabytes of Shannon information. Indeed, in a sample recording of 20 000 video frames from typical television programs, presumably of interest to millions of watchers, we measured only 0.25 megabytes of Shannon information per second once compressed to constant-quality MPEG4 to eliminate redundancy. In contrast, in matched MPEG4-compressed uniform snow clips, probably of interest only to a few engineers, we measured nearly 20 times more Shannon information (4.90 megabytes/s). The situation was reversed when we measured that snow clips carried about 17 times less surprise per second than the television clips. Note that this result is not dependent upon the technique utilized to focus on non-redundant information (here, MPEG-4): it simply reflects the fact that natural scenes (or scenes which you may observe on a television set) form a very small subset of all the possible images, while random snow entirely spans the space of all possible images. Thus, the Shannon entropy of natural scenes ought to be smaller than the Shannon entropy of snow.

11.2.3   Unit of surprise

To define a unit of surprise, we parallel the approach of Shannon when defining the bit. The Shannon information contained in a dataset D is $-\log P(D)$ bits (here and throughout this chapter, the logarithm should be taken in base 2 for all numerical applications). An outcome observation with probability 0.5 corresponds to one bit of information. Thus the bit is defined *before* averaging over all possible datasets to yield Shannon entropy. Likewise, we can measure surprise contained in D for a single model M before the integration over models, by $\log(P(M|D)/P(M))$. A unit of surprise – a *"wow"* – may then be defined as the amount of surprise corresponding to a two-fold variation between prior and posterior probabilities for the model M of interest. A positive wow is experienced when data are received which double belief in the model under consideration, and a negative wow when data halve that belief. After integration over the model family $\mathcal{M}$, if data are observed which does not change the observer's beliefs about which models or hypotheses are probable, those data yield no surprise, no matter how improbable or informative it may be; conversely, data which cause a significant redistribution of beliefs over the observer's model family yield surprise. Surprise is always computable numerically, but also analytically in many practical cases, in particular those involving probability distributions in the exponential family (Brown, 1986) with conjugate or other priors (Baldi, 2005).

11.2.4   Kullback–Leibler, machine learning, and surprise

The Kullback–Leibler divergence (KL) has been used extensively, at least since Shannon with the mutual information between two random variables X and Y defined as $KL(P(X, Y), P(X)P(Y))$. In particular, there is a rich history of using KL in machine learning, Boltzmann machines, and neural networks, especially in the context of computing the gradient of the KL, and using gradient descent on the KL for learning

(Ackley *et al.*, 1985).

Here, however, we use it in a different way. In neural networks, for instance, training is often done to maximize the likelihood $P(D|M) = P(D|w)$, or, when there is a prior on the weight vector w, to maximize the posterior $P(w|D)$. (Note that the data vector D may include target values in the case of supervised learning.) The KL often then appears in the expression of the error function, usually the negative log likelihood. In a typical multinomial classification problem, learning is done by gradient descent on the negative log likelihood associated with the KL between the data distribution $P(D)$ and the distribution produced by the network $P(D|w)$. That is, one tries to minimize the mismatch between $P(D)$ and $P(D|w)$ by adjusting w. Clearly this is different from the KL between the posterior $P(w|D)$ and the prior $P(w)$, which is surprise: surprise requires integration over the model space (or weights w) while previous methods integrate over the space of data D.

11.2.5 A simple example of surprise computation

Maybe the simplest class of examples where surprise can be computed exactly consists of contingency tables of any size. Consider for instance a parent who has two competing internal models or hypotheses about a new television channel, the first, M, according to which that new channel is appropriate for children, and the second, $\overline{M}$, according to which it is not. Assume that initially our observer is undecided and equally split across both models, that is, $P(M) = P(\overline{M}) = 1/2$. Next consider two possible data observations, D_1, a TV program that contains some nudity, and D_2, one that does not, with, for instance, $P(D_1) = P(D_2) = 1/2$. Finally, assume that the observer initially believes that observing nudity is three times more likely on a channel that is inappropriate for children.

The initial beliefs of our observer may thus be tabulated as follows:

	D_1	D_2
M	$a = 1/8$	$c = 3/8$
$\overline{M}$	$b = 3/8$	$d = 1/8$

where the table verifies the above specifications, in that $P(D_1) = a + b = 1/2$, $P(D_2) = c + d = 1/2$, $P(M) = a + c = 1/2$, $P(\overline{M}) = b + d = 1/2$, and $P(D_1, \overline{M}) = b = 3 \times P(D_1, M) = 3 \times a$. Assume that D_1 is observed (a program with some nudity). Since $P(D_1) = 1/2$, this observation carries $-\log P(D_1) = 1$ bit of Shannon information (remember that the logarithm should be taken in base 2 for all numerical applications). The posterior probabilities of M and $\overline{M}$ are

$$P(M|D_1) = \frac{P(M, D_1)}{P(M, D_1) + P(\overline{M}, D_1)} = \frac{a}{a+b} = \frac{1}{4} \quad \text{and} \quad (11.3)$$

$$P(\overline{M}|D_1) = \frac{P(\overline{M}, D_1)}{P(M, D_1) + P(\overline{M}, D_1)} = \frac{b}{a+b} = \frac{3}{4} \quad (11.4)$$

That is, observing D_1 (a program with some nudity) shifted the observer's initial indecision between M and $\overline{M}$, now favoring $\overline{M}$ (the new TV channel is inappropriate for children) over M (it is appropriate) by a factor 3. The amount of surprise resulting from this shift, first considering only model M, is $S(D_1, M) = \log(P(M|D_1)/P(M)) = -1.00$ wow. Similarly, with respect to $\overline{M}$, the surprise is $S(D_1, \overline{M}) = \log \frac{P(\overline{M}|D_1)}{P(\overline{M})} = 0.58$ wows. After averaging over the model family $\mathcal{M} = \{M, \overline{M}\}$ weighted by the posterior (11.2), the total surprise experienced by the observer is

$$S(D_1, \mathcal{M}) \quad = \quad P(M|D_1)S(D_1, M) + P(\overline{M}|D_1)S(D_1, \overline{M}) \tag{11.5}$$

$$= \quad \frac{a}{a+b} \log \frac{a}{(a+b)(a+c)} + \frac{b}{a+b} \log \frac{b}{(a+b)(b+d)} \tag{11.6}$$

$$\approx \quad 0.19 \text{ wows}. \tag{11.7}$$

The new beliefs of the observer may hence be tabulated as follows, using the posterior resulting from our above observation as new prior:

	D_1	D_2
M	$a' = 1/16$	$c' = 3/16$
$\overline{M}$	$b' = 7/16$	$d' = 5/16$

Consider next what happens if D_1 is observed once more. We intuitively expect this second observation to carry less surprise than the previous one, since our observer now already fairly strongly believes that the new TV channel is inappropriate, and observing nudity once again should only incrementally consolidate that belief. Indeed, proceeding as above, the total surprise now experienced by the observer is $S(D_1, \mathcal{M}) \approx 0.07$ wows, nearly three times less than on the previous observation.

11.3   Computational model

In this section we describe how the definition of surprise can be implemented into an image processing algorithm. Further, we describe five additional algorithms for comparison with surprise. To calibrate the time-constant at which surprise is computed, we use neural recordings from monkey primary visual cortex (Müller *et al.*, 1999). Once so calibrated, the model is used in the following section for comparison to human eye movement data.

11.3.1   Surprise model

Armed with our theoretical framework, we can revisit our previously proposed model of saliency-based visual attention, where activity in a topographic master saliency map guides attention bottom-up (Itti *et al.*, 1998; Itti and Koch, 2000). The master map (40×30 lattice of temporally low-pass leaky integrator artificial neurons, given 640×480 stimuli) receives inputs from five center-surround feature channels, operating in parallel over the visual field at six spatial scales and thought to guide human attention (Itti and Koch, 2001; Wolfe, 1998): intensity contrast (six feature maps), red/green and

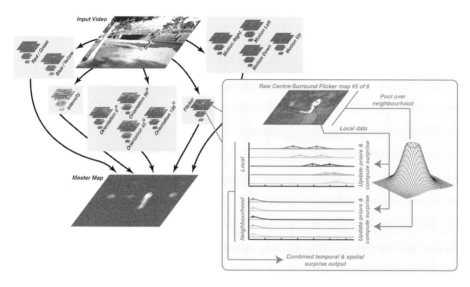

Figure 11.1. Architecture of the computational model of surprise in video streams. Incoming 640×480-pixel video frames are processed by up to five feature channels for color, flicker, etc. In each channel, 6, 12 or 24 feature maps are computed using center-surround linear filters. After rescaling all maps to 40×30 pixels, in the surprise model a cascade of five surprise detectors (inset) is attached to every pixel in each of the 72 feature maps, and the resulting surprise values sum across feature channels, spatial, and temporal scales into the master map. Simulation takes ≈ 30 s/frame on a typical computer. Further detail is available with our source code, distributed freely at http://iLab.usc.edu/toolkit/ and on the accompanying CD-ROM.

blue/yellow color opponencies (12 maps), four orientation contrasts (24 maps), temporal onset/offset (six maps) and motion energy in four directions (24 maps), totalling 72 feature maps.

Here we retain the raw center-surround features of that model, but attach local surprise detectors to every location in each of the model's 72 neural feature maps (Figure 11.1). To reproduce phenomena of attention capture and pop-out in visual search (Wolfe, 1998), we additionally introduce below a second, spatial, type of surprise detectors. As individual biological neurons are unlikely to learn multimodal distributions of inputs (Maffei *et al.*, 1973), we consider unimodal model families, but several operating at different timescales.

In our implementation, image patches are described by a 72D feature vector representing the responses from the 72 low-level feature channels (color, motion, etc., at six spatial scales). A model of an image patch, then, is a 72D Poisson random variable, under the assumption that low-level feature detectors output trains of Poisson-distributed spikes in response to visual stimulation (Softky and Koch, 1993). We consider the model family that comprises all possible such 72D Poisson models, parameterized by a 72D Poisson rate vector. The conjugate prior on Poisson rate is the Gamma distribution, and under these assumptions surprise can be computed in closed form. For instance, patches of motionless vs. trembling foliage correspond to two different models, described by two vectors of 72 Poisson firing rates (with, among other differences, lower rates for motion features in the motionless foliage model). Note that with these simple models, there is no single explicit model M_{snow} that can capture random snow. Rather, when snow is observed, the prior quickly becomes uniform, indicating that every model is believed to be equally bad and that the observer does not have any strong belief in favor of any one model. More complex models (Doretto *et al.*, 2003) could be used as well, without affecting the theory.

Consider a neuron at a given location in one of the 72 feature maps, receiving Poisson spikes as inputs from low-level feature detectors. We thus consider in that feature map and at that location a family of models which are all the Poisson distributions for all possible firing rates $\lambda > 0$.

Using the theory of surprise outlined above, we consider conjugate priors, whereby the posterior belongs to the same functional family as the prior. In such case, the posterior at one video frame can directly serve as prior for the next frame, as is customary in Bayesian learning. Thus, we use for $P(M)$ a functional form such that $P(M|D)$ has the same functional form when D is Poisson-distributed. It is easy to show that $P(M)$ satisfying this property is the Gamma probability density

$$P(M(\lambda)) = \gamma(\lambda; \alpha, \beta) = \frac{\beta^\alpha \lambda^{\alpha-1} e^{-\beta\lambda}}{\Gamma(\alpha)} \qquad (11.8)$$

with shape $\alpha > 0$, inverse scale $\beta > 0$, and $\Gamma(.)$ the Euler Gamma function. Given an observation $D = \overline{\lambda}$ at one of our surprise detectors and prior density $\gamma(\lambda; \alpha, \beta)$, the posterior $\gamma(\lambda; \alpha', \beta')$ obtained by Bayes' theorem is also a Gamma density, with:

$$\alpha' = \alpha + \overline{\lambda} \quad \text{and} \quad \beta' = \beta + 1. \qquad (11.9)$$

To prevent these from increasing unboundedly over time, we add a forgetting factor $0 < \zeta < 1$, yielding:

$$\alpha' = \zeta\alpha + \overline{\lambda} \quad \text{and} \quad \beta' = \zeta\beta + 1. \qquad (11.10)$$

ζ preserves the prior's mean α/β but increases its variance α/β^2, embodying relaxation of belief in the prior's precision (our simulations use $\zeta = 0.7$, based on a reproduction of neural recordings from Müller *et al.* (1999); see Figure 11.2). Local temporal surprise S_T resulting from the update is computed exactly using the KL divergence to quantify the differences between posterior and prior distributions over models

$$\begin{aligned} S_T(D, \mathcal{M}) &= KL(\gamma(\lambda; \alpha', \beta'), \gamma(\lambda; \alpha, \beta)) \\ &= \alpha \log \tfrac{\beta'}{\beta} + \log \tfrac{\Gamma(\alpha)}{\Gamma(\alpha')} + \beta \tfrac{\alpha'}{\beta'} + (\alpha' - \alpha)\Psi(\alpha'), \end{aligned} \qquad (11.11)$$

with $\Psi(.)$ the digamma function. For example, local temporal surprise arises when new observations are received such that an image patch previously well modeled as stationary-black becomes better modeled as flickering-red. Similarly, a bush that suddenly starts trembling is for a moment locally surprising, as priors at the visual location of the bush rapidly shift from a motionless model to a trembling model.

Spatial surprise S_S is computed similarly. For every t, (x, y), f and i, a Gamma neighborhood distribution of models is computed as the weighted combination of distributions from the next-faster local models, over a large neighborhood with two-dimensional Difference-of-Gaussians profile ($\sigma_+ = 20$ and $\sigma_- = 3$ feature map pixels). As new data arrives, spatial surprise is the KL divergence between prior neighborhood distribution and the posterior after update by local samples from the neighborhood's center. For example, spatial surprise arises when a model of the entire image as stationary-black must be reconsidered at some locations better modeled as flickering-red. Thus, a bush that trembles like many others in a windy savannah elicits no spatial surprise, but one that trembles differently from its neighbors yields spatial surprise and pops out.

To model the interaction between local and spatial surprises, we turn to single-unit recordings of complex cells in striate cortex of anesthetized monkey (Müller *et al.*, 1999). From Figure 11.2, total surprise S is

$$S = \left[S_T + \frac{S_S}{20} \right]^{\frac{1}{3}}. \tag{11.12}$$

We posit that surprise combines multiplicatively across timescales, such that an event is surprising only if at all timescales, allowing the model to learn periodic stimuli of various frequencies. We finally assume that surprise sums across features, such that a location may be surprising by its color, motion, or other. The sum is passed through a saturating sigmoidal nonlinearity to enforce plausible neuronal firing dynamics, then provides input to the master map. Figure 11.3 illustrates the model's internal functioning on simple stimuli.

11.3.2 Models compared

We test six computational models, encompassing and extending the state-of-the-art found in previous studies. The first three quantify static image properties: (local intensity variance in 16×16 image patches (Reinagel and Zador, 1999); local oriented edge density as measured with Gabor filters (Itti and Koch, 2001); and local Shannon entropy in 16×16 image patches (Privitera and Stark, 2000). The remaining three models are more sensitive to dynamic events (local motion (Itti and Koch, 2001); saliency (Itti and Koch, 2001); and surprise (Itti and Baldi, 2005)).

More specifically, the local intensity variance model $V(x, y)$ is simply computed as the variance of the 8-bit grey levels of pixels in 16×16 image patches (Parkhurst and Niebur, 2003; Reinagel and Zador, 1999). The input to each pixel (x, y) in the 40×30 master map was thus computed from the corresponding 16×16 patch in the luminance image I at the original frame resolution of 640×480

$$V(x, y) = \sum_{(i,j) \in [16x...16x+15] \times [16y...16y+15]} \left[I(i, j) - \overline{I}(x, y) \right]^2 \tag{11.13}$$

where

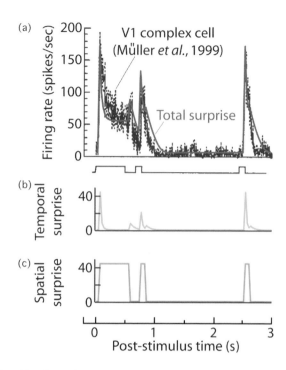

Figure 11.2. Combination of temporal and spatial surprises. We calibrate our model against single-neuron monkey data, then will test it against behavioral human data. (a) Extracellular mean firing rate (solid-black curve, ±S.D. dashed-black) of a macaque V1 complex cell during three successive brief presentations of an isolated grating stimulus demonstrates rapid adaptation (from first to second presentations) and recovery (from second to third; Müller *et al.*, 1999). This suggests that cortical neurons do not passively signal Shannon information, which here would directly follow the stimulus (some information when stimulus on, none otherwise), but instead are actively affected by prior exposures to a stimulus. (b) Temporal surprise signals in real-time how rapidly the neuron's adapting "belief" in the presence or absence of a stimulus is changing as the stimulus is flashed on and off. Hence temporal surprise here follows stimulus transients within the receptive field, more weakly when temporally closer. (c) Spatial surprise signals how much a local model which hypothesizes in real-time the presence or absence of a grating stimulus disagrees with a broader model by which the display overall is blank. Hence spatial surprise here follows the stimulus. A reasonable fit of the neuron's mean firing rate (a; line plotted through data) is obtained with the additive temporal/spatial surprise combination rule of eqn. (11.12): spatial surprise provides a sustained component of the firing rate while the stimulus is on, and temporal surprise provides firing transients at stimulus onsets and offsets. This yields the fastest of our five timescales. While certainly many other interpretations of this particular neuron's behavior are possible, it is intriguing that the data quite naturally fits our theoretical framework.

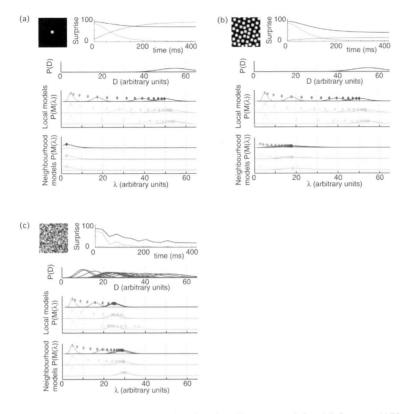

Figure 11.3. Model behavior with simple stimuli presented for 15 frames (450 ms). A feature map is considered (image insets) corresponding to: (a) a small stationary isolated stimulus on black background, (b) a stationary array of small stimuli, or (c) uniform random noise refreshed at every frame. Behaviors of local and neighborhood models at the center location are shown. In each panel, the top graph shows normalized local temporal surprise (cyan), spatial surprise (green) and total surprise (red) over time. $P(D)$ represents the Poisson data distributions received at the center location (one black curve per frame; all identical for stationary stimuli). The Gamma prior distributions $P(M(\lambda))$ over local and neighborhood models are shown, considering $n = 3$ cascaded surprise detectors for clarity although our full model uses $n = 5$ (fastest in orange, second in purple, third in blue; more saturated colors correspond to later frames; only four Gamma distributions for frames 1, 5, 10, and 15 are plotted for clarity, with means of the others plotted as small ellipses; initial condition is a black-image prior). (a) Local priors quickly adapt towards the mean of the locally received data samples, generating decaying local temporal surprise. Neighborhood priors remain unchanged given the black background, generating increasing spatial surprise, as local and neighborhood priors increasingly differ. (b) The local situation is identical but neighborhood priors now quickly adapt towards an average data value. Hence, spatial and total surprises are lower than in (a), allowing the model to predict pop-out. (c) Both local and neighborhood priors quickly adapt towards a broad average data value, rapidly yielding lowest total surprise and demonstrating how surprise does not suffer from the white snow paradox.

$$\bar{I}(x,y) = \frac{1}{256} \sum_{(i,j)\in[16x...16x+15]\times[16y...16y+15]} I(i,j) \qquad (11.14)$$

is the average image luminance over the patch of interest.

The Shannon entropy model $E(x,y)$ was as proposed by Privitera and Stark (2000). The input to each pixel (x,y) in the master map (corresponding to a 16×16 patch in original frames) was

$$E(x,y) = - \sum_{i\in G(x,y)} F_i(x,y) \log F_i(x,y) \qquad (11.15)$$

where $F_i(x,y)$ is the frequency of occurrence of grey level i (quantized into 32 levels) within the 16×16 patch of interest, and $G(x,y)$ is the set of all grey levels present in the patch. While we found elevated entropy at human fixations, highly entropic regions were typically numerous over the visual field (Figure 11.4), making this model poorly specific and yielding lower KL distance between humans and random.

The saliency model was as previously described (Itti and Koch, 2001). It was tested either in full form (including all feature types), or in reduced form where a single feature type was computed (orientation contrast, or motion energy contrast).

11.4   Experimental validation results

We compare spatiotemporal distributions of surprise in the model's master map to eye-movement recordings from four naïve human observers watching 50 video clips, including outdoors scenes, video games, television newscast, sports, and others. Obviously, bottom-up sensory processing may only contribute a fraction among all competing influences on attentional allocation (Henderson and Hollingworth, 1999; Noton and Stark, 1971; Rensink, 2000). Nevertheless, models computing local image information in Shannon's sense predict human gaze fixations significantly more reliably than chance (Parkhurst *et al.*, 2002; Privitera and Stark, 2000; Reinagel and Zador, 1999), providing a challenging baseline for our model. Gaze was recorded with a 240 Hz infrared-video-based eye-tracker (ISCAN, Inc. model RK-464), with experimental protocol as previously (Itti, 2004) (Figure 11.4), yielding 10 192 saccadic gaze shifts. To determine whether humans preferentially oriented towards surprising stimulus elements, at onset of every human saccade we sampled (circular aperture, diameter $6°$) model-predicted master map activity around the saccade's future endpoint, and around a random endpoint (uniform probability). Saccade initiation latency was assumed accounted for by the master map's leaky integrators.

We quantify differences between distributions of master map samples from human and random saccades using the KL distance: models which better predict human scanpaths exhibit higher distances from random, as observers non-uniformly gaze towards a minority of regions with highest model responses. Six models were compared. Three are illustrated in Figure 11.4: Shannon entropy (Privitera and Stark, 2000), saliency, and surprise.

For all models, humans saccaded towards image locations of higher model-predicted response than expected by chance (nonparametric sign test, $p < 10^{-100}$ or better). KL distances between human and random (Figure 11.4) were all significantly higher than zero, which would indicate a model not predicting human saccades better than chance (t-test, $p < 10^{-100}$ or better). KL distances all differed significantly from one another (Bonferroni-corrected t-tests, $p < 10^{-100}$ or better), indicating significantly different performance levels and a strict ranking of all models. Because KL is nonlinear, attempting to interpret the magnitudes of differences between models may be hazardous. Yet, among all six models tested in total, the suprise model significantly outperformed all others by a large margin (20% better than the second best, saliency).

11.5   Discussion and conclusion

Much research has employed Shannon entropy to analyze neuronal processing (Atick, 1992; Barlow, 1959; Simoncelli and Olshausen, 2001). However, even casual observation suggests that entropy alone fails to capture neural response transients and adaptation (Figure 11.2). By explicitly considering observer models and changing beliefs, surprise may be better suited to studying neuronal function and behavior. We argue that, indeed, there is not much point for information *communication* or *transmission* in a biological brain, beyond initial sensory transduction; if information is available at some stage, why not directly use it there, in original or transformed form? Instead, there is much need – as most studies of attention show – for information *pruning*, that is, irremediably discarding a large fraction of the available nonredundant information, so that later processing resources can more efficiently be focused on the little that remains. While previous research has shown with static scenes that humans preferentially fixate information-rich locations (Parkhurst *et al.*, 2002; Privitera and Stark, 2000; Reinagel and Zador, 1999), here, developing new tools to quantify bottom-up influences on attention in dynamic scenes, we find that humans fixate surprising locations even more reliably, making surprise the strongest of all algorithmic models tested. These results provide a quantitative confirmation to a number of previous behavioral observations that what you see is what you need (Triesch *et al.*, 2003), and, conversely, that information which has no current behavioral relevance, no matter how rich in Shannon's sense, will be lost.

Interesting extensions of our modeling and experiments may compare our data to monkey eye-tracking, possibly exhibiting lower or different top-down biases, or introduce additional top-down priors into the model, based on higher-level expectations and beliefs. In this respect, top-down guided search (Wolfe, 1994) could well involve modulating from the top adaptive priors learned bottom-up.

Our model exhibits desirable properties for computer vision. For example, it resembles background subtraction algorithms that isolate moving objects from backgrounds whose statistics are learned (Friedman and Russell, 1997), although these algorithms lack our notion of spatial surprise. While surprise certainly is not a new concept, it had lacked a formal definition, broad enough to capture the intuitive meaning of the term, yet quantitative and computable in a principled manner. The advantage of our definition is its generality which results in widespread applicability not limited to early

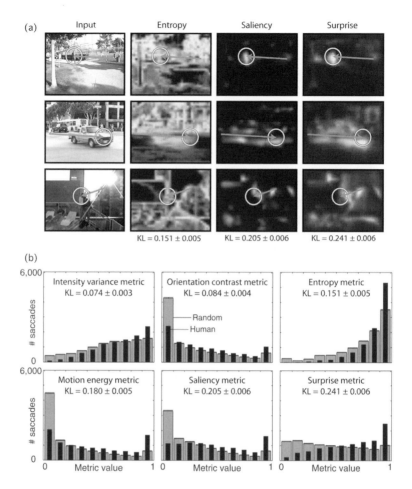

Figure 11.4. (a) Sample video frames, with corresponding human saccades and predictions from the entropy, saliency, and surprise models. Entropy maps, like intensity variance and orientation maps, exhibited many locations with high responses, hence had low specificity and were poorly discriminative. In contrast, motion, saliency, and surprise maps were much sparser and more specific, with surprise significantly more often on target. For three example frames (first column), saccades from one subject are shown (arrows) with corresponding apertures over which master map activity at the saccade endpoint was sampled (circles). (b) KL scores for these models indicate significantly different performance levels, and a strict ranking of variance < orientation < entropy < motion < saliency < surprise. KL scores were computed by comparing the number of human saccades landing onto each given range of master map values (narrow blue bars) to the number of random saccades hitting the same range (wider green bars). A score of zero would indicate equality between the human and random histograms, i.e. humans did not tend to hit various master map values any differently from expected by chance, or, the master map could not predict human saccades better than random saccades. Among the six computational models tested in total, surprise performed best, in that surprising locations were relatively few yet reliably gazed at by humans.

vision or attention. For example, surprise may be computed on auditory, olfactory, gustative, somatosensory or other features similarly. Detecting surprise in neural spike trains does not require semantic understanding of the data carried by the spike trains.

Under a small set of axioms (Cox, 1964; Jaynes, 2003; Savage, 1972) the Bayesian definition of probability provides the only consistent approach to inference and learning. Likewise, in the same framework, surprise is the only consistent measure of novelty and saliency. Previous measures of novelty and saliency, for instance defining important stimuli as spatial and/or temporal outliers to the learned distribution of observed data values (Itti and Koch, 2001; Markou and Singh, 2003), at best can be viewed as approximations to surprise, but can be flawed in some extreme cases. Consider, for instance, a case where a datum d has very small probability both for a model or hypothesis M and for a single alternative hypothesis $\overline{M}$. Although d is a strong outlier, it carries very little information regarding whether M or $\overline{M}$ is the better model, and therefore very little surprise. Thus an outlier detection method would strongly focus attentional resources onto d, although d is a false positive and is irrelevant, in the sense that it carries no useful information for discriminating between the two alternative hypotheses M and $\overline{M}$.

At higher abstraction levels, informal ideas of novelty and surprise have been proposed that could capture attention and trigger learning (Ranganath and Rainer, 2003), which may now be formalized in terms of priors and posteriors. For example, a projectile's sudden trajectory deviation may elicit surprise that could be computed from distributions of trajectory models. Beyond biology, computable surprise could guide the development of future data mining and compression systems, to find surprising agents in crowds, surprising sentences in books or speeches, surprising sequences in genomes, surprising medical symptoms, surprising documents on the world-wide-web, or to design surprising advertisements.

Acknowledgments

Supported by HFSP, NSF and NGA (L. I.), NIH and NSF (P. B.). We thank UCI's Institute for Genomics and Bioinformatics and USC's Center High Performance Computing and Communications (www.usc.edu/hpcc) for access to their computing clusters. The authors affirm that the views expressed herein are solely their own, and do not represent the views of the United States government or any agency thereof.

Supplementary videos

The videos should be played in the Quicktime player and may not play at the correct frame rate (about 30 frames/s) in the Windows Media Player. From left to right, videos show three panels.

(1) The original video clip frames (downscaled; original size was 640×480)

(2) The original video clip plus eye position from one subject (C. Z.) indicated by small cyan squares (up to eight squares/frame since we track eyes at 240 Hz and play video at 30.13 frames/s). During saccadic gaze shifts, the squares turn purple. At onset of each human saccade, master map activity is sampled once

around the saccade's future endpoint (circles flashed during clips indicate aperture over which samples were taken). At the same time, another sample is taken at a random location (not shown), for comparison.

(3) The model's dynamic master map. Brighter values indicate higher model response.

- *ittivideo1.mpg* - Shannon entropy model (Privitera and Stark, (2000). While humans certainly avoid low-entropy regions, the rather low score for this model comes from the fact that entropy is always high over large portions of the image (many false positives). Thus it would be difficult to pick just one best location towards which to point a pair of eyes based on the entropy map.

- *ittivideo2.mpg* - Saliency model. This model more strongly highlights the players and ball, which also captured the attention of the human observers. However, this model also yields substantial responses to the strong textures in the grass and background scenery, owing to the rapid camera motion which prevents trivial adaptation by constantly changing the inputs.

- *ittivideo3.mpg* - Surprise model. Much sparser maps that well predict human gaze yield a better score. Note how the model is little perturbed by the strong textures in the background and the strong motion transients elicited by rapid camera motion.

Source code

The source code for all models tested here is freely available on our web site at http://iLab.usc.edu/toolkit/

References

Abrams, R. A. and Christ, S. E. (2003). Motion onset captures attention. *Psychol. Sci.*, **14**, 427–432.

Ackley, D. H., Hinton, G. E. and Sejnowski, T. J. (1985). A learning algorithm for boltzmann machines. *Cogn. Sci.*, **9**, 147–169.

Atick, J. J. (1992). Could information theory provide an ecological theory of sensory processing? *Network*, **3**, 213–251.

Baldi, P. (2002). A computational theory of surprise. In M. Blaum, ed., *Information, Coding, and Mathematics*, pp. 1–25.

Baldi, P. (2005). Surprise: A shortcut for attention? In L. Itti, G. Rees, and J. Tsotsos (Eds), *Neurobiology of Attention*, pp. 24–28, San Diego, CA: Elsevier.

Baldi, P. and Itti, L. (2005). Attention: Bits versus wows. *Proc. IEEE International Conference on Neural Networks and Brain*, Beijing, China.

Barlow, H. B. (1959). Sensory mechanisms, the reduction of redundancy and intelligence. In D. V. Blake and A. M. Utlley, eds., *Proc. Symposium on the Mechanization of Thought Processes*, Vol. 2. London: HM Stationery Office, pp. 537–574.

Brown, L. D. (1986). *Fundamentals of Statistical Exponential Families*. Hayward, CA: Institute of Mathematical Statistics.

Cox, R. T. (1964). Probability, frequency and reasonable expectation. *Am. J. Phys.*, **14**, 1–13.

Doretto, G., Chiuso, A., Wu, Y. and Soatto, S. (2003). Dynamic Textures. *Int. J. Comp. Vis.*, **51**, 91–109.

Fecteau, J. H. and Munoz, D. P. (2003). Exploring the consequences of the previous trial. *Nat. Rev. Neurosci.*, **4**, 435–443.

Friedman, N. and Russell, S. (1997). Image segmentation in video sequences: A Probabilistic Approach. *Annual Conference on Uncertainty in Artificial Intelligence*, pp. 175–181.

Hayhoe, M. M., Shrivastava, A., Mruczek, R. and Pelz, J. B. (2003). Visual memory and motor planning in a natural task. *J. Vis.*, **3**, 49–63.

Henderson, J. M. and Hollingworth, A. (1999). High-level scene perception. *Ann. Rev. Psychol.*, **50**, 243–271.

Itti, L. (2005). Quantifying the contribution of low-level saliency to human eye movements in dynamic scenes. *Visual Cogn.*, **12**, 1093–1123.

Itti, L. and Baldi, P. (2005). A principled approach to detecting surprising events in video. *Proc. IEEE Conference on Computer Vision and Pattern Recognition (CVPR)*, pp. 631–637.

Itti, L. and Baldi, P. (2006). Bayesian surprise attracts human attention. *Advances in Neural Information Processing Systems*, **19**: 1–8. Cambridge, MA: MIT Press.

Itti, L. and Koch, C. (2000). A saliency-based search mechanism for overt and covert shifts of visual attention. *Vis. Res.*, **40**: 1489–1506.

Itti, L. and Koch, C. (2001). Computational modeling of visual attention. *Nature Reviews Neurosci.*, **2**: 194–203.

Itti, L., Koch, C. and Niebur, E. (1998). A model of saliency-based visual attention for rapid scene analysis. *IEEE PAMI*, **20**, 1254–1259.

James, W. (1890). *The Principles of Psychology*. Cambridge, MA: Harvard University Press.

Jaynes, E. T. (2003). *Probability Theory. The Logic of Science*. Cambridge: Cambridge University Press.

Kullback, S. (1959). *Information Theory and Statistics*. New York: Wiley.

Maffei, L., Fiorentini, A. and Bisti, S. (1973). Neural correlate of perceptual adaptation to gratings. *Science*, **182**, 1036–1038.

Markou, M. and Singh, S. (2003). Novelty detection: a review - part 1: statistical approaches. *Signal Processing*, **83**, 2481–2497.

Müller, J. R., Metha, A. B., Krauskopf, J. and Lennie, P. (1999). Rapid adaptation in visual cortex to the structure of images. *Science*, **285**, 1405–1408.

Noton, D. and Stark, L. (1971). Scanpaths in eye movements during pattern perception. *Science*, **171**, 308–311.

Parkhurst, D. J. and Niebur, E. (2003). Scene content selected by active vision. *Spat. Vis.*, **16**, 125–154.

Parkhurst, D., Law, K. and Niebur, E. (2002). Modeling the role of salience in the allocation of overt visual attention. *Vis. Res.*, **42**, 107–123.

Privitera, C. M. and Stark, L. W. (2000). Algorithms for defining visual regions-of-interest: comparison with eye fixations. *IEEE PAMI*, **22**, 970–982.

Ranganath, C. and Rainer, G. (2003). Neural mechanisms for detecting and remembering novel events. *Nat. Rev. Neurosci.*, **4**, 193–202.

Reinagel, P. and Zador, A. M. (1999). Natural scene statistics at the centre of gaze. *Network*, **10**, 341–350.

Rensink, R. A. (2000). The dynamic representation of scenes. *Vis. Cogn.*, **7**, 17–42.

Savage, L. J. (1972). *The foundations of statistics*. New York: Dover. (First edition in 1954.)

Shannon, C. E. (1948). A mathematical theory of communication. *Bell Sys. Tech. J.*, **27**, 379–423, 623–656.

Simoncelli, E. P. and Olshausen, B. A. (2001). Natural image statistics and neural representation. *Ann. Rev. Neurosci.*, **24**, 1193–1216.

Softky, W. R. and Koch, C. (1993). The highly irregular firing of cortical cells is inconsistent with temporal integration of random EPSPs. *J. Neurosci.*, **13**, 334–50.

Tatler, B. W., Baddeley, R. J. and Gilchrist, I. D. (2005). Visual correlates of fixation selection: effects of scale and time. *Vis. Res.*, **45**, 643–659.

Theeuwes, J. (1995). Abrupt luminance change pops out; abrupt color change does not. *Percept. Psychophys.*, **57**, 637–644.

Triesch, J., Ballard, D. H., Hayhoe, M. M. and Sullivan, B. T. (2003). What you see is what you need. *J. Vis.*, **3**, 86–94.

Vinje, W. E. and Gallant, J. L. (2000). Sparse coding and decorrelation in primary visual cortex during natural vision. *Science*, **287**, 1273–1276.

Wolfe, J M. (1994). Guided search 2.0: a revised model of visual search. *Psychonom. Bull. Rev.*, **1**, 202–238.

Wolfe, J. (1998). Visual Search. In H. Pashler, ed., *Attention*. London: University College London Press.

Part III

Stereo

12 Global stereo in polynomial time

Carlo Tomasi

12.1 Introduction

Stereo vision is one of the most thoroughly studied problems in computer vision. In a survey of the state of the art (Scharstein and Szeliski, 2002) and more recently on the accompanying Middlebury stereo vision web page, Scharstein and Szeliski categorize and compare a wide array of algorithms that follow approaches ranging from window-level correlation to dynamic programming, to combinatorial optimization, to belief propagation.

This survey shows that the problem of stereo matching is relatively easy to formulate, but hard to solve. More than thirty years after the first attempts on computers (Hannah, 1974; Marr, 1974), and in spite of the existence of several experimental or commercial hardware systems that match stereo image pairs (Point Grey, undated; Woodfill *et al.*, 2004; Kanade, 1994; Konolige, 1997) most computer vision conferences still have entire sessions on this thriving topic. If the problem were solved, this would not be the case.

A public data benchmark like the Middlebury web site is a precious resource for comparing approaches, coalescing efforts, and eventually advancing the state of the art. We need more work in this direction. Because of this benchmark, whether one algorithm is better than another is not a matter of judgement, but can be measured by the number of correct matches for the two methods on the same image pairs.

One clear lesson learned from past work is that stereo is best formulated as a global problem, in which an entire image is matched to another one as the result of a single optimization problem. The two common alternatives are to match one point at a time (the favorite hardware solution), or two corresponding epipolar lines at a time. The latter is a reasonable compromise between the greediest solution and the completely global one, and has been traditionally addressed with dynamic programming (see, for example, Arnold and Binford, 1980; Belhumeur and Mumford, 1992; Birchfield and

Computational Vision in Neural and Machine Systems, ed. L. Harris and M. Jenkin. Published by Cambridge University Press. © Cambridge University Press 2007.

Tomasi, 1998; Cox *et al.*, 1996; Ohta and Takeo, 1985; Van Meergergen *et al.*, 2002).

The great advantage of dynamic programming is its conceptual and algorithmic simplicity. This has allowed recasting stereo matching into a Bayesian formulation (Belhumeur and Mumford, 1992) and a Maximum-likelihood approach (Cox *et al.*, 1996) as mathematical sophistication in computer vision progressed, to propose variations based on different similarity metrics (Birchfield and Tomasi, 1998), and to explore efficient multi-scale implementations (Van Meergergen *et al.*, 2002). Less tangibly, but perhaps not less importantly, when a problem that is simple to state has a solution that is simple to explain, we feel that we are on the right track: if something goes wrong it is easier to fix, and when things go right we know why and what to retain when attempting improvements. Good performance in the experiments is of course the ultimate indicator of a good idea, but until we can claim perfect performance an improvement that comes at the expense of understanding is of somewhat reduced heuristic value.

This is why I have not been able to experience the same sense of satisfaction with the completely global solutions that perform best on the Middlebury web page, whether I contributed to them (Birchfied and Tomasi, 1999; Lin and Tomasi, 2004) or not (Kim *et al.*, 2003; Kolmogorov and Zabih, 2001; Vesker *et al.*, 1999; Sun *et al.*, 2003). These solutions are all complex in two ways. First, the exact problem in all these formulations is NP hard, and approximations (still relatively expensive) must be used. Second, algorithms that use sophisticated heuristics to search for an approximate optimum in a large space are difficult to understand intimately. When something goes wrong, it is often hard to tell whether the culprit is in the necessary approximations introduced for tractability or rather an inappropriately defined optimization target. When things go well, it is not clear if a small modification to the algorithm, meant to improve some aspect of its solution, would retain good performance in other aspects.

Fortunately the dilemma between a simple but line-by-line solution to stereo and a more global solution can be resolved in a different way, through a formulation based on maximum flows in networks. This solution has been shown in the literature in somewhat different versions (Buehler *et al.*, 2002; Ishikawa and Geiger, 1998; Roy, 1999; Roy and Cox, 1998). The version in Roy and Cox (1998) was even featured on the Middlebury web page, where it performed respectably (2.98% of pixels with disparity wrong by more than one pixel on the Tsukuba image), although not among the "stars."

In a nutshell, as shown most elegantly in Buehler *et al.* (2002), instead of finding a shortest path on the usual graph used in the dynamic programming formulations, one first transforms this graph into its graph-theoretical dual, and *voilà*, the shortest path becomes a minimum cut. As well known, a minimum cut can be found by computing a maximum flow through the graph. If one considers one scan line at a time, this problem transformation is just an exercise in graph theory. However, if the two images in the stereo pair are considered in their entirety, the dynamic programming solution ceases to be applicable, while the minimum cut formulation still admits a polynomial-time solution. This is also practically very fast, thanks to Cherkassky and Goldberg's implementation (Cherkassky and Goldberg, 1997) of the Goldberg–Tarjan max-flow algorithm (Goldberg and Tarjan, 1988).

The max-flow/min-cut solution to the stereo correspondence problem has not received the attention that it deserves. Few others work on it, and the approach is rarely taught in computer vision courses or books. Part of the reason may be the method's good but not stellar performance on the benchmarks. Another part may have to do with the fact that the network flow formulation is apparently less flexible than the one based on dynamic programming, as it seems more difficult to incorporate some of the heuristic constraints that we are used to seeing in stereo vision algorithms. A third part of the explanation may be that previous formulations based on network flow may be more complex than they need to be.

The goal of this contribution is to introduce an even simpler max-flow/min-cut formulation of stereo correspondence than previously published, in the hope that the very simplicity of the approach will spur the types of studies of this method that have been devoted to dynamic programming for the line-by-line case. Specifically, section 12.2 shows why dynamic programming cannot be applied to the global stereo corre-spondence problem. Section 12.3 then introduces the proposed formulation of global correspondence as a max-flow/min-cut problem, and compares it to previous ones. Fi-nally, Section 12.4 shows anecdotal evidence of good performance, and Section 12.5 gives some indications for future work.

12.2 Dynamic programming stereo and its limits

Assume that pixels in a given scan line of the left image always correspond to pixels in the same scan line of the right image, and viceversa. This assumption entails no loss of generality, because stereo images can be always rectified so that this is the case (Trucco and Verri, 1998). Figure 12.1 shows the standard graph used in dynamic-programming formulations of the line-to-line stereo correspondence problem.

If the pixels of the right scan line are listed at integer positions along the horizontal axis of a Cartesian reference frame and those of the left scan line are listed at integer positions along the vertical axis, as shown in Figure 12.1, then a match between two pixels can be represented by a point on the plane with integer coordinates. Thus, the integer grid on the plane is the set of all possible matches. In the rectified camera configuration, a pixel in the left scan line can only match a pixel in the right scan line that has a lower horizontal image coordinate: points in the image from the right camera are shifted to the left relative to where they are in the left camera. This restriction eliminates all points of the grid that are above the main diagonal, labeled "disparity 0" in Figure 12.1. Points on this diagonal have a disparity of zero, which means that their horizontal image coordinates are equal. The ones on the next diagonal have a disparity of one, that is, their coordinates differ by one pixel, and so forth. Greater disparity corresponds to points that are closer to the camera, so disparities can also be bounded from above if one assumes that no object in the world can come closer than a given distance from the two cameras. This results in the trapezoidal shape of the grid in Figure 12.1.

A list of all the actual matches between the two scan lines yields a *path* on the grid, like the thick blue line in Figure 12.1, which is assumed to start at the top left of the grid, and end at the bottom right (dummy, compulsory matches can be added at the corners to enforce this). Not all paths correspond to valid solutions to the stereo matching problem. For instance, some paths may represent surfaces that hide themselves or each

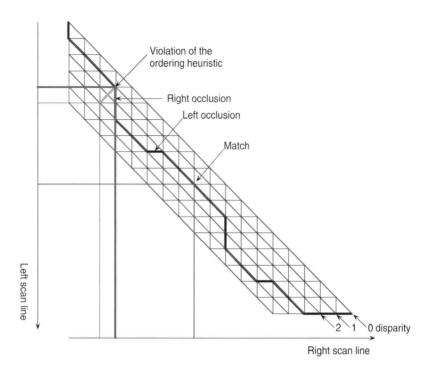

Figure 12.1. The standard graph used in dynamic-programming formulations of the line-to-line stereo correspondence problem. See text for explanation.

other from either camera, a situation that cannot occur in reality. To eliminate these impossible paths from the set of solution, valid paths are often constrained to only go monotonically from top left to bottom right. Thus, the blue path in Figure 12.1 is valid, because it is only made of segments that when the path is traversed from top to bottom go vertically down, horizontally to the right, or diagonally down and to the right. In contrast, the short, thick, orange segment would not be a valid path segment, because it goes diagonally down and to the left. Physically, this segment would connect two matches in which the order of the two points in the left image is opposite to the order of the two points in the right image (see the order of the thick and thin lines at the endpoints of the segment). Such pairs of matches are not impossible, but they are rare. Forbidding them results into the *ordering constraint*, which restricts the set of solution somewhat more than necessary, but in a way that is very easy to enforce, especially when using dynamic programming.

A horizontal segment of the path corresponds to right pixels that have no corresponding left pixels, that is, to a point in the left image where disparity changes abruptly. This is called a *left occlusion*. A *right occlusion* is defined similarly, with the role of the two images reversed.

When formulating the stereo correspondence problem within the framework of dynamic programming, one typically defines a *cost* for each candidate match, which is an increasing function of the difference in the pixel values at the two image points being

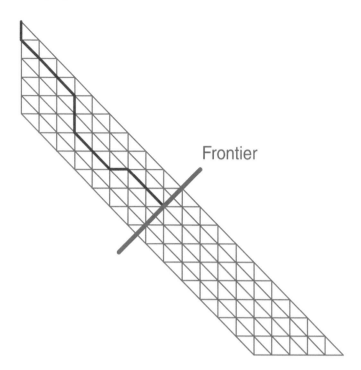

Figure 12.2. Dynamic programming moves a frontier (thick, red line) from top left to bottom right, and updates the costs of the best (blue) path up to each grid point on the frontier. Only a small number of such cost values must be maintained on the frontier.

matched: similar pixels are more likely to match than dissimilar ones. A cost is also typically charged to occlusions, both left and right, according to the observation that most surfaces in the world are smooth, that is, that disparity changes only slowly from point to point most of the time. One can then look for a path that satisfies the ordering constraint and has overall minimum cost. This is done very efficiently with *dynamic programming*.

In this style of solution, sketched in Figure 12.2, a frontier (some curve that splits the start point from the end point of the path) is moved down the grid one step at a time. *For each position of the frontier, dynamic programming records the cost of the least expensive path up to each of the grid points on the frontier.* Because of the associative nature of the measure of the cost of a path (equal to the sum of the costs incurred along the path), the path costs recorded on the frontier can be updated efficiently when the frontier is moved. Once the frontier meets the bottom right of the grid, the cost of the best path from start to end is known. Additional information stored during the procedure allows to quickly reconstruct the best path that leads to this optimal cost.

The details of dynamic programming are not important for our purposes. The crucial observation is highlighted in the previous paragraph: a temporary variable is associated to each point on the frontier in order to store the cost of the best path up to that point. This is feasible because both the frontier and any path are polygonal curves

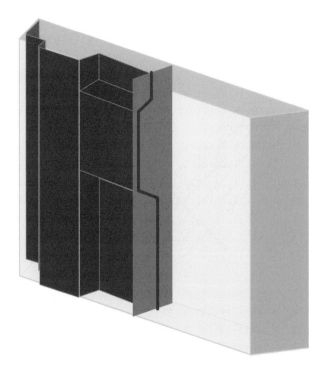

Figure 12.3. The blue path has now become a match *surface* that intersects the red frontier (another surface) along a curve.

on the plane, whose vertices are the integer coordinates of the grid points: two curves intersect at a point, and any frontier has a small number of possible intersection points.

If we now were to extend this principle of solution to full images, the match grid would become three-dimensional, since the two-dimensional grids for every scan line pair would have to be stacked on top of each other. Both curves involved in dynamic programming, the path and the frontier, would become surfaces: the path would be replaced by a family of paths, one per scan line pair, and this would form a match *surface*. Similarly, the frontier would have to be a surface as well in order to separate the top left from the bottom right of the three-dimensional grid. The new situation is illustrated in Figure 12.3.

This is why dynamic programming becomes infeasible for full image pairs: the intersection of a match surface and a frontier is no longer a point but a curve, and *the number of possible curves on any one frontier is too great*. We cannot store or update the cost of each possible match surface up to some frontier. The computational complexity makes dynamic programming infeasible.

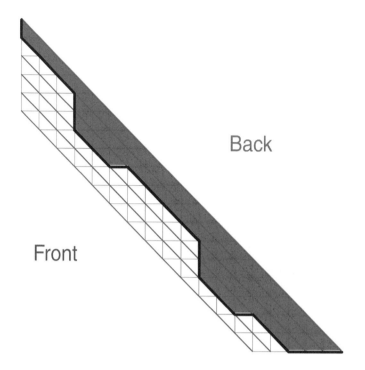

Figure 12.4. The path in Figure 12.1 can be viewed as a *cut* that separates what is in front of the surface (higher disparity) from what is behind.

12.3 The max-flow/min-cut formulation

What is unfeasible in Section 12.2 is the solution method, not the problem itself. In fact, to come up with a feasible solution, we just need to look at Figure 12.1 in a different way. The blue curve in that figure has been described so far as a *path* that connects the top left corner of the match grid to its bottom right corner. Figure 12.4 shows the same curve interpreted differently, as a boundary or *cut* that separates the empty space in front of the surface, where disparities are higher, from that behind the surface, where disparities are lower.

Finding a good match then turns into the problem of separating front from back with a minimum cut, where the "size" of a cut is measured by the cost of the matches that lie along the cut. However, cutting the grid as drawn would entail removing nodes from it (the nodes on the solution cut). Minimum-cut problems are instead cast in terms of removing edges of a graph.

As explained in Buehler *et al.* (2002), since the graph is planar, all we need to do is to replace the original one with its dual, in which each region (triangle) in the original graph becomes a node, and edges are drawn between nodes of adjacent regions. Figure 12.5 shows this transformation. From here on, the details of graph construction are different from those in previous papers, and make the resulting graph simpler.

Since the original graph is undirected, so is its dual. The resulting graph is made

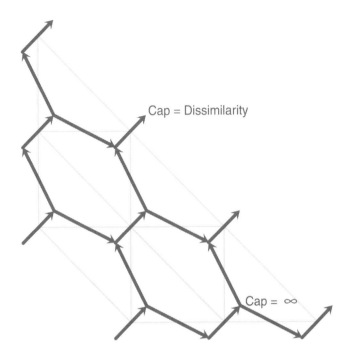

Figure 12.5. The thick, red and green arrows form the dual of the graph drawn in thin, yellow lines. We made the graph directed by having all arrows point from the front of the graph (higher disparities) to the back.

to be directed by making all arrows point from high to low disparity. This will become useful a little later, when the ordering constraint is enforced.

There is one green, short edge for each match in the original (primal) grid, and the capacity of these edges equals the match cost that was charged to each node in the primal graph. The other, red edges have infinite capacity. Because of this, they cannot be cut without incurring an infinite penalty, so they will never be part of any minimum cut. Since the red edges are in series with the green ones, it is still possible to cut the graph by cutting only green edges.

To make the graph into a traditional flow network, we need to add a source and a sink node, and some plumbing to connect these to the rest of the graph. This is shown on a very small dual graph in Figure 12.6. From now on, we can forget the original (primal) graph.

The resulting graph can be cut with paths that are not valid, in that they do not satisfy the ordering constraint. To enforce the latter, we add one more set of edges, as shown in Figure 12.7. These also have infinite capacity, so they cannot be part of any minimum cut. The role of the ordering edges can be understood by referring to Figure 12.8, in which the small-scale details of a cut (blue curve) have been suppressed and only a few of the ordering edges have been drawn, for greater clarity. Note that whether the ordering edges traverse a cut from front to back of the cut or from back to

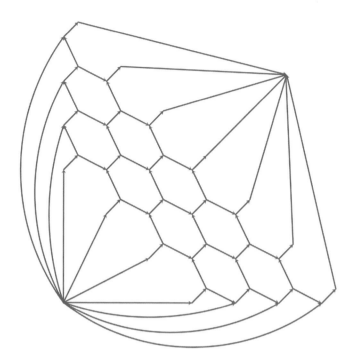

Figure 12.6. Adding a source and a sink, together with the necessary plumbing, makes a complete dual graph for a standard, single-source max-flow/min-cut problem.

front depends on the local orientation of the path. Solid arrows are edges that traverse the cut from front to back, and they occur in parts of the cut that are oriented in the direction forbidden by the ordering constraint, that is, generally from south–east to north–west when walking along the path starting from the top left of the diagram.

Dotted arrows, on the other hand, traverse parts of the cut that run in the valid direction, compatible with the ordering constraint, and they carry flow from back to front.

Because of this arrangement, any path that violates the ordering constraint must also cut ordering edges that carry flow forward (the solid arrows). Because these have infinite capacity, no minimum cost cut can have sections that run in the forbidden direction. On the other hand, cutting ordering edges where the cut has a valid direction is harmless, as these edges only carry flow from back to front, and do not contribute to the total flow from source to sink. Thus, these edges appropriately enforce the ordering constraint.

We are now ready for the last and crucial step, that is, the insertion of additional edges that connect adjacent pairs of scan lines for a completely global formulation of the stereo correspondence problem. The main constraint added by a global solution is the *connectedness* of the resulting match surface. This requires vertically adjacent pixels to have similar disparities most of the time, a constraint of considerable heuristic power.

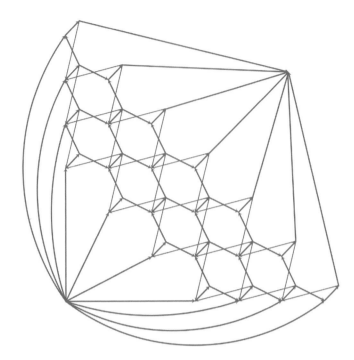

Figure 12.7. This is the complete graph for the two-dimensional matching problem. The extra, infinite-capacity edges enforce the ordering constraint, as explained in the text and in Figure 12.8.

In previous work within the max-flow/min-cut framework, this constraint has invariably been implemented by the addition of tunable smoothness terms between vertically adjacent pixels. The resulting networks all have a large number of edges (17 have been found by both Ishikawa and Geiger (1998), and by Buehler *et al.* (2002)), and parameters. While parameters provide flexibility, they must be tuned, and it is hard to think of matching algorithms that can tune their parameters automatically as a function of the input images.

Instead, we propose a simpler version of connectedness, in which vertically adjacent pixels are merely required to have disparities that differ by at most one pixel. We handle discontinuities in depth by waiving this requirement whenever there are great changes in brightness between vertically adjacent pixels in either image, corresponding to the assumption that depth discontinuities come usually with brightness discontinuities.

Of course, this assumption is not always true. Also, constraining vertical disparity changes to at most one pixel might in some circumstances smooth over a very slanted surface. However, in both cases a (rare) violation of the heuristic merely costs a local blurring of the match surface with respect to truth. The great advantage of making this assumption is that the only parameter in the proposed method is a threshold implied by the edge detector that determines when a brightness discontinuity has occurred between

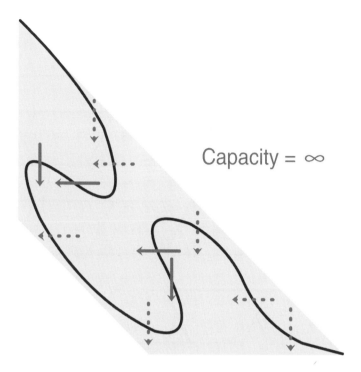

Figure 12.8. A conceptual view of the edges added in Figure 12.7. These enforce the ordering constraint by preventing cuts that would also have to cut infinite-capacity edges carrying flow from front to back of the cut. Solid arrows are examples of these. Dashed arrows are harmless because they carry flow from back to front, and therefore do not contribute to the cost of a cut.

two vertically adjacent pixels. Edge detection is well understood, including methods for selecting parameters (Canny, 1986).

Connectedness is enforced by a cross-connection, again with infinite-capacity edges, between vertically adjacent match edges (the green edges in Figure 12.7). Figure 12.9 shows these edges for a vertical slice through the three-dimensional graph obtained by stacking the two-dimensional graphs for all the scan line pairs. The slice is taken so that horizontally adjacent green edges correspond to disparities that differ by one pixel. The caption of this Figure explains why this arrangement enforces the proposed version of connectedness.

In summary, the formulation of the stereo correspondence problem proposed here is essentially parameter-free (except for the well-understood parameters implied by the edge detector), and has seven edges per node, shown in Figure 12.10. Figure 12.11 shows a network for a very small matching problem.

The optimal disparity surface is found with an entirely off-the-shelf algorithm, Cherkassky and Goldberg's implementation (Cherkassky and Goldberg, 1997) of the Goldberg–Tarjan max-flow algorithm (Goldberg and Tarjan, 1988). This algorithm was designed to compute the maximum flow that can be pushed through a network.

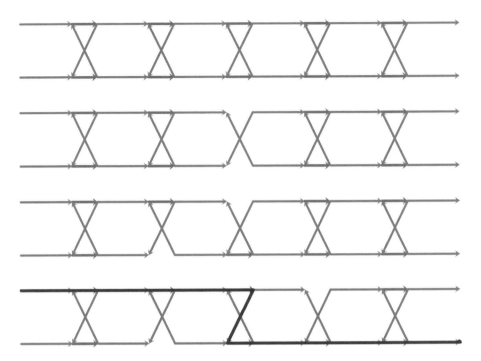

Figure 12.9. The top diagram shows the cross-edges added to enforce connectedness between rows for a slice of the complete, three-dimensional graph for the global stereo matching problem. To obtain a genuine cut, one must cut two vertically adjacent green edges (second diagram), or two diagonally adjacent green edges (third diagram), corresponding to disparity differences of zero or one pixel. The bottom diagram shows that removing green edges in violation of connectedness (two or more pixels of disparity difference) does not lead to a cut, as the blue flow can still make its way through the network.

As well known (Ford Jr. and Fulkerson, 1962), there exists a minimum cut of the network whose capacity is exactly the maximum flow, and finding the maximum flow also yields the minimum cut.

The asymptotic complexity of Goldberg and Tarjan's algorithm is $O(mn \log(n^2/m))$, where n is the number of vertices in the network and m is the number of edges. In our case, $m = 7n$ (see Figure 12.10), so m is $O(n)$, and the resulting bound is $O(n^2 \log n)$. To relate this to image size, let p be the number of pixels in the image and d the maximum disparity allowed. Then, $n = pd$. As image resolution increases, the maximum disparity must increase proportionally, so that d is $O(\sqrt{p})$. In summary, the asymptotic complexity is $O(p^3 \log p)$. In practice, the constants are small, and matching a 512×512 image takes of the order of one minute on a standard personal computer.

Both the goals of computational and conceptual simplicity have been achieved, albeit at the cost of a simplification of the underlying heuristics. The next section

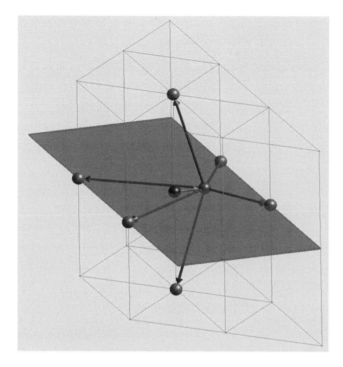

Figure 12.10. A node in the full network has seven edges. Of these, one (short, in gold) has a finite capacity that is an increasing function of the cost of the match corresponding to the node. The other six edges have infinite capacity.

shows that at least in one non-trivial case practical results are good. More experiments are left for future work.

12.4 An experiment

The Middlebury web page provides among others the stereo pair shown in Figure 12.12, for which students at Tsukuba University have determined the correct matches by hand. Figure 12.13 shows the result computed by the max-flow/min-cut method described in the previous Section, and Figure 12.14 gives a different view of the left map of Figure 12.13. Images were processed at a resolution of 384×288 pixels, and matching required 40 s on a 1.4 MHz Pentium personal computer. No parameters had to speci-fied, except for the values for Canny's edge detector when determining intensity edges in the two images. These values are $\sigma = 1$ for the standard deviation of the detector's gradient operator, and $\theta_h = 0.14$ for the high threshold in the non-maximum suppres-sion stage of the detector. The low threshold is then automatically set to $0.4\theta_h$. The two thresholds are referred to a range of image values normalized to $[0, 1]$. Please see Canny (1986) for the detailed meaning of these parameters. All these parameter values are the default values in the Matlab implementation of Canny's edge detector.

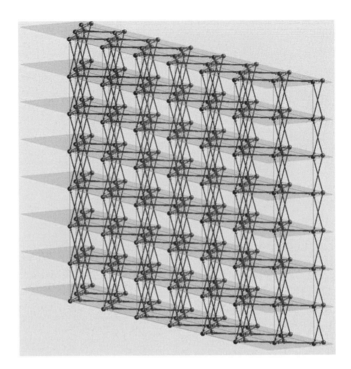

Figure 12.11. The three-dimensional network for a small matching problem. Source and sink edges have been omitted for clarity. Each of the shaded planes corresponds to a different pair of scan lines.

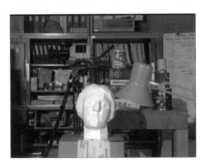 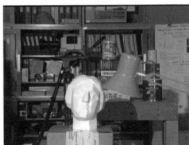

Figure 12.12. The Tsukuba stereo pair.

The fraction of correct disparity values is about 97%, similarly to Roy and Cox (1998). This places this algorithm among the "relatively good" ones in the Middlebury competition, in which the absolute best reach just above 99% (if we take the hand-determined correspondences as the absolute truth). Note, however, that the proposed algorithm achieved these results without setting any parameters in the matcher. This out-of-the-box performance is rather unusual for stereo algorithms which typically require extensive parameter tuning to yield good results.

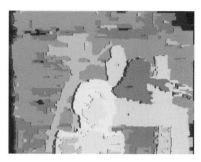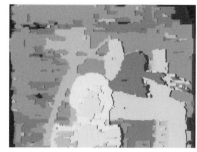

Figure 12.13. Color-coded view of the disparity surface mapped to the left and right image. Occlusions can be seen in magenta on the color version of this figure on the CDROM.

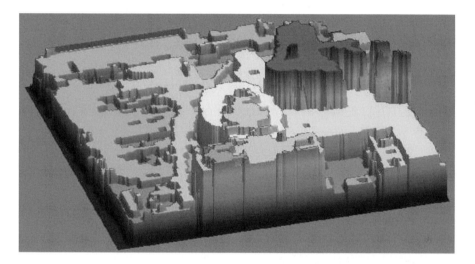

Figure 12.14. A three-dimensional display of the left view of the disparity surface.

12.5   Conclusions and future work

The main goal of this contribution has been to champion a global (i.e., image-to-image) formulation of stereo matching that is equivalent to determining the minimum cut in a flow network. The resulting problem is essentially parameterless and can be solved by efficient, off-the-shelf algorithms. This approach has been proposed a few times in the past eight years, and this paper provides a simpler instantiation of essentially the same idea.

The single experiment in the previous section is not sufficient to establish the performance of the proposed algorithm. A systematic evaluation would run the algorithm on a series of image pairs of real scenes for which accurate ground truth is available. We are setting up an experimental facility with funding from the National Science Foundation of the USA for acquiring just this type of images.

All the same, the hope is that good performance achieved on a difficult image in the first run of the code will entice more researchers into studying and developing an approach to stereo that has the same features of simplicity of dynamic programming, but is applicable to entire images rather than just one pair of scan lines at a time.

In addition to working on alternative formulations within this framework, it may be useful to examine implementations that take advantage of the regular structure of the network in Figure 12.11 to achieve greater practical efficiency. This may be particularly useful for parallel implementations of the algorithm.

Acknowledgements

This material is based upon work supported by the National Science Foundation under Grant No IIS-0222516 and by a research gift from Science Applications International Corporation (SAIC). Any opinions, findings, conclusions or recomendations expressed in this material are those of the author and do not necessarily reflect the views of the National Science Foundation (NSF) or of SAIC.

References

Arnold, R. D. and Binford, T. O. (1980). Geometric constraints in stereo vision. *Technical report, Computer Science Department, Stanford University*.

Belhumeur, P. N. and Mumford, D. (1992). A Bayesian treatment of the stereo correspondence problem using half-occluded regions. *Proc. IEEE CVPR*, pp. 506–512.

Birchfield, S. and Tomasi, C. (1998). Depth discontinuities by pixel-to-pixel stereo. *Proc. ICCV*, Bombay, India, pp. 1073–1080.

Birchfield, S. and Tomasi, C. (1999). Multiway cut for stereo and motion with slanted surfaces. *Proc. ICCV*, Kerkyra, Greece, pp. 489–495.

Buehler, C., Gortler, S. J., Cohen, M. F. and McMillan, L. (2002). Minimal surfaces for stereo. *Proc. ECCV*, Vol. 3, pp. 885–899.

Canny, J. (1986). A computational approach to edge detection. *IEEE PAMI*, **8**, 679–698.

Cherkassky, B. V. and Goldberg, A. V. (1997). On implementing the push–relabel method for the maximum flow problem. *Algorithmica*, **19**, 390–410.

Cox, I. J., Hingorani, S. L., Rao, S. B. and Maggs, B. M. (1996). A maximum likelihood stereo algorithm. *CVIU*, **63**, 542–567.

Ford, Jr., L. R. and Fulkerson, D. R. (1962). *Flows in Networks*. Princeton: Princeton University Press.

Goldberg, A. V. and Tarjan, R. E. (1988). A new approach to the maximum-flow problem. *J. Assoc. Comput. Mach.*, **35**, 921–940.

Hannah, M. J. (1974). *Computer matching of areas in stereo imagery*. PhD thesis, Computer Science Department, Stanford University, Stanford, CA.

Ishikawa, H. and Geiger, D. (1998). Occlusions, discontinuities, and epipolar lines in stereo. *Proc. ECCV*, **1**, pp. 232–249.

Kanade, T. (1994). Development of a video-rate stereo machine. *Proc. ARPA Image Understanding Workshop*, Monterey, CA, pp. 549–557.

Kim, J., Kolmogorov, V. and Zabih, R. (2003). Visual correspondence using energy minimization and mutual information. *Proc. ICCV*, pp. 1033–1040.

Kolmogorov, V. and Zabih, R. (2001). Computing visual correspondence with occlusions using graph cuts. *Proc. ICCV*, pp. 508–515.

Konolige, K. (1997). Small vision systems: hardware and implementation. *Proc. Eighth Int. Symp. Robot. Res.*, pp. 111–116.

Lin, M. H. and Tomasi, C. (2004). Surfaces with occlusions from layered stereo. *IEEE PAMI*, 26: 1073–1078.

Marr, D. (1974). A note on the computation of binocular disparity in a symbolic, low-level visual processor. *Technical Report 327, MIT A.I. Lab.*, Cambridge, MA.

Ohta, Y. and Takeo, T. (1985). Stereo by intra- and inter-scanline search using dynamic programming. *IEEE PAMI*, **7**, 139–154.

Point Grey. The Digiclops stereo vision camera system. http://www.ptgrey.com.

Roy, S. (1999). Stereo without epipolar lines: a maximum-flow fomulation. *Int. J. Comp. Vis.*, **34**, 147–161,

Roy, S. and Cox, I. (1998). A maximum-flow formulation of the N-camera stereo correspondence problem. *Proc. ICCV*, pp. 492–499.

Scharstein, D. and Szeliski, R. (2002). A taxonomy and evaluation of dense two-frame stereo correspondence algorithms. *Int. J. Comp. Vis.*, **47**, 7–42. See also www.middlebury.edu/stereo.

Sun, J., Zheng, N. N. and Shum, H. Y. (2003). Stereo matching using belief propagation. *IEEE PAMI*, **25**, 787–800.

Trucco, E. and Verri, A. (1998). *Introductory techniques for 3-D computer vision.* Upper Saddle River, NJ: Prentice Hall.

Van Meerbergen, G., Vergauwen, M., Pollefeys, M. and van Gool, L. (2002). A hierarchical symmetric stereo algorithm using dynamic programming. *Int. J. Comp. Vis.*, **47**, 275–285.

Veksler, O., Boykov, Y. and Zabih, R. (1999). Fast approximate energy minimization via graph cuts. *Proc. ICCV*, pp. 377–384.

Woodfill, J., Gordon, G. and Buck. R. (2004). Tyzx DeepSea high speed stereo vision system. *Proc. IEEE Workshop on Real Time 3-D Sensors and their use, CVPR*, Washington, DC.

13 Computational analysis of binocular half occlusions

Mikhail Sizintsev and
Richard P. Wildes

13.1 Introduction

13.1.1 Motivation

Spatially displaced views of the world support the recovery of the 3D geometry of an imaged scene. Of possible viewing configurations, binocular imaging has been a particularly well researched situation as it provides the minimal multiview situation. Further, since binocular imaging reflects biological design, there is potential for cross fertilization between research in artificial and natural binocular stereo.

Significant strides have been made in the investigation of artificial (Brown *et al.*, 2003; Scharstein and Szeliski, 2002) as well as natural (Howard and Rogers, 2002) binocular stereo. Still, outstanding problems persist. From a computational point of view areas of particular concern include poor speed-accuracy trade-offs, reliance on precise a priori calibration and poor reconstruction in the vicinity of 3D object boundaries. In this chapter, the concern is with improving reconstruction in the vicinity of 3D object boundaries. While humans appear to be able to make precise depth estimates in such situations (Howard and Rogers, 2002), artificial systems are not capable of similar performance (Brown *et al.*, 2003; Scharstein and Szeliski, 2002). Improved computational analysis of reconstruction near 3D object boundaries will shed light on how natural systems operate and also make 3D information practical for a variety of artificial vision system applications, e.g., precision robot manipulation, shape-based recognition and new view synthesis. A valuable source of information about 3D boundaries is provided by half occlusion, where one view in a pair sees surface features that are occluded to the other view, see Figure 13.1. Half occlusion usually occurs around object boundaries and other 3D scene discontinuities. As such, these points have great

Computational Vision in Neural and Machine Systems, ed. L. Harris and M. Jenkin. Published by Cambridge University Press. © Cambridge University Press 2007.

potential to aid in accurate reconstruction near 3D boundaries.

As early as Euclid, the basic geometric relationship that gives rise to half cclusion was documented (Burton, 1945). Further, the potential perceptual significance of binocular half occlusion has been known at least since the time of Leonardo Da Vinci (Richter, 1977). Much more recently, the fact that humans actually do exploit half occlusions in making depth inferences was documented (Lawson and Mount, 1967). Subsequently, a great number of psychophysical studies of half occlusion have supported their use by humans (see, e.g., Howard and Rogers, 2002, for review); however, the enabling computations remain unclear.

To forward understanding of half occlusions, this chapter presents research that distills their analysis and detection from other aspects of binocular stereo. That is, constraints are isolated that are indicative of half occlusions, while making only generic assumptions about other aspects of the problem, e.g. calibration, correspondence and reconstruction. The two constraints of study concern the change of disparity across a region of half occlusion and the expected quality of match within a region of half occlusion. It is argued that these two constraints are complementary and their spatial conjunction is highly indicative of half occlusion. Moreover, they encompass information that has been exploited across a significant number of previous approaches, that variously consider measurements of disparity gradient and poor match quality as indicative of half occlusion. The practical efficacy of the combined constraints for half occlusion detection is illustrated via post-processing applied to the output of a simple area-based stereo matcher, as it allows the utility of the constraints to be studied apart from other aspects of binocular stereo and facilitates comparison to a recent empirical study of half occlusion detection methods (Egnal and Wildes, 2002). More generally, however, the constraints could be employed within other approaches to binocular analysis, e.g., as an integral component of local or global correspondence algorithms.

13.1.2   Related research

Early work on computational stereo ignored half occlusion or treated it as noise in the matching process (Barnard and Fischler, 1982). Subsequently, a number of approaches to dealing with half occlusions have emerged (see, e.g., Brown *et al.*, 2003; Egnal and Wildes, 2002, for reviews and empirical comparison). Significantly, empirical comparison suggest that none of the compared approaches reliably identify the majority of half occlusions while keeping false positives modest and no one approach is superior to the others.

Several more recent contributions to the literature of half occlusions can be noted. The use of adaptive spatial support for match windows can ameliorate issues arising in attempts to match half occluded regions by shaping windows to avoid poorly defined matches (Kanade and Okutokmi, 1994); recent extensions increase the accuracy and efficiency of such processing (Fusiello and Roberto, 1997; Hirschmuller *et al.*, 2002; Veksler, 2003). Further, with more than two views, such adaptive processing can define which scene points are visible to which views (Kang *et al.*, 2001; Okutomi *et al.*, 2002). Other recent additions to the literature are based on the expected behavior of disparity gradient in the vicinity of half occlusions (Grammalidis and Strintzis, 1998;

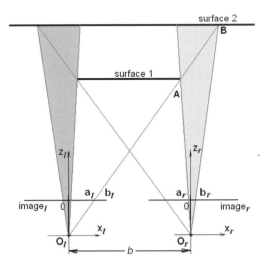

Figure 13.1. Geometry of binocular half occlusion. Interposition of surface 1 between surface 2 and the images causes portions of surface 2 that intersect the shaded regions to be visible to only one of the two views, i.e. half occluded.

Hirschmuller *et al.*, 2002; Ishikawa and Geiger, 1998; Sun *et al.*, 2005), for example the fact that occlusions in a left-based disparity map correspond to occluded regions in the right-based disparity map and vice versa (the "occlusion constraint"). The importance of disparity gradient as a constraint on allowable stereo matches has been known for some time (see Burt and Julesz, 1980; Pollard *et al.*, 1985); however, its specific interpretation in terms of half occlusion is relatively recent. Yet another approach rejects matches that are ambigous (in having rival candidates of similar cost) to diagnose occlusion (Sara, 2002). Occlusion detection also has been bolstered by constraining occlusion boundaries to align with those of uniform color segments (Deng *et al.*, 2005). Another recent addition to the literature involves interleaved processes of layered disparity estimation and assignment to layers, with the option of pixel assignment to no layer, so that half occlusions are dealt with as assignment outliers (Lin and Tomasi, 2004). Interleaved calculation of correspondences and occlusions also has been cast within an expectation maximization framework (Dempster *et al.*, 1977), with high cost matches rejected as arising from occlusion (Strecha *et al.*, 2004). Finally, previous Bayesian approaches to binocular stereo have been documented (see Belhumeur, 1996; Geiger *et al.*, 1995; Read, 2002; Strecha *et al.*, 2004), which to varying degrees have dealt explicitly with half occlusions.

In the light of previous efforts, the major contributions of the present research are as follows. (i) A novel, complementary combination of constraints for binocular half occlusion detection is presented. The constraints arise from consideration of disparity change and match score in the vicinity of half occlusions. While previous research has considered instances of both types of constraint for half occlusion detection, the current work appears to be the first to recognize explicitly their complementarity to yield a combined approach. (ii) The isolated constraints are embodied in a Bayesian estimation framework, which has been implemented in software with qualitative and quantitative evaluation on a standard set of seven binocular test sets. The results show that, where direct comparison is possible, the developed method outperforms all others presented in a recent empirical comparison of half occlusion detection methods (Egnal and Wildes, 2002).

13.1.3   Chapter outline

Section 13.1 of this chapter has served to establish motivation for the study of binocular half occlusion and place the work in the context of previous research. Section 13.2 will detail the technical approach that has been developed for half occlusion analysis and recovery. Section 13.3 will document empirical evaluation of the developed approach. Finally, Section 13.4 will provide a brief summary and conclusions.

13.2   Technical approach

13.2.1   Overview

In this section of the chapter the developed approach to binocular half occlusion detection is delineated. The presentation begins by isolating two constraints that, when taken in tandem, tend to be highly indicative of half occlusions. The first constraint comes in terms of an analytic relationship between the difference in disparities on either side of a half occluded region and the region width. The second constraint stems from the observation that a region that is visible to one view but occluded to the other view has no physically defined match; hence, any attempted match is likely to have a poor match score (e.g., low correlation value). To deal in a principled fashion with uncertainties and the combination of the isolated constraints, half occlusion inference is cast in a Bayesian formulation to yield a probabilistic approach to detection. The section culminates by presenting the details of the resulting estimation procedure that, given disparity and match score maps that result from binocular image matching, produces a map of probability of half occlusion.

13.2.2   Image formation

The operative geometric model of image formation is expressed in terms of Figure 13.1, which shows a top down view of parallel axis (or otherwise rectified) binocular images formed under perspective projection with, e.g., left and right Euclidean coordinate systems defined at the centers of projection, O_l and O_r (respectively), and separated by baseline, b. The Z-axes are taken parallel to the optical axes and increasing toward the orthogonal image planes, located at distance $f = 1$ along these axes. X-axes are parallel to the stereo baseline, increasing to the right and Y-axes are mutually orthogonal to the X and Z axes to yield right handed systems. Let world points be given as $\mathbf{A} = (X, Y, Z)$ and subscripts l and r used to reference points to the left and right coordinates systems, respectively, e.g. $\mathbf{A}_l$ references $\mathbf{A}$ to the left system. Image coordinates are similarly denoted using lower case letters; further, since ensuing developments concentrate on relationships along horizontal scan lines, image coordinates will be restricted correspondingly, so that perspective yields, e.g., $\mathbf{a}_l = X_l/Z_l$ as the left image coordinate of $\mathbf{A}$. Given the binocular imaging model, the right image coordinate for $\mathbf{A}$ is given as $\mathbf{a}_r = X_r/Z_r = (X_l - b)/Z_l$. Correspondingly, disparity (right-based) is given as

$$d_r(\mathbf{A}) = \mathbf{a}_l - \mathbf{a}_r = \frac{b}{Z}. \tag{13.1}$$

Notice that for surfaces of constant Z (fronto-parallel surfaces) disparity is constant.

13.2.3 Constraints

Two sources of constraint for half occlusion detection are considered, which will be shown to be complementary in nature. The first constraint relates disparities that arise from the binocularly visible parts of the surfaces that border the half occluded region. The second constraint is concerned with a property of the half occluded region itself.

The first constraint comes in terms of an analytic relationship between the difference in disparity on either side of a half occluded region and the region width. This relationship can be derived with reference to the geometry illustrated in Figure 13.1. With respect to the right image, consider the shaded region on the right side of the figure and let world point $\mathbf{A}$ be the left-most point that is binocularly visible, while the world point $\mathbf{B}$ is the right-most half occluded point (visible only to the right image). The width of the half occluded region projected to the right image is given as

$$\Omega_r^w(\mathbf{B}, \mathbf{A}) = \mathbf{b}_r - \mathbf{a}_r. \tag{13.2}$$

The disparity values for points $\mathbf{A}$ and $\mathbf{B}$ are

$$\begin{aligned}
d_r(\mathbf{A}) &= \mathbf{a}_l - \mathbf{a}_r \\
d_r(\mathbf{B}) &= \mathbf{b}_l - \mathbf{b}_r \\
&= \mathbf{a}_l - \mathbf{b}_r,
\end{aligned}$$

with $\mathbf{b}_l = \mathbf{a}_l$ because $\mathbf{A}$ and $\mathbf{B}$ lie along the same line through O_l, the left optical center, by construction. Correspondingly, the change in disparity across the half occluded region is given as

$$\begin{aligned}
\Delta d_r(\mathbf{B}, \mathbf{A}) &= d_r(\mathbf{B}) - d_r(\mathbf{A}) \\
&= \mathbf{a}_l - \mathbf{b}_r - (\mathbf{a}_l - \mathbf{a}_r) \\
&= \mathbf{a}_r - \mathbf{b}_r \tag{13.3}
\end{aligned}$$

Now, taking the ratio of disparity change (13.3) to occlusion width (13.2) it is found that

$$\frac{\Delta d_r(\mathbf{B}, \mathbf{A})}{\Omega_r^w(\mathbf{B}, \mathbf{A})} = \frac{\mathbf{a}_r - \mathbf{b}_r}{\mathbf{b}_r - \mathbf{a}_r} = -1. \tag{13.4}$$

Interestingly, it is seen that this ratio is equal to the disparity gradient limit (Burt and Julesz, 1980). Further consideration of the geometry illustrated in Figure 13.1 shows that relationship (13.4) between disparity change and occlusion width also holds for regions visible only to the left view of a binocular pair. In the following, (13.4) will be referred to as the *disparity-change/width constraint* (see, Grammalidis and Strintzis, (1998), where this constraint is used, albeit differently, to define legal state transitions for dynamic programming disparity estimation).[1]

The second constraint utilized for half occlusion detection is based on the observation that, by definition, a region of half occlusion, e.g. as delimited by $\mathbf{A}_+$ and $\mathbf{B}$ in Figure 13.1, projects to only one of the two images in a pair. Therefore, in attempting to match points, x, in a region visible to one image only, (e.g. the region spanned by $\mathbf{a}_{r+}$ and $\mathbf{b}_r$), the match goodness resulting from match score, $\rho(x)$, is expected to be poor, since there is no physically defined match, i.e.

$$\rho(x \in \mathcal{R} = occl) \in \{poor\ match\ scores\}, \tag{13.5}$$

with $\mathcal{R} = occl$ symbolizing that a region, $\mathcal{R}$, is half occluded and $\{poor\ match\ scores\}$ match scores indicative of poor performance for a given matcher. In the following, this constraint will be referred to as the *poor match constraint* and will be used in tandem with the disparity-change/width constraint to detect half occlusions.

Prior to embedding the isolated constraints in a method for half occlusion detection, it is worth briefly noting their relationships to other approaches (see Brown *et al.*, 2003; Egnal and Wildes, 2002) for extended discussion of alternatives and note that for space reasons explicit citations in the remainder of this section focus on more recent contributions). The disparity-change/width constraint is derived by an analysis that explicitly considers both the occluding and occluded surfaces. Therefore, it is most closely related to other approaches that consider the disparities of both occluded and occluder. The "occlusion constraint" states that a discontinuity in disparity in a right-based disparity map corresponds to a half occluded region in a left-based disparity map and vice versa (Hirschmuller *et al.*, 2002; Ishikawa and Geiger, 1998). In comparison, the disparity-change/width constraint is more precise than the occlusion constraint in that it gives a particular relationship between disparity change and occlusion region width; furthermore, it is defined with respect to one view only, which may make it more natural to exploit without performing two-way matching.

The "ordering constraint" also considers disparity of occluder and occluded, as it imposes strict ordering of matched points in left and right images (essential to dynamic programming-based matchers, see Criminisi *et al.*, 2003) and as a result can disallow matching in half occlusion regions. However, ordering can be violated in physically realizable view conditions (e.g. involving thin objects) (Krol and van der Grind, 1980), in particular, in situations that do not involve half occlusion. With respect to any given point in a binocularly viewed scene, the "forbidden zone" is that which contains points that will appear as violations of the ordering constraint (Krol and van der Grind, 1982), e.g. the zone bounded by lines through $\mathbf{A}, \mathbf{a}_l$ and $\mathbf{A}, \mathbf{a}_r$ in Figure 13.1. The loci of points that yield the value of -1 for the disparity gradient lie along a boundary of the forbidden zone (Yulle and Poggio, 1984), e.g., the line through

---

[1]While definition of the disparity-change/width constraint appeals to the disparity of a half occluded point, e.g. $\mathbf{B}$, this should not pose a problem in practice: Let subscript $+$ applied to a point refer to a point immediately to the right, e.g. $\mathbf{B}_+$ refers to the point immediately to the right of $\mathbf{B}$. If the surface about $\mathbf{B}$ is taken as locally fronto-parallel, then its disparity is constant in that local region and can be estimated from, e.g. $\mathbf{B}_+$, which by definition is binocularly visible.

A, a_l (and hence **B**). The disparity-change/width constraint captures a subset of a foreground point's (e.g. **A**'s) forbidden zone as delimited by a background point (e.g. **B**) that lies along the foreground point's forbidden zone boundary, e.g. that portion of the forbidden zone that intersects the region bounded by lines through **A**, a_r and **B**, b_r, i.e., that portion relevant to labeling the interval $[a_{r+}, b_r]$ as half occluded. While the disparity-change/width constraint and disparity gradient limit share the same critical value, -1, for developments in this paper the disparity-change/width formulation and nomenclature are better suited as they provide an explicit link to occlusion width, which is exploited in detection.

Other approaches that explicitly consider both surfaces involved in half occlusion are "bimodality tests," which rely on the observation that histogrammed disparity in the vicinity of half occlusions can show bimodal distributions as both foreground and background surfaces are captured. Again, the disparity-change/width constraint is tighter, explicitly stating the relationship between disparity values of the surfaces which are covered by the aggregation window.

The poor match constraint arises from consideration of expected match score within a half occluded region. Previously, such consideration has been used in half occlusion detection in two ways. (i) Unidirectionally defined (e.g. right-to-left) match scores are examined for patterns indicative of match failure; in some cases patterns of interest involve rapid change in match score. Some global match methods (e.g. dynamic programming, graph cut; Brown *et al.*, (2003) and Scharstein and Szeliski (2002)), make use of match scores to set occlusion cost. A recent cooperative matcher (Ztinick and Kanade (2000), an extension of Marr and Poggio (1976)) also uses poor matches to filter out half occlusions (as well as other matching errors). Poor matches defined by color differences at aligned image locations also have been used to diagnose half occlusion (Strecha *et al.*, 2004). The poor match constraint is an instance of this type of approach as it simply looks for locally bad matches. (ii) Inconsistencies between bidirectional matches are detected, i.e., "left-right checking", a method that requires two matching processes and therefore more expensive that unidirectional approaches. While both approaches can detect half occlusions, they are not specific to this situation; rather, they more generally diagnose problems in matching (e.g. arising from various sources of noise).

Significantly, the two broad classes of approach to half occlusion detection discussed in the previous paragraphs are complementary: Methods based on analysis of half occlusion geometry predict the relationship between disparities that arise on either side of a half occluded region; whereas, methods based on considerations of match quality predict what is expected within a region of half occlusion. From this perspective, the present work encompasses a wide range of approaches (including all five compared in Egnal and Wildes, (2002)), even as it yields a method that is more specific to half occlusion than other approaches, which often are more generally aimed at diagnosing errors in matching. In the following these observations will be exploited to yield a method for half occlusion detection that relies on a particular pattern of disparity across a region (as given by the disparity-change/width constraint, since it is particularly tight) as well as analysis of match scores in the intervening region (observation of the poor match constraint, owing to its simple, yet proven to be effective nature).

13.2.4 Bayesian formulation

To deal rigorously with uncertainties in inference, the disparity-change/width (13.4) and poor match (13.5) constraints are cast in a Bayesian framework. Let $\mathcal{R}$ be a region of interest, moving left-to-right along a scan-line, defined within the interval $[x_1, x_2]$. Let $\mathbf{D} = (D_\Delta, D_\rho)$ be a data vector, comprised of two terms, where D_Δ provides data relevant to the disparity-change/width cue (13.4) and D_ρ provides data relevant to the poor match queue (13.5).

Let x_{1-} and x_{2+} stand for points immediately to the left and right (respectively) of $\mathcal{R}$ and d_{1-}, d_{2+} be the associated disparities, then D_Δ is given as

$$D_\Delta = (d_{2+} - d_{1-})/(x_{2+} - x_{1-}) \qquad (13.6)$$

(see the disparity-change/width constraint (13.4)). Here D_ρ is given as the set of match scores for each point in the region of concern

$$D_\rho = \{\rho(x) : x_1 \leq x \leq x_2\}. \qquad (13.7)$$

The posterior probability, P, of some region $\mathcal{R}$ being half occluded, $\mathcal{R} = occl$, given data, $\mathbf{D}$, is expressed via Bayes rule (Leonard and Hsu, 1999) as

$$P(\mathcal{R} = occl \mid \mathbf{D}) = \frac{P(\mathbf{D} \mid \mathcal{R} = occl) P(\mathcal{R} = occl)}{P(\mathbf{D})} \qquad (13.8)$$

with evidence calculated according to

$$P(\mathbf{D}) = P(\mathbf{D} \mid \mathcal{R} = occl) P(\mathcal{R} = occl) + P(\mathbf{D} \mid \mathcal{R} = vis) P(\mathcal{R} = vis) \qquad (13.9)$$

where $\mathcal{R} = vis$ stands for the region $\mathcal{R}$ being visible to both views (as opposed to half occluded).

The likelihood $P(\mathbf{D} \mid \mathcal{R} = occl)$ depends on both terms of the data vector $\mathbf{D}$. For present purposes, these two terms are taken as independent. This assumption is justified by the observation that spatial change in disparity and match score can vary independently of one another. Empirically, the assumption is supported by the test data used in Section 13.3. Correlation coefficients between disparity gradient and match score goodness data have values of -0.09 and -0.04 for occluded and visible regions, respectively. Under the independence assumption, the likelihood of a region being occluded is

$$P(\mathbf{D} \mid \mathcal{R} = occl) = P(D_\Delta \mid \mathcal{R}) = occl) P(D_\rho \mid \mathcal{R} = occl). \qquad (13.10)$$

Similarly, the likelihood of a region being visible is

$$P(\mathbf{D} \mid \mathcal{R} = vis) = P(D_\Delta \mid \mathcal{R} = vis) P(D_\rho \mid \mathcal{R} = vis). \qquad (13.11)$$

The Bayesian formulation has led to the introduction of various distributions that must be instantiated for inference to ensue in practice. Based on the disparity-change/width constraint (13.4), the expected value of the ratio of disparity change to width across which change is calculated is -1 for regions of half occlusion. In contrast, if surfaces are assumed to be locally fronto-parallel (an implicit assumption of standard area-based stereo matchers), then the locally expected value for a binocularly visible region is 0. In either case, noise in disparity estimation will lead to values both larger and smaller than the expected values, with the possibility that values further away from those expected are less likely to be encountered. Based on these observations, the likelihood of a region being half occluded based on the disparity-change/width constraint, $P(D_\Delta|\mathcal{R} = occl)$, has been modeled as a normal distribution (Hoel, 1984), with a mean of -1 and variance estimated from a subset of data used in the empirical validation of the overall approach (see Section 13.3). Similarly, $P(D_\Delta|\mathcal{R} = vis)$, also is modeled as a normal distribution, but with a mean of 0 and variance estimated from a subset of data used in the empirical validation of the overall approach.

The validity of the normal distribution model fits to $P(D_\Delta|\mathcal{R} = occl)$ and $P(D_\Delta|\mathcal{R} = vis)$ was evaluated via the χ^2 goodness-of-fit test (Hoel, 1984), which suggests that the observed data sets do not differ significantly from the normal distribution fits.

Based on the poor match constraint (13.5), two additional distributions must be instantiated to realize the Bayes formulation, the probability of match score given that a region is (half) occluded, $P(D_\rho|\mathcal{R} = occl)$, and the probability of match score given that a region is (binocularly) visible, $P(D_\rho|\mathcal{R} = vis)$. To evaluate these distributions, the individual match scores, $\rho(x)$, comprising D_ρ, (13.7), are taken as independent, based on the local winner-take-all nature of the matching technique used in empirical evaluation (Section 13.3), which does not explicitly enforce relationships (e.g. smoothness) between nearby matches. Under independence alone, the likelihood of a region being half occluded based on match scores would be the product of likelihoods of each pixel in the region being half occluded. However, some weighting of the product is appropriate in the present context as different sized regions will contribute sets of match scores, D_ρ, of different cardinality. Without weighting, larger regions would have effectively more match score likelihood terms, which would lower the relative weight of the disparity-change/width cue. In this respect, the product of w likelihood terms can be weighted by taking its w-root to yield the geometric mean of the D_ρ components, leading to

$$P(D_\rho|\mathcal{R} = occl) = \sqrt[w]{\prod_{x \in \mathcal{R}} P(\rho(x)|x = occl)}, \qquad (13.12)$$

with w the width of region $\mathcal{R}$. Similar reasoning yields an analogous definition for $P(D_\rho|\mathcal{R} = vis)$.

To instantiate the distributions of $P(\rho(x)|x = occl)$ and $P(\rho(x)|x = vis)$ the particular metric used to produce the match scores, $\rho(x)$, must be considered. For empirical evaluation (Section 13.3), an SAD match metric (Brown *et al.*, 2003; Trucco and Verri, 1998) is used

$$match_{SAD}(d; x) = \Sigma_{x \in W}|I_r(x) - I_l(x + d)| \qquad (13.13)$$

which evaluates th cost of associating disparity, d, with location, x, in the right image, I_r, with location $x + d$ in the left image, I_l, and W the match window support. For simple cases where surface patches in the world yield the same image intensity patterns to two views (excepting shift by disparity, d), the expected SAD match score is 0, with a systematic bias (e.g. photometric difference between the images) yielding some off-set. In either case, noise in image formation and/or the matching process will perturb match scores from the expected value, with larger perturbations less likely than smaller. So, ignoring the effects of the absolute value, one might consider a normal distribution to model match scores. Applying the absolute value remaps differences yielding negative values by reflecting them about zero, back to positive values, i.e. letting I denote images, $\forall m = I_r(x) - I_l(x + d) < 0, m \mapsto -m$. Correspondingly, the distribution for probability of match score (SAD), given that a pixel is (binocularly) visible, $P(D_\rho|\mathcal{R} = vis)$, or half occluded, $P(D_\rho|\mathcal{R} = occl)$, is modeled as a "mirrored-about-zero-normal" distribution, i.e., as normal, but with negative valued observations reflected back along the positive axis

$$P(\rho) = \begin{cases} (\sqrt{2\pi}\sigma)^{-1} \left(e^{-\frac{1}{2}\left(\frac{\rho-\mu}{\sigma}\right)^2} + e^{-\frac{1}{2}\left(\frac{-\rho-\mu}{\sigma}\right)^2} \right); \rho > 0 \\ (\sqrt{2\pi}\sigma)^{-1} e^{-\frac{1}{2}\left(\frac{-\mu}{\sigma}\right)^2}; \rho = 0 \\ 0; \rho < 0 \end{cases} \qquad (13.14)$$

with μ and σ the mean and standard deviation of the underlying normal distribution.

Separate parameters sets (μ, σ) for fits to (13.14) for $P(\rho(x)|x = occl)$ and $P(\rho(x)|x = vis)$ were estimated from a subset of test data of Section 13.3. As before, the validity of these model fits was evaluated through the χ^2 goodness-of-fit test, which suggests that the observed data sets do not differ significantly from the mirrored-normal distribution fits (probability > 0.95 that rejection of the null hypothesis would be in error, with the null hypothesis now being that the data are mirror-normally distributed).[2]

Finally, it is difficult to analytically define priors for a region being half occluded, $P(\mathcal{R} = occl)$, and a region being binocularly visible, $P(\mathcal{R} = vis)$. For present purposes, these have been defined empirically, based on the ground-truth associated with a subset of the test data used in Section 13.3, to yield $P(\mathcal{R} = occl) = 0.08$ and $P(\mathcal{R} = vis) = 0.92$ with standard error of 0.03 between different ground-truth images.

13.2.5   Estimation

Having observed data $\mathbf{D} = (D_\Delta, D_\rho)$ for a region $\mathcal{R}$, it is straightforward to evaluate the probability that the region is half occluded $P(\mathcal{R} = occl \mid \mathbf{D})$ by solving the Bayes relation (13.8) with appropriate substitutions for evidence (13.9) and combined likelihoods (13.10 and 13.11) and making use of the instantiated model distributions and priors given in Section 13.2.4.

Input to the estimation process is taken to be a disparity map and an associated map of match scores, which for convenience are assumed to be rectified. Along each horizontal scan-line, the probability of half occlusion, $P(\mathcal{R} = occl \mid \mathbf{D})$, given by (13.8)

---

[2] In formulating the match score distributions it has been necessary to make a commitment to a particular matching metric, SAD. Other match metrics that avoid negative values, e.g. sum of squared differences, might yield to a similar analysis; although, formulations that deal with symmetric distributions would be more appropriate in other situations, e.g. correlation-type metrics.

is calculated for each region, $\mathcal{R}$, with widths ranging from 1 pixel to the largest magnitude disparity observed along the line. For each width of interest, the data vector, $\mathbf{D}$ is calculated by applying the formulae for its components, (13.6) and (13.7), to the disparity and match score maps, which provides the necessary fodder for calculation of $P(\mathcal{R} = occl \mid \mathbf{D})$. Any given pixel along a scan-line can be associated with a number of regions of varying widths. To make a final probability of half occlusion assignment to any given pixel, it is associated with the largest posterior probability of being half occluded out of all regions that could possibly cover it. Completion of this calculation for all pixels along a scan-line assigns a probability of occlusion to each pixel. Iteration across scan-lines yields a map of half occlusion probability in spatial registration with the input disparity and match score maps.

13.3   Empirical evaluation

13.3.1   Methodology

To evaluate the efficacy of the combined constraints for half occlusion detection, two considerations are critical. (i) It is desirable to document the utility of the constraints independent of other aspects of stereo processing. (ii) Comparison to previous empirical evaluation of half occlusion detection methods must be supported (see Egnal and Wildes, 2002).[3] For both reasons the current approach is evaluated in terms of postprocessing on disparity and match-score maps recovered via a simple area-based stereo matcher. Use of a simple matcher forces half occlusion detection to deal with a range of difficult situations (e.g., foreground fattening, poorly resolved thin structures, mismatches in low texture, etc). Post-processing allows for clear separation of the effects of the half occlusion constraints from other aspects of stereo processing. Moreover, this methodology matches that of Egnal and Wildes (2002), which makes direct comparison possible. While operation in conjunction with a more sophisticated matcher or as a more integral component of a matcher has potential to yield better results (suggesting interesting future directions), such options are less well suited to the goal of understanding the current approach in comparison to others and with independence from other aspects of stereo processing.

Two classes of test data have been used to evaluate an algorithmic instantiation of the half occlusion probability estimation procedure described below. First, a set of laboratory images with associated ground truth is used to allow for quantitative evaluation. Second, a set of natural, outdoor images is used to allow for evaluation of performance in more realistic scenes, albeit without quantitative analysis as ground truth is not available. The laboratory images are selected from the Middlebury test suite (Middlebury College, 2005). For these cases, ground truth half occlusion was constructed by labeling any unmatched pixel according to the ground truth disparity as a half occlusion. The particular data sets used were *Tsukuba*, *Map*, *Venus* and *Sawtooth* (as they were used in previous empirical comparisons) (see Egnal and Wildes, 2002;

---

[3]Results reported in conjunction with the Middlebury test suite (Middlebury College, 2005; Scharstein and Szeliski, 2002) are not directly comparable as they do not show results for half occlusion detection per se; they focus on disparity.

Scharstein and Szeliski, 2002) and *Cones* (as it provides greater scene complexity). Natural outdoor images selected were *Pentagon* (Carnegie Mellon University, 2004) and *Flower Garden* (Brown University, 2004) as they are standard and provide very different viewing scenarios, aerial and terrestrial, respectively.

For the majority of test cases, tests are performed with input disparity and match-score maps recovered by an area-based matching algorithm (Trucco and Verri, 1998) using the SAD match metric (13.13), fixed squared aggregation windows (7×7), winner-take-all and operating in a hierarchical, coarse-to-fine framework (Quam, 1984) using Gaussian pyramids (Jahne, 1993). During half occlusion evaluation, one set of matching parameters was used across the entire test suite (hand selected to yield good overall performance), except for search range, which was set to the maximum disparity present for each test case. The exception to these specifications is *Tsukuba*: To facilitate direct comparison with previous results (Egnal and Wildes, 2002), the correlation and plane-plus-parallax-based disparity and match score maps (and ground truth half occlusion) used in the previous study were employed (courtesy of G. Egnal). In all cases, the recovered disparity and match score maps are input to the half occlusion detection procedure, as described in Section 2.5. Currently, algorithmic instantiation in software produces a half occlusion map for 384×288 images in approximately 1 second, running in unoptimized C under Linux on a Xeon 3.06GHz processor with 1MB cache. Only right-based results are reported for reasons of space; left-based results are similar.

13.3.2   Results

For laboratory scenes (Figures 13.2 and 13.4), the algorithm generally gives consistently good qualitative results. Both wide and narrow half occlusion regions are detected; although, localization can be imprecise due to disparity errors near object boundaries – a known weakness of area-based matchers (Brown *et al.*, 2003; Scharstein and Szeliski, 2002).

Quantitative analysis derives from comparison of the obtained occlusion maps to ground truth. Results are presented as ROC plots, percentage of hits and false positives (relative to the entire image) along the ordinate and responses along the abscissa. It is found that the vast majority of true half occlusions can be detected while keeping the false positive rate in the $10\% - 20\%$ range. While current state-of-the-art stereo matchers can yield impressive performance in the vicinity of 3D boundaries (Scharstein and Szeliski, 2002), these methods make use of constraints and heuristics beyond those embodied in the matcher used in the current study. With respect to a comparable matcher (Egnal and Wildes, 2002), all half occlusion detection methods considered yielded a higher rate of false positives for similar hit rates. Also of note, performance is reasonably stable to variation in algorithm parameters, e.g. even extremes of changing half occlusion and visible priors to equiprobable and changing match window size by a factor of two yield less than 2% change in the areas under the ROCs.

The relative contributions of the disparity-change/width and poor match score constraints are shown in Figure 13.3 using *Tsukuba*. While both constraints are seen to be preferentially indicative of half occlusion, individually they yield lower hit-to-false-positive ratios than their combination, with poor match score alone being the worst in this regard. Inspection of the probability maps shows that the false signals from one constraint tend not to correspond to those in the other; whereas hits do tend to correspond. Hence the constraints are complementary; their combination yields the best result.

For *Tsukuba*, direct comparison can be made to five standard approaches (Egnal and Wildes, 2002). Here, it is found that for both correlation-based (Figure 13.2) and plane-plus-parallax-based matching (Figure 13.4) the current approach outperforms all of the five standard approaches, as its ROC tends to the upper left of the ROCs for the alternative ones. In certain cases, the difference is dramatic, e.g., in the low false positive regions under correlation, the current method can improve on hits by as much as approximately 75% over the best previous results. The closest rival appears to be the occlusion constraint under plane-plus-parallax matching; although even here the current methods wins out beyond approximately 10% false positives, ultimately improving on hits by approximately 15% for a given false positive rate.

Outdoor scene testing also shows strong performance in the test cases considered (Figure 13.5). For *Pentagon*, the major half occlusion regions on the right side of the building's inner and outer sides are correctly located, as well as many of the interior corridors; whereas, the number of false positives is small. For *Flower Garden*, the right side of the tree and the narrow inclined bar in the background are correctly detected as half occluded. The algorithm also gives strong response, albeit poorly localized, in the vicinity of clustered tree branches and associated thin half occlusions. There are few false positives in the flower field itself, with greatest spurious signal tending to coincide with sharp disparity gradient associated with poor match score.

Overall the developed algorithm performs well in detecting half occlusions across a wide variety of scenes while keeping false positives relatively low. The apparent weakness arises in fine localization of half occluded regions: The offset from ground truth is noticeable and the width of detection regions is inexact. Also, false positives are often detected near non-half occlusion 3D boundaries. Both of these phenomena can be attributed to the fact that the area-based matcher performs poorly near 3D boundaries, resulting in poor match scores and spurious disparity gradient patterns, which mimic the utilized constraints.

13.3.3 Application

In practice the proposed method for half occlusion detection could be used as post-processing for a fast area-based method of disparity estimation, or incorporated directly into either local or global methods to find disparity and occlusion simultaneously. Here option one is demonstrated: improvement of the initial disparity produced by the SAD-based matcher in the vicinity of 3D boundaries, especially half occlusions. The originally recovered disparity map has been refined in regions that are marked as half occluded by repeating the matching process while making use of adaptively defined windows that conform in spatial support to avoid half occlusions; non-half occluded regions are not altered; results are shown in Figure 13.6. Statistics are given across all test pairs shown in Figure 13.2, with *Tsukuba* disparity maps given as a visual example. It is seen that disparity estimates in the vicinity of 3D boundaries, especially half occlusion, are improved without damaging results in other difficult areas (e.g., textureless),

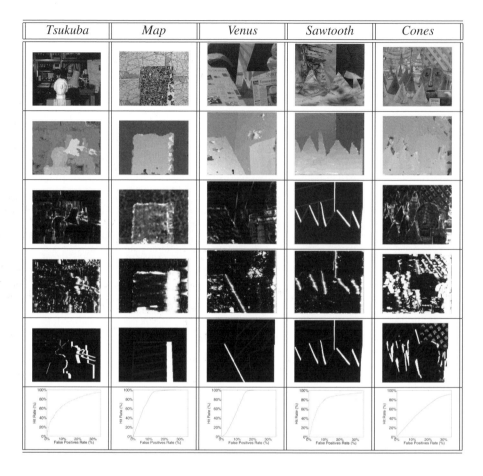

Figure 13.2. Half occlusion results for laboratory imagery with ground truth. For five stereo pairs (left-to-right) shown are left image, estimated disparity (brighter is closer), match scores (brighter is poorer), probability of half occlusion (brighter is higher), ground-truth half occluded regions (white), and detection ROC (top-to-bottom).

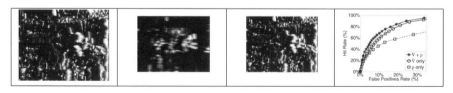

Figure 13.3. Half occlusion constraint comparison for *Tsukuba*. Shown are disparity-change/width ($\bigtriangledown$), poor match score (ρ), combination ($\bigtriangledown + \rho$, repeated from Figure 13.2) probability of half occlusion and detection ROCs (left-to-right). Input disparity and match score maps are as in Figure 13.2.

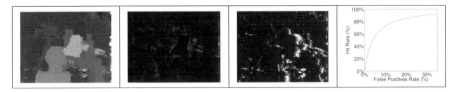

Figure 13.4. Half occlusion results for *Tsukuba* under plane-plus-parallax. Shown are disparity, match scores, probability of half occlusion and detection ROC (left-to-right). ROCs for five previous methods under Plane-Plus-Parallax can be found in Egnal and Wildes (2002).

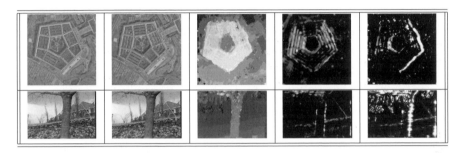

Figure 13.5. Half occlusion results for outdoor imagery. For two standard stereo pairs, *Pentagon* and *Flower Garden* (top-to-bottom), shown are left and right images, estimated disparity, associated match scores, and probability of half occlusion (left-to-right).

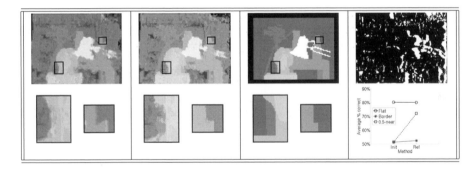

Figure 13.6. Application of detected half occlusions. Left to right: *Tsukuba* initial, refined and ground truth disparity maps; thresholded half occlusion probability, $P \geq 0.5$; comparative plot of good-pixels in textureless regions (Flat), near general 3D boundaries, i.e., discontinuities not including half occlusions (Border), and near half occlusions (0.5-near) for initial (Init) and refined (Ref) disparity maps. Percentage correct given according to standard criteria of estimated disparity being within 1 of ground truth disparity taken as a good pixel (Scharstein and Szeliski, 2002) and percentage relative to an entire image. Averages taken across all test images used in Figure 13.2. Insets highlight a few selected improvements.

as adaptive matching also operates at false positives. Improvements are most noticeable in reducing fattening of foreground objects and increased precision of boundary details. Significantly, while the utility of adaptive windows has been documented previously (Brown *et al.*, 2003; Scharstein and Szeliski, 2002), here improvement is had without the need to apply adaptive processing everywhere as effort is concentrated in regions of half occlusion.

13.4   Summary and conclusions

A novel approach to binocular half occlusion detection has been presented. The approach is based on two complementary constraints derived from binocular matching data (disparities and match scores) that arise in the vicinity of half occluded regions. The first constraint concerns disparity change across a region of half occlusion. In particular, the ratio of disparity change to width is equal to -1 in the ideal case. The second constraint concerns the expected behavior of a binocular matcher operating within a region of half occlusion. In particular, since there is no physically defined match in such regions, any recovered match is expected to have a poor match score (e.g. large SAD). To allow for uncertainty in inference, the constraints have been combined in a Bayesian formulation. To understand applicability of the approach, a corresponding algorithm for detecting half occlusions provided input maps of disparity and match score has been developed. To isolate the effects of half occlusion constraints from other aspects of stereo processing and to facilitate comparison to previous empirical studies of half occlusion analysis, the presented instantiation of the approach works as post-processing on precomputed disparities and match scores. Empirically, the algorithm yields strong performance on standard test data; indeed, performance is superior to all approaches evaluated in the most comparable study to date (Egnal and Wildes, 2002).

The computational analysis presented in this chapter can be applied in a number of ways. Application to correcting inappropriate matches near three-dimensional boundaries via disparity post-processing has been illustrated in this chapter. Alternatively, the approach could be embedded within a matching procedure, be it local or global (Brown *et al.*, 2003), to inhibit bad correspondences as they emerge. Finally, the developed computational framework can be used to guide efforts aimed at modeling the recovery of half occlusions and otherwise processing disparity information in biological systems (Wilcox *et al.*, 2005).

Acknowledgments

This reseach was supported in part by a grant jointly funded by CRESTech, the Ontario Centres for Excellence and Macdonald-Detweiller Associates, Space Missions.

References

Barnard, S. and Fischler, M. (1982). Computational stereo. *ACM Computer Surveys (CSUR)*, **14**, 553–572.

Belhumeur, P. (1996). A Bayesian approach to binocular stereopsis. *Int. J. Comp. Vis.*, **19**, 237–260.

Bolles, R., Baker, H. and Hannah, M. (1993). The JISCT stereo evaluation. *Proc. April DARPA Image Understanding Workshop*, pp. 263–274.

Brown, M., Burschka, D. and Hager, G. (2003). Advances in computational stereo. *IEEE PAMI*, **25**, 993–1008.

Brown University (2004). *Image Sequences*, http://www.cs.brown.edu/ people/black/images. html, current 2004.

Burt, P. and Julesz, B. (1980). A disparity gradient limit for binocular fusion. *Nature*, **208**, 615–617.

Burton, H. (1945). The optics of Euclid. *J. Opt. Soc. Am.*, **35**, 357–372.

Carnegie Mellon University (2004). *VASC Image Database*, http://www.vasc.ri.cmu.edu/idb, current 2004.

Criminisi, A., Shotton, J., Blake, A. and Torr, P. (2003). Gaze manipulation for one-to-one teleconferencing. *Proc. IEEE ICCV*, **2**, 191.

Dempster, A., Laird, N. and Rubin, D. (1977). Maximum likelihood from incomplete data. *J. Roy. Stat. Soc.*, B **39**, 1–38.

Deng, Y., Yang, Q., Lin, X. and Tang, X. (2005). A symmetric patch-based correspondence model for occlusion handling. *Proc. ICCV*.

Egnal, G. and Wildes, R. (2002). Detecting binocular half-occlusions: empirical comparisons of five approaches. *IEEE PAMI*, **24**, 1127–1133.

Fusiello, A. and Roberto, V. (1997). Efficient stereo with multiple windowing. *Proc. IEEE CVPR*, pp. 885–863.

Geiger, D., Ladendorf, B. and Yuille, A. (1995). Occlusion and binocular stereo. *Int. J. Comp. Vis.*, **14**, 211–226.

Grammalidis, N. and Strintzis, M. (1998). Disparity and occlusion estimation and their coding for the communication of multiview image sequences. *IEEE Trans. Circuits Sys. for Video Tech.*, **8**, 328–344.

Hirschmuller, H., Innocent, P. and Garibaldi, J. (2002). Real-time correlation-based stereo vision with reduced border errors. *Int. J. Comp. Vis.*, **47**, 229–246.

Hoel, P. (1984). *Introduction to Mathematical Statistics (Fifth Edition)*. John Wiley and Sons. Toronto, Ontario.

Howard, I. and Rogers, B. (2002). *Seeing in Depth. 1*. Thornhill, Ontario: Porteous Press.

Ishikawa, H. and Geiger, D. (1998). Occlusions, discontinuities and epipolar lines in stereo. *Lecture Notes in Computer Science*, **1406**, 232–248; Proc. ECCV pp. 1–14.

Jahne, B. (1993). *Digital Image Processing: Concepts, Algorithms and Scientific Applications*. Berlin: Springer-Verlag.

Kanade, T. and Okutomi, M. (1994). A stereo matching algorithm with an adaptive window: theory and experiment. *IEEE PAMI*, **16**, 920–932.

Kang, S., Szeliski, R. and Chai, J. (2001). Handling occlusions in dense multi-view stereo. *Proc. IEEE CVPR*, pp. 103–110.

Krol, J. D. and van der Grind, W. A. (1980). The double nail illusion. *Percept.*, **9**, 651–659.

Krol, J. D. and van der Grind, W. A. (1982). Rehabilitation of a classical notion of Panum's fusional area. *Percept.*, **11**, 615–619.

Lawson, R. and Mount, D. (1967). Minimum condition for stereopsis and anomalous contour. *Science*, **158**, 804–806.

Leonard, T. and Hsu, J. (1999). *Bayesian Methods*. Cambridge: Cambridge University Press.

Lin, M. and Tomasi, C. (2004). Surfaces with occlusion from layered stereo. *IEEE PAMI*, **26**, 1073–1078.

Marr, D. and Poggio, T. (1976). Cooperative computation of stereo disparity. *Science*, **194**, 283–287.

Middlebury College (2005). *Stereo Vision Research Page*, http://www.middlebury.edu/stereo, current 2005.

Okutomi, M., Katayama, Y. and Oka, S. (2002). A simple stereo algorithm to recover precise object boundaries and smooth surfaces. *Int. J. Comp. Vis.*, **47**, 261–273.

Pollard, S., Mayhew, J. and Frisby, J. (1985). PMF: a stereo correspondence algorithm using a disparity gradient limit. *Percept.*, **14**, 449–470.

Quam, L. (1984). Hierarchical warp stereo. *DARPA Image Understanding Workshop*, pp. 149–155.

Read, J. (2002). A Bayesian approach to the stereo correspondence problem. *Neural Comp.*, **14**, 1371–1392.

Richter, J. (1977). *Selections from the Notebooks of Leonardo da Vinci*. (Ed.) Oxford: Oxford University Press.

Sara, R. (2002). Finding the largest unambiguous component of stereo matching. *Proc. ECCV*, Part III, pp. 900–914.

Scharstein, D. and Szeliski, R. (2002). A taxonomy and evaluation of dense two-frame stereo correspondence algorithms. *Int. J. Comp. Vis.*, **41**, 7–42.

Strecha, C., Fransens, R. and van Gool, L. (2004). Wide-baseline stereo from multiple views: A probabilistic account. *Proc. IEEE CVPR*, Vol. 1, pp. 718–725.

Sun, J., Li, Y., Kang, S. and Shum, H. (2005). Symmetric stereo matching for occlusion handling. *Proc. IEEE CVPR*, Vol. 2, pp. 399–406.

Szeliski, R. (1990). Bayesian modeling of uncertainty in low-level vision. *Int. J. Comp. Vis.*, **5**, 271–301.

Trucco, E. and Verri, A. (1998). *Introductory Techniques for 3-D Computer Vision*. Upper Saddle River, NJ: Prentice-Hall.

Veksler, O. (2003). Fast variable window for stereo correspondence using integral images. *Proc. IEEE CVPR*, Vol 1. pp. 556–561.

Wilcox, L., Wildes, R., Lakra, D. and Spengler, R. (2005). The contribution of binocular and monocular texture elements to depth ordering. *J. Vision*, **5**, 722a.

Yuille, A. and Poggio, T. (1984). A Generalized Ordering Constraint for Stereo. *AI Lab Memo* 777, Cambridge, MA: MIT.

Zitnick, L. and Kanade, T. (2000). A cooperative algorithm for stereo matching with occlusion detection. *IEEE PAMI*, **22**, 675–684.

14 Speed versus quality – measuring and optimizing stereo for telepresence

Jane Mulligan

14.1 Stereo reconstruction of the human form

Acquiring high fidelity representations of humans as they perform in unconstrained settings is a challenging task. In particular I have worked extensively in dense computational stereo for reconstruction of people in 3D (three dimensional) telepresence environments. Telepresence is the idea that human users feel at some level present in an environment from which they are physically remote (Azuma, 1977; Schloerb, 1995). This is generally achieved through a combination of audio, video and networking technologies. Immersive telepresence seeks to provide a compelling 3D viewing environment which in turn requires an augmented capture system to create 3D models for rendering. The demands for such a capture system include the following.

- Low lag: the viewer wants to see what is happening now, not five minutes ago.

- High throughput: if the model is not updated at a fast rate movement will appear jerky and disconnected.

- Models must be of high quality to facilitate the *sense of presence* and subtleties of communication such as nuances facial expression.

These requirements for speed and quality tend to be at odds when building a 3D reconstruction system. A range of systems are possible varying from pure reconstruction as described below, to various combinations of modeling, prediction and reconstruction. At the other extreme avatars, or predefined graphical models (Leigh *et al.*, 1999), can be animated to reflect the motion and posture of the real person in the loop. We

Computational Vision in Neural and Machine Systems, ed. L. Harris and M. Jenkin. Published by Cambridge University Press. © Cambridge University Press 2007.

have chosen to use multicamera stereo to reconstruct the user in real-time in order to more directly transcribe his appearance and actions.

Working on stereo reconstruction in the specific context of telepresence causes us to prefer certain solutions over others based on performance constraints. We have worked to evaluate our systems with respect to our specific application and the tradeoffs necessary to meet its demands for speed and quality. We have previously examined the task related performance of real-time stereo for robot manipulation (Mulligan, 1996, 1998).

Speed and quality of reconstructed 3D models is the key tradeoff for the telepresence task. The goal is to achieve performance perceptually like our real world experience but mediated by cameras, depth calculation, network transmission and immersive rendering. In order to evaluate and improve our systems we need to be able to measure and compare performance. Time measurement is straightforward, but the question of measuring the quality of a 3D reconstruction is more challenging. Generally speaking, evaluating depth reconstruction requires obtaining image sets with known (ground truth) depth, and deciding on a metric to meaningfully measure and compare the output of the system.

Reconstructing a single stereo frame gives us a shell of visible surface fragments. When rendering these surfaces in a high end graphical environment they may appear disconnected and incomplete. Reconstructing a continuous temporal stream of stereo pairs allows us to exploit the temporal persistence of the human user in the scene. We have been working on high-speed human pose estimation based on tracking and reconstructing the user's hands and face. This skeletal pose can be used to cluster and propagate dense stereo depth data from frame to frame, and accrue a denser more compelling model over multiple frames.

In this chapter we will look at the basics of stereo reconstruction and survey our efforts to measure and achieve the speed and quality of reconstruction necessary for Immersive Telepresence.

14.2 Stereo, depth and surfaces

Just as our eyes provide two slightly different views of the world, in computational stereo we use two or more camera views of a scene to calculate the distances to surfaces (Figure 14.1). Stereo reconstruction is based on knowing the relative positions of the cameras, and *correspondence* – determining the positions in each view which represent the same world point.

The two critical issues for stereo reconstruction are then: acquiring the viewing geometry (Hartley and Zisserman, 2003), and computing correspondence (Atzpadin and Mulligan, 2005). Multiview geometry and methods for acquiring or calibrating the relative pose of camera views based on features or targets has been studied extensively in the past decade (Hartley and Zisserman, 2003). Correspondence is a subject of greater debate and there are many competing techniques for matching points from an image pair. These involve a variety of image features, similarity metrics, assumptions about the scene and search techniques.

The basic parallel binocular reconstruction geometry is depicted in Figure 14.1. A

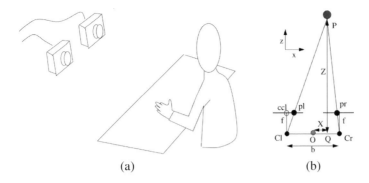

(a)   (b)

Figure 14.1. (a) Multiple cameras provide differing views of the scene, similar to our eyes. (b) Plan view (X, Z) of a pair of cameras observing the world point P. The triangle $cc_lC_lp_l$ is similar to QPC_l.

world point $P = (X, Y, Z)$ is projected into the image planes of the right and left camera at points $p_l = (u_l, v_l)$ and $p_r = (u_r, v_r)$ respectively. We observe that the triangles $cc_lC_lp_l$ and QPC_l are similar, which tells us that the ratios of corresponding sides are equal, thus

$$\frac{\frac{b}{2} + X}{Z} = \frac{p_l}{f} \text{ and } \frac{\frac{b}{2} - X}{Z} = \frac{-p_r}{f}$$

adding we have

$$\frac{b}{Z} = \frac{p_l - p_r}{f},$$
$$d = (u_l - u_r),$$
$$Z = \frac{bf}{d}.$$

Here f is the focal length (assumed identical) for the cameras, and b is the baseline or distance between the two camera centers C_l and C_r. O is the origin at the midpoint of the baseline. The value d is usually referred to as *disparity* and describes the difference in image position of the projection of the point P in the two cameras. This is the quantity we seek to compute during correspondence search.

For more details on more general multiview geometry, reconstruction and epipolar geometry the reader is referred to Hartley and Zisserman (2003). Computational stereo has a long history and a huge number of papers have been published in the literature. Some representative texts and surveys can be found in (Brown *et al.*, 2003; Trucco and Verri, 1998; Scharstein *et al.*, 2001; Dhond and Aggarwal, 1989).

In our systems we use fixed, strongly calibrated cameras. That is to say our cameras are rigidly mounted relative to each other and we have used a system such as the MATLAB calibration toolbox to estimate the internal (focal length, camera center) and external (position and orientation) camera parameters. As described above, knowledge of these parameters makes computation of the world positions of corresponding points possible. Each pixel in the reference image defines a ray from the world through the pixel to the camera center, along which light must have entered the camera. The projection of this ray into the other image gives us the *epipolar line* on which the corresponding image feature must appear. Our correspondence search then is only along one dimension. We can use our knowledge of calibrated camera parameters to warp or *rectify* the image pairs so that the epipolar lines lie along the scanlines of the images, emulating the parallel camera configuration of Figure 14.1. This makes memory access and image manipulation somewhat more efficient.

The first question in stereo correspondence is what feature to use for matching. Many early systems which attempted to achieve real-time performance used sparse features such as edges in order to reduce the cost of matching (Ayache, 1991). Having only sparse correspondences however makes it difficult to construct dense surfaces for rendering in a 3D telepresence environment. As a result our work has focussed on area or correlation-based approaches, which directly compare image intensities in a window around each pixel, rather than extracting sparser features. The implicit assumption is that depth (and therefore disparity) does not vary across the window. This assumption is violated at discontinuities and for surfaces tilted away from the camera. As desktop computers become faster these approaches achieve 20–30 stereo frames per second for images with 320×240 pixel images.

Correspondence search can also be implemented as a local or global process (Brown *et al.*, 2003). Area and feature-based approaches are typically local, where only the local image neighbourhood is considered during matching. Global search techniques such as dynamic programming, graph cuts or belief propagation, incorporate global constraints on the smoothness and continuity of the disparity surface. The price of smoother, more complete surfaces however is greater computational complexity. As a result we have not considered these techniques for the telepresence application.

14.2.1   Matching metrics

The next question is what form of similarity metric to use for correspondence matching. The most common and fastest area based or block matching techniques for stereo are Sum of Absolute Differences (SAD) and Sum of Squared Differences (SSD). Essentially for each pixel in the reference image we move along the epipolar line in the other image comparing each pixel and its surrounding window. The pixel distance along the line is the disparity. It should be noted that we can choose the range of disparity values we will search based on our expectations about the scene. The time required for computing area-based stereo disparity maps is highly dependent on the size of the disparity search range. We can think of the correspondence search as constructing a plot of correlation value for each tested disparity and choosing the peak which is the minimum (or maximum depending on the metric) of the curve.

For each disparity in the search range SAD has the form:

$$\text{SAD}(x, y, \mathbf{d}) = \sum_{(i,j)} \mid I_L(x + j, y + i) - I_R(x + d_x + j, y + d_y + i) \mid;$$

SSD has the form:

$$\text{SSD}(x, y, \mathbf{d}) = \sum_{(i,j)} \{I_L(x + j, y + i) - I_R(x + d_x + j, y + d_y + i)\}^2,$$

where x and y are image coordinates, I_L and I_R are the left and right images respectively, and d is the disparity.

Both of these metrics directly compare raw intensities (although a variety of pre-processing steps are possible), but if the two cameras have slightly different responses to light the observed differences between correctly matched pixels can be large. A normalized metric is somewhat more robust to such overall variations but is more costly in terms of computation time. Normalized Cross-Correlation is one such metric, but we prefer Modified Normalized Cross Correlation (MNCC) which is normalized by the sum of variances of the right and left windows, rather than the product. The result is that MNCC ranges from -1 to 1 rather than infinity.

$$\text{MNCC}(x, y, \mathbf{d}) = \frac{2\sigma_{lr}^2(x, y, \mathbf{d})}{\sigma_l^2(x, y) + \sigma_r^2(x + d_x, y + d_y)}$$

where σ_{lr}^2 is the covariance of the image windows in the right and left images, σ_l^2 is the variance of intensities in the left image window and σ_r^2 is the variance for the right image window.

Examining these metrics we can see that in areas where there is no intensity variation the plot of correlation versus disparity will be flat with no distinct peak. This is a key failing of local correspondence techniques: in low texture regions where all pixels match equally well we cannot distinguish a correct match.

There are numerous variations on area based matching techniques such as zero mean metrics (Atzpadin and Mulligan, 2005), rank transforms (Zabih and Woodfill, 1994) and hierarchical techniques. However, we will focus on the common, fast techniques described above for our evaluations.

We can use these metrics to accumulate evidence for matching with more than two images. Okumtomi and Kanade (1993) proposed a Sum of SSD (SSSD) metric for combining evidence from multiple views. We have used a Sum of MNCC (SMNCC) metric in our work on reconstruction from three views (trinocular stereo). Using more images provides more evidence for correspondence calculations. Given a calibrated camera setup, if we have a proposed match in two views, we can calculate the position in a third view where a match should occur if the proposed match is correct.

14.3   Quality and empirical evaluation

Our work on empirical evaluation of stereo systems (Mulligan *et al.*, 2002, 2003) began with the goal of evaluating our design for a real-time telepresence system. In particular we wanted objective measures of the relative quality of our reconstructions for different correspondence methods and binocular versus trinocular correspondence. We also wanted to compare trinocular configurations where the cameras were on a horizontal plane (inline) and the classic L-shape: "one camera up, 2 down." In other work we have also examined relationship between image gradient (a measure of texture) and depth error (Mulligan *et al.*, 2001) and the effect of large correlation windows on boundary errors (Mulligan *et al.*, 2003).

When we began this work stereo images with known scene depth (ground truth data) were not readily available. Since that time a number of datasets have be-

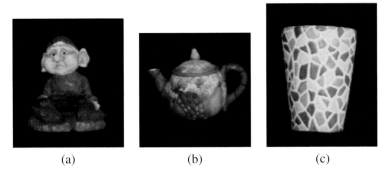

(a)   (b)   (c)

Figure 14.2. Three of the captured ground truth objects: (a) the elf statue; (b) the teapot; and (c) the vase.

come standard measures of algorithm performance. Currently the primary form of evaluation is to use the image sets provided on the Middlebury Stereo Page (http://www.middlebury.edu/stereo/) (Scharstein *et al.*, 2001). The metric used to rank algorithms on this page is percentage of bad pixels:

$$\frac{\sum_{i=1}^{N} (\hat{d}_i - d_i) > 1}{N} \times 100, \qquad (14.1)$$

for a reference test image with N pixels, estimated disparity $\hat{d}_i$ at pixel i, and ground truth disparity d_i. The metric can be computed for the entire image or independently for nonoccluded, discontinuity and low texture regions.

A comprehensive review of best practices in performance evaluation for computer vision can be found in Thacker *et al.* (2005). The authors emphasize not only evaluating technologies on particular test sets, but understanding the characteristics of the application domains under which the system must work reliably. They recommend a white-box approach to performance evaluation including rigorous statistical modeling of input, algorithm and, by propagation, output. An interesting question in the context of Middlebury Stereo evaluation is to what degree the test images provided, reflect tasks and environments in which a stereo system might be expected to perform?

We constructed our own ground truth datasets by registering scans from a laser scanner to our camera coordinate frame (see Figure 14.2). The scanner used was a Cyberware Head and Face 3D Color Scanner (Model 3030) which rotates around the subject to be scanned in a $360°$ circle, to capture a cylinder of range values. Registration requires a 3D target with both visible markings and identifiable shape (three intersecting planes). Visible targets on the planes are extracted and reconstructed by the stereo system. Independent planes are hand selected from the laser data. The transformation from laser scanner to camera frame is computed using the corresponding equations for the three planes in each frame. For details on the registration process see Mulligan *et al.* (2001).

Aside from the significant challenges of building accurate and workable calibration targets and actually achieving correct transforms from laser to camera coordinate

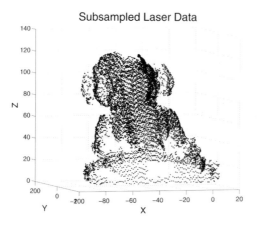

Figure 14.3. Plot of the (subsampled) laser scan of the elf from Figure 14.2a. See the accompanying CD-ROM for a color version.

frames, laser range data has its own set of inadequacies. It suffers from occlusions, and when light is not sufficiently reflected from dark or black regions gap occur in the data much like low texture regions for stereo. After registration we are left with two point sets in the same coordinate frame (laser and reconstructed stereo depth points) and we need to consider the most meaningful metric for error or difference between the two. When we project the laser data into the image, we discover that it is not "dense enough," so some pixels inside the object silhouette have no projected point. To evaluate the Middlebury bad-pixel metric in Eq. (14.1) we would have to construct a disparity map, but to fill the empty pixels we would have to construct a surface triangulation of the laser point set and determine the intersection of rays from pixels with the triangle set. We have settled on simply using the root mean squared and median nearest neighbor (NN) distance between stereo and laser points. Nearest neighbor distance is defined as

$$d_i = \forall_j \min(||l_j - s_i||_2) \tag{14.2}$$

for stereo depth point s_i and laser depth point l_j. The root mean squared NN distance is

$$\mathrm{RMS_{NN}} = \sqrt{\frac{\sum_{i=1}^N d_i^2}{N}} \tag{14.3}$$

for N stereo depth points.

We set out to collect ground truth data to evaluate our design for a real-time telepresence system. We tried to scan objects which had interesting surface detail, since we are interested in high quality reconstruction of people and faces. We were limited objects which were small enough to fit within our laser scanner. Our data captures individual objects on an easily segmented background (Figure 14.2). It differs in this regard from other ground truth datasets. Thacker *et al.* (2005) emphasize understanding algorithm performance under different viewing and scene conditions, so ideally one

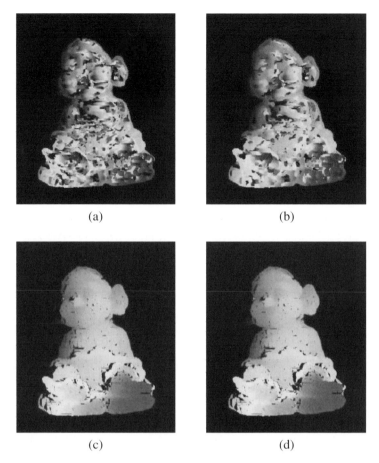

Figure 14.4. Disparity maps for (a) SAD, (b) SSD, (c) MNCC and (d) SMNCC correlation metrics. Figure 14.3 is a plot of the (subsampled) laser scan of the elf from figure 14.2(a). For a color version see the CD-ROM.

would use the full range of datasets available.

Our first goal was to compare the accuracy of various correspondence metrics with respect to the laser ground truth. Figure 14.3 is a plot of the elf laser depth data (subsampled for display). Figure 14.5 shows disparity images calculated for the elf data (Figure 14.2a) using SAD (Figure 14.5a), SSD (Figure 14.5b), MNCC (Figure 14.5c), and the trinocular SSSD (Figure 14.5d). Binocular MNCC produces a much smoother disparity map, than SAD or SSD. The trinocular SMNCC disparity image is somewhat smoother than MNCC.

To visualize the effects of various parameters and thresholds on the performance of algorithms with respect to ground truth error, we evaluate error at various levels of output density as proposed by Barron *et al.* (1994). By $n\%$ disparity density we denote the *best* $n\%$ of reconstructed points as determined by a quality metric. In the

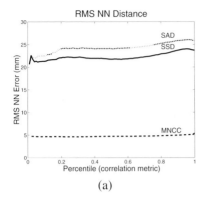 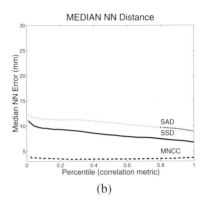

(a)   (b)

Figure 14.5. Density plots for (a) root mean squared NN distance error and (b) median NN distance for binocular similarity metrics. For the elf data SAD and SSD have consistently higher RMS and median NN distance.

following we sort depth points according to the correlation score computed during correspondence, select the top n% and compute error metrics for the selected points.

Figure 14.5 uses density plots to compare the error profiles for the binocular similarity metrics. The plots depict the error for decreasing proportions of the data according to their correlation score for SAD, SSD and MNCC for the registered elf data. Figure 14.5a plots root mean squared (RMS) nearest neighbour distance between reconstructed and laser depth points. Figure 14.5b shows the density plots for median NN distance. RMS distance tends to overweight outliers and thus gives much higher error values. Median distance gives more consistent error across the densities. Clearly the quality of normalized correlation metric disparity is superior to the faster SAD and SSD metrics.

Figure 14.6 shows RMS and median density plots illustrating the performance of the inline and L-shape trinocular stereo systems as well as the binocular MNCC system, for comparison. Under RMS error the trinocular systems behave similarly, while the binocular system has consistently higher error. The results for median NN distance look anomalous since the best 10% of the points according to the correlation metrics have the highest error. This is the result of the problems local correspondence methods have at occlusion boundaries. Erroneous depth points at the boundary tend to have high correlation scores and high error. At low proportions of the data these bad depth points affect the median. Under median error the MNCC and inline depth have similar accuracy while the L-shape configuration is superior.

The results of our work on empirical evaluation clearly demonstrate that our normalized MNCC correlation metric is markedly superior to SAD and SSD, sufficiently better to justify the added cost of computation. Similarly the added constraint of trinocular correspondence produced results with lower error and somewhat greater stability. Our measurements also demonstrate that the L-shape camera configuration produces more accurate and less volatile depth estimates than those obtained by placing all cameras on the same horizontal plane (inline).

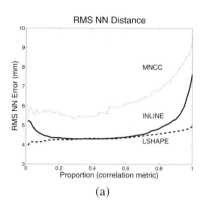
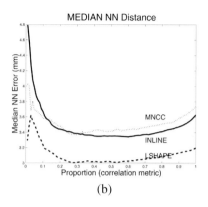

(a)   (b)

Figure 14.6. Density plots for (a) root mean squared NN distance error and (b) median NN distance for binocular versus trinocular correspondence. For the elf data the trinocular system is better for denser plots, but in the mid range the behavior of the two systems is similar.

14.4   Temporal coherence

Online stereo offers dense depth frames at 10–20 frames per second. These large volumes of evolving points should allow us to seed local depth estimates as well as improve our models over time. Our earlier work on temporal stereo focused mainly on the former (Mulligan and Daniilidis, 2000). Our more recent efforts have attempted to use models of human motion to compensate for frame to frame motion and integrate depth frames into better models of the person in the frame (Mulligan, 2005).

14.4.1   Computing flow to predict disparity

The first approach to exploiting temporal coherence is the general idea of predicting what will appear in the next frame based on previous frames. The simplest form of this is to restrict correspondence search at each pixel to a range of disparity values about the last estimated value (Mulligan *et al.*, 2003). This provides significant speedup when the overall disparity search range for the scene is large. Problems occur when the user moves to cover or uncover parts of the background causing large changes in the depth at these pixels.

We proposed a more sophisticated approach to predicting disparity using sparse optical flow to estimate motion in the scene (Mulligan and Daniilidis, 2000). The key to the approach is a disparity segmentation step which takes an initial full disparity image, and uses a seed fill technique to cluster regions of similar disparity. The regions are bounded by overlapping windows (see Figure 14.7b). Optical flow is calculated per *disparity window* to allow us to predict the image position of the propagated window in the next frame (Figure 14.7c). In other words we do a course estimation of the motion of our segmented depth patches and use it to predict the disparity in the next frame. To verify the disparity for the next frame we perform a window-based correspondence

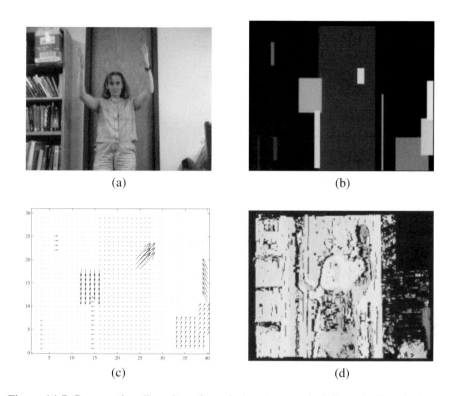

Figure 14.7. Propagating disparity using window-base optical flow. A disparity image (b) is segmented in to overlapping windows with narrow disparity ranges; optical flow velocities are computed per window (c) and used to propagate the disparity range to the next frame. Window based correspondence (d) produces a disparity map comparable to full frame correspondence. For a color version see the CD-ROM.

with a narrow range of disparity for each window (Figure 14.7d). Predicting image motion reduces the problem of user motion resulting in the wrong disparity search range for a region.

Optical flow approximates the motion field of objects moving relative to the cameras, based on the *image brightness constancy equation*: $I_x v_x + I_y v_y + I_t = 0$, where I is the image intensity and I_x, I_y and I_t are the partial derivatives of I with respect to x, y and time (t), and $v = [v_x, v_y]$ is the image velocity. We use a standard local weighted least square algorithm (Lucas and Kanade, 1981; Trucco and Verri, 1998) to calculate values for v based on minimizing

$$e = \sum_{W_i} (I_x v_x + I_y v_y + I_t)^2 \qquad (14.4)$$

for the pixels in the current disparity window W_i.

The steps are as follows

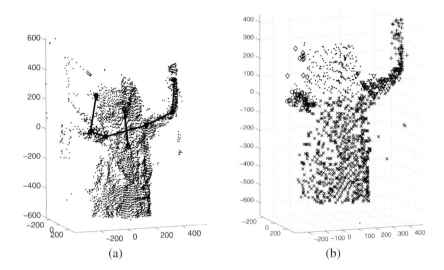

Figure 14.8. We estimate the upper body pose for the user based on color segmentation based face and hand position estimation and initial pose for the sequence (a). Pose estimate allows us to refine and segment reconstructed depth points based on proximity to skeleton segments (b). For color version see the CD-ROM.

- Compute full disparity map for first image of the sequence.

- For each new frame:

  - segment disparity map into regions of similar depth;

  - calculate optical flow for each window for the right and left images;

  - propagate window positions and disparity ranges'

  - window based correspondence search with predicted disparity.

Our goal of course is to improve the speed of our algorithms without sacrificing the quality of our reconstructions. In this case we are reducing the range of disparity we search for each pixel, but we are adding significant computation to determine the flow parameters. Our experiments have demonstrated that depth calculation with disparity windows and flow prediction reduce computation about 50% over full dense correlation matching (Mulligan and Daniilidis, 2000). The disparity maps achieved (Figure 14.7d) are of similar quality, and in some cases are cleaner than the full calculation. In Figure 14.7 the textureless white wall cannot be matched with the MNCC metric we use. Since no coherent disparity region or flow is found, the upper right part of the region is ignored.

14.4.2   Adding domain knowledge – human pose models

The work described in this chapter is all based on tuning and evaluating stereo reconstruction for the Telepresence task. This implies some strong assumptions about what the content of our scenes will be. Essentially we are concerned with looking at people.

The reconstructions we have investigated to this point are essentially surface fragments which are visible to all camera views. They tend to be disconnected and of course they are like a shell with nothing behind them. To achieve compelling 3D rendering of the imaged person in a remote immersive display we should ideally compute a richer, more complete model. In the theme of exploiting the stream of reconstructions available, we are working on explicitly modeling the human in the scene and accruing depth and appearance over time (Mulligan, 2005).

The first step in this process is to be able to track and identify the pose of the user over time. This gives us the ability to propagate and combine reconstructed depth over time. As a preprocessing step for detailed real-time surface reconstruction, pose estimation and tracking must be very fast. In a desktop telepresence setting we can further restrict our model to upper body pose, primarily head, torso and arm pose.

Extensive work on hand and face extraction is described in the literature and we will not attempt to improve on these approaches. If we can identify the face and hand positions in multiple views based on color, we can reconstruct their 3D position. This is the first step to identifying the user's pose. We use the simplest approach, exploiting color segmentation of fleshtones in normalized RGB space, which has proved fast and effective (Wren *et al.*, 1997; Yang and Ahuja, 1999).

Psychophysical research by Soechting and Flanders (Soechting and Flanders, 1989a, b) examines human subjects and how their performance in pointing to visible and obscured targets relates to target position. They describe a kinematic model which uses linear functions of the components of target endpoint position to generate the angles required to define the arm pose. Our experiments with motion capture data have demonstrated that given an initial pose estimate we can accurately predict pose from frame to frame. Figure 14.8a illustrates an extracted pose skeleton plotted with the reconstructed stereo depth points for the frame in Figure 14.7. Figure 14.8b is the segmentation of the depth points based on proximity to the skeleton segments.

Fast pose estimation and depth map segmentation give us the data we need to refine the frame-to-frame alignment for components of the body model. Figure 14.9a plots the segmented right arm points from three frames in a reconstructed stereo sequence. The obvious first step is to align the data based on the estimated arm pose at each frame, and render them as illustrated in Figure 14.9b. The result is still noisy and not prefectly aligned but it is more complete and dense that the unregistered data. We are currently exploring fitting conics to body components at each frame in order to refine the pointset and iterating based on color and shape to create an improved model. Iterating to achieve a better quality merging of the data in turn provides a more exact pose estimate. In a telepresence setting a refined and persistent model of the user and a tracked estimate of his pose allows us to interpolate in a seemless way across lost frames or through degraded network service.

Right Arm (Frame 26 to 28)

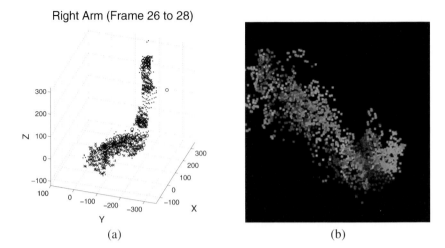

(a)   (b)

Figure 14.9. Registering body components over multiple frames. (a) Right arm pose over three stereo frames. (b) Initial registration of depth points based on pose estimates only. Color versions on the CD-ROM.

14.5   Conclusion

In this chapter we have briefly described the basic concepts of computing depth from multiple camera views. We emphasize that methods for computational stereo must be designed and evaluated with respect to the task to which they will be applied. Our goal is to build Immersive Telepresence systems based on transmitting and rendering 3D models captured in real-time using stereo. This imposes two competing demands on our systems: the stereo reconstructions must be of high quality to create a compelling experience when rendered in a stereoscopic graphical environment, and they must be computed fast enough to allow natural communication. In order to optimize our tradeoffs of speed and quality we have undertaken ground truth accuracy evaluation for a variety of binocular and trinocular stereo correspondence metrics, and the more subtle issue of camera configuration in the form of L-shape versus coplanar camera placement. We demonstrated that normalized correlation metrics for L-shape trinocular camera configurations produced the best accuracy results.

Real-time area based stereo reconstruction produces dense depth frames at 10–20 frames per second. Exploiting the temporal coherence from frame to frame can allow us to optimize our correspondence search and create richer, more compelling models of the human in the scene. We have described a method for propagating disparity estimates based on segmenting the disparity image and computing optical flow per segment window. This approach allows us to reduce our computational load by approximately 50%, thus addressing our requirement for increased speed. Finally we have described current work on exploiting the large available volumes of depth data over time to create better, more complete models of the user. We use fast color-based hand and face tracking to estimate a skeletal upper body pose. Estimated pose allows us to segment and roughly register body components which are further refined by fitting conic components and optimizing the pose estimate.

References

Atzpadin, N. and Mulligan, J. (2005). Methods for disparity estimation. In O. Schreer, P. Kauff, and T. Sikora, eds., *3D Videocommunication*, Chapter 7. New York: Wiley.

Ayache, N. (1991). *Artificial Vision for Mobile Robots: Stereo Vision and Multisensory Perception*. Cambridge, MA: The MIT Press.

Azuma, R. T. (1977). A survey of augmented reality. *Presence: Teleoperators and Virtual Environments*, **7**, 355–385.

Barron, J. L., Fleet, D. J. and Beauchemin, S. S. (1994). Performance of optical flow techniques. *Int. J. Comp. Vis.*, **12**, 43–78.

Brown, M., Burschka, D. and Hager, G. D. (2003). Advances in computational stereo. *IEEE PAMI*, **25**, 993–1008.

Dhond, U. and Aggarwal, J. (1989). Structure from stereo – a review. *IEEE SMC*, **19**, 1489–1510.

Hartley, R. and Zisserman, A. (2003). *Multiple View Geometry in Computer Vision*, Second Edition. Cambridge: Cambridge University Press.

Leigh, J., Johnson, A. E., Brown, M., Sandin, D. J. and DeFanti, T. A. (1999). Visualization in teleimmersive environments. *Computer*, **32**, 66–73.

Lucas, B. D. and Kanade, T. (1981). An iterative image registration technique with an application to stereo vision. Proc. *IJCAI'81*, pp. 674–679, Vancouver, BC.

Mulligan, J. (1996). Fast calibrated stereo vision for manipulation. *Proc. IEEE ICRA*, **3**, 2326–2331, Minneapolis, Minnesota.

Mulligan, J. (1998). Empirical modeling and comparison of robotic tasks. *Proc. IEEE-RSJ IROS*, Victoria, Canada.

Mulligan, J. (2005). Upper body pose estimation from stereo and hand-face tracking. *Proc. 2nd Can. Conf. on Comp. and Robot Vis.*

Mulligan, J. and Daniilidis, K. (2000). Predicting disparity windows for real-time stereo. *Proc. ECCV*, Dublin, Ireland.

Mulligan, J. Isler, V. and Daniilidis, K. (2001). Performance evaluation of stereo for tele-presence. *Proc. IEEE Int. Conf. Comp. Vis.*, **2**, 558–565, Vancouver, Canada.

Mulligan, J., Isler, V. and Daniilidis, K. (2002). Trinocular stereo: a real-time algorithm and its evaluation. *Int. J. Comp. Vis.*, **47**, 51–61, 2002.

Mulligan, J., Zampoulis, X., Kelshikar, N. and Daniilidis, K. (2003). Stereo-based environment scanning for immersive telepresence. *IEEE Trans. Circ. Sys. Video Technol.*, **14**, 304–320.

Okutomi, M. and Kanade, T. (1993). A multiple-baseline stereo. *IEEE PAMI*, **15**, 353–363.

Scharstein, D., Szeliski, R. and Zabih, R. (2001). A taxonomy and evaluation of dense two-frame stereo correspondence algorithms. *Proc. IEEE Workshop on Stereo and Multi-Baseline Vision*, Kauai, HI.

Schloerb, D. W. (1995). A quantitative measure of telepresence. *Presence*, **4**, 64–80.

Soechting, J. F. and Flanders, M. (1989a). Sensorimotor representations for pointing to targets in three-dimensional space. *J. Neurophysiol.*, **62**, 582–594.

Soechting, J. F. and Flanders, M. (1989b). Errors in pointing are due to approximations in sensorimotor transformations. *J. Neurophysiol.*, **62**, 595–608.

Thacker, N. A., Clark, A. F., Barron, J. *et al.* (2005). *Performance characterisation in computer vision: A guide to best practices.* Tina Memo 2005-009, Medical School, University of Manchester, Manchester.

Trucco, E. and Verri, A. (1998). *Introductory Techniques for 3-D Computer Vision.* Upper Saddle River, NJ: Prentice Hall Inc.

Wren, C., Azarbayejani, A., Darrell, T. and Pentland, A. (1997). Pfinder: Real-time tracking of the human body. *IEEE PAMI*, **19**, 780–785.

Yang, M. and Ahuja, N. (1999). Recognizing hand gesture using motion trajectories. *Proc. IEEE CVPR*, **1**, 466–472.

Zabih, R. and Woodfill, J. (1994). Non-parametric approach to visual correspondence. *IEEE PAMI*.

15 Binocular combination: measurements and a model

Jian Ding and George Sperling

15.1 Introduction

15.1.1 Cyclopean image

When different stimuli are presented to the left and right eyes, only a single, combined image is perceived, often called the *cyclopean image* after Cyclops, the one-eyed mythological monster. When the images in the left and right eyes are similar (compatible), the cyclopean image is a combination of the two. This chapter is concerned with the early visual processes that determine the proportion that each eye's image contributes to the cyclopean image. When the images in the left and right eyes are dissimilar (incompatible), such as a vertical grating in one eye and a horizontal grating in the other, or a positive image in one eye and its negative in the other, then typically within any small area of the visual field, only one of the two images is perceived. This phenomenon is called *binocular rivalry*. Although the processes of binocular combination and binocular rivalry share early stages of visual processing, we are here concerned only with the laws governing binocular combination.

Vector summation of same-wavelength monocular sinewave gratings

To obtain experimental data that yield the quantitative parameters of binocular combination, we take advantage of a simple mathematical fact. The arithmetic sum of two sine waves of the same wavelength is again a sine wave whose amplitude and phase are dependent on the phases and amplitudes of the two component sine waves. As shown in Figure 15.1, a sine wave can be represented as a vector, and the arithmetic summation of two sine waves of the same wavelength can be represented by vector summation. If $\vec{L}_\phi$ and $\vec{R}_\phi$ represent two sinewave gratings (in this example, images in the left and right eyes, respectively), the vector sum, $\vec{B}_\phi$, represents the sum of the two

Computational Vision in Neural and Machine Systems, ed. L. Harris and M. Jenkin. Published by Cambridge University Press. © Cambridge University Press 2007.

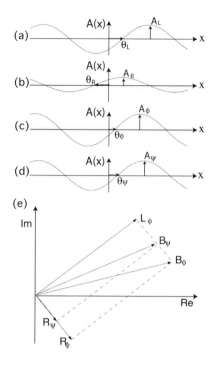

Figure 15.1. Vector presentations of sine waves and their arithmetic summation in the complex plane. (a) Representation of a horizontal sinewave grating presented to the left eye with modulation amplitude A_L and phase θ_L. The abscissa represents the vertical direction x and the ordinate is amplitude $A(x)$. (b) A horizontal grating presented to the right eye with modulation amplitude A_R and phase θ_R. (c) The physical, algebraic sum of gratings (a) and (b) has modulation amplitude A_ϕ and phase θ_ϕ. (d) The (perceived) cyclopean grating has modulation amplitude A_ψ and phase θ_ψ. (e) The complex plane. The abscissa is the real axis and the ordinate is the imaginary axis. Vector $\vec{L}_\phi$ and vector $\vec{R}_\phi$ represent the sine waves presented to the left and right eyes, respectively. The vector components of $\vec{L}_\phi$, (A_L, θ_L), are shown as vectors (arrows) in (a). Other vectors in (e) are similarly derived from the components shown in (b, c, d). Vector $\vec{B}_\phi$ is the vector sum: $\vec{B}_\phi = \vec{L}_\phi + \vec{R}_\phi$. Vector $\vec{B}_\psi$ is drawn with a phase angle that represents the psychophysically measured phase of the (perceived) cyclopean sine wave. Vector $\vec{R}_\psi$ represents a reduced right-eye contribution to the cyclopean sine wave that would account for the (perceived) cycopean phase.

sine waves. It is both reasonable to assume and empirically observed that the cyclopean image of two parallel monocular sinewave gratings of the same wavelength is indeed, to a very close approximation, a sinewave grating of the same wavelength. Therefore, in this instance, predicting the combined cyclopean image is equivalent to predicting the apparent phase and amplitude of the cyclopean sinewave grating.

Consider two monocular images, parallel sinewave gratings, that differ in phase and amplitude. If the binocular combination were linear, the apparent phase of the cyclopean sinewave grating would be predicted by a simple vector summation of the monocular sine waves. Our experimental results indicate that the apparent phase of the cyclopean sinewave grating, relative to vector summation, is biased toward the eye with the higher-contrast stimulus. For example, in Figure 15.1, the left eye is presented with a higher-contrast sinewave grating $\vec{L}_\phi$ and the right eye with a lower-contrast sinewave grating $\vec{R}_\phi$. Linear vector summation is $\vec{B}_\phi = \vec{L}_\phi + \vec{R}_\phi$. The observed cyclopean image is $\vec{B}_\psi$, which is biased toward the left (higher-contrast) eye relative to vector summation.

Binocular combination implies attenuation of a weaker signal relative to a stronger signal

We interpret the observed failure of vector summation in predicting cyclopean images by assuming: (1) there is vector summation of left- and right-eye same-wavelength sinewave gratings and (2) prior to the site of binocular combination, the physically weaker (lower contrast) monocular image is attenuated relative to the stronger (higher-contrast) monocular image. In the example of Figure 15.1, if the physical right monocular image ($\vec{R}_\phi$) were attenuated to precisely $\vec{R}_\psi$, it would reproduce precisely the experimentally observed cyclopean phase. The contrasts of the physical stimuli are in a ratio of 2:1; the observer acts as though the ratio were 4:1. This assumed perceptual attenuation of the lower-contrast relative to the higher-contrast monocular grating is the critical derived measurement that we subsequently use to construct our theory of binocular combination.

Outline

In this chapter, we offer a procedure for measuring the apparent phase of a cyclopean sinewave grating. The observer's task is to judge the center position of the black stripe that corresponds to the minimum in the cyclopean sinewave grating relative to the position of an adjacent reference line. We present a gain-control model to fit our data. The model accounts for over 97% of the variance of the experimental data in the sense of successfully predicting the apparent phase of the cyclopean sinewave grating. In our experiments, we measure only the phase, not amplitude of the cyclopean sine wave. To determine whether the model can predict amplitude as well as phase, we rely on the contrast-matching data of Legge and Rubin (1981). By means of model simulations, we find that the model does indeed give a united explanation of binocular combination data derived from simple stimuli. The model does not deal with complex binocular combinations that involve faces and other meaningful stimuli (see Blake, 2003) in which higher-order visual processes are probably involved.

15.1.2 Empirical manipulations in the sinewave summation experiments

Figure 15.2 outlines the principles used to derive the relative contribution of the left- and right-eye images to the cyclopean image. Basically, given the physically presented

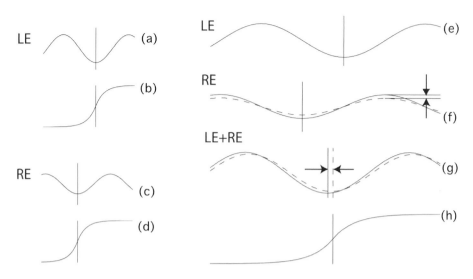

Figure 15.2. Control conditions, experimental conditions, and their interpretations. (a, c) Only one eye is presented with a sinewave grating (as illustrated). (b,d) Psychometric functions. The fraction of trials on which the reference lines are judged above the dark stripe of the sinewave grating as a function of the vertical position of the reference lines. The midpoint of a psychometric function (indicated by the vertical bar) is taken as the perceived phase of the presented sinewave. The right column shows binocular conditions. The scale is magnified to better illustrate the results. (e) A high-contrast sine wave presented to the left eye (LE). The solid vertical line indicates the midpoint of the dark stripe. (f) The solid curve represents a low-contrast sine wave presented to the right eye (RE). (g) The algebraic sum of (e) and (f) is shown as a solid line. (h) The perceived phase of cyclopean sine wave is measured by a psychometric function. It is closer to the phase of the left eye's stimulus than would be expected from the algebraic sum (g). An attenuated lower-contrast sine wave is shown as a dotted line in (f). Using this attentuated lower-contrast sine wave to form the left-plus-right-eye sum (dashed line in (g)) causes the algebraic sum of the original left-eye sinewave and the attentuated right-eye sine wave to match the phase of the cyclopean sine wave. The change from physical contrast of the stimulus to effective contrast at the point of binocular combination is here expressed as a reduction in effectiveness of the lower-contrast sinewave grating. However, for a given pair of left- and right-eye sinewave grating phases, the phase of the cyclopean sine wave is determined entirely by the *ratio* of left- to right-eye effective contrasts.

phases of the two monocular stimuli, and the phase of the perceived cyclopean image, we calculated the attenuation of the lower-contrast stimulus that would be required to reproduce the observed cyclopean phase. In control conditions, on each trial only one randomly chosen eye was presented with a sinewave grating. The other eye was simultaneously presented a blank screen with the same mean luminance as the sinewave grating. These control stimuli were interleaved in a sequence of experimental displays.

Indeed, observers could not distinguish control from experimental conditions, and were unaware that occasionally only one eye had received a grating stimulus.

Psychometric functions

To measure a psychometric function, the position of the reference line relative to the sine wave was varied from trial to trial using a staircase procedure described below. On each trial, the observer judged whether the reference line was "above" or "below" the center of the black stripe in the cyclopean sinewave grating. The position of the reference line that was equally likely to be judged as "above" and "below" was taken as the Point of Subjective Equality (PSE), i.e. the median perceived position of the center of the black stripe of the cyclopean sinewave grating.

Figures 15.2 a-d illustrate the control trials. Figure 15.2a illustrates the stimulus for control trials with a left-eye stimulus, and Figure 15.2c illustrates the right-eye stimulus. Figures 15.2 b,d illustrate psychometric functions derived from presentations of these stimuli and the estimated positions of the PSEs. Typically, the measured value of apparent phase $\hat{\theta}_L$ of the PSE differed slightly but significantly from the physical value of θ_L, indicating a small bias of the measurement. When two psychometric functions for $\hat{\theta}_R$ and $\hat{\theta}_L$ are obtained in the same session, the position bias would be expected to be the same and therefore canceled by considering the difference $\hat{\theta}_L - \hat{\theta}_R$. The phase difference between the perceived phases of the left- and right-eye control sine stimuli would be expected to be identical to the phase difference between the input sines, i.e. $\hat{\theta}_L - \hat{\theta}_R = \theta_L - \theta_R$. Satisfaction of this constraint within a small measurement error was verified for each observer before each experimental session.

In experimental sessions, staircases for control conditions were interleaved with the staircases for measurement conditions. As noted above, observers did not discriminate monocular from binocular trials. In experimental trials, observers view sinewave gratings that might differ between eyes in both spatial phase and contrast. Figures 15.2e and f illustrate stimuli in which the left eye was presented with a higher-contrast sinewave grating with phase θ_L (Figure 15.2e) and the right eye was presented a lower-contrast sinewave grating with phase θ_R (Figure 15.2f). The linear summation of these two sine waves is again a sine wave, illustrated by the solid line of Figure 15.2g. The location of its minimum is indicated by a solid vertical line.

The perceived binocular combination of the left- and right-eye's gratings, the cyclopean image, is assumed to be a sinewave grating whose apparent phase is measured by a psychometric function (Figure 15.2h). To arrive at an arithmetic summation of the left and right eyes' sinewave gratings that has the same phase as the cyclopean sinewave grating, we assume that the signal from the right eye (the lower-contrast stimulus) was attenuated prior to binocular combination. This assumed-attenuated right-eye input to binocular combination is shown by the dashed line in Figure 15.2f. The combination of the unattenuated higher-contrast input and the attenuated lower-contrast input is illustrated by the dashed line in Figure 15.2g. The minimum of this combination now precisely matches the observed position derived from the emprical psychometric function Figure 15.2h.

Many observers exhibit some eye dominance. That is, in binocular combination, the input from one eye (the dominant eye) is given greater weight than that from the other eye. To cancel biases of measurement related to eye dominance, the experiment was repeated with the stimuli to the two eyes interchanged. The average of these two measured phase shifts was taken as the phase shift for the cyclopean condition. Additionally, to cancel biases related to vertical position, all the above procedures were repeated with the stimuli mirror-reflected around the horizontal midline, and all the results were averaged.

15.1.3   Outline of the experiments

Six experiments were performed. In all experiments, observers judged the vertical position (phase) of a horizontal sinewave grating that was presented to both eyes. In experiment 1, no external noise or mask was superimposed and simple sinewave gratings were presented to the left and right eyes in various different phases and with various different contrasts. The data of experiment 1 are accounted for by the gain-control model described below with just one free parameter.

Experiment 2 investigated the prediction that reducing contrast energy reduces the nonlinearity of (i.e. linearizes) binocular combination. The stimuli and procedure were similar to experiment 1 except the fixed duration of 1000 ms in experiment 1 was varied in the range from 50 ms to 1000 ms, creating stimuli ranging from very low contrast energy (50 ms $\times$ 0.1) to very high energy (1000 ms $\times$ 0.2). This experiment defines the temporal parameters of interocular gain control in binocular combination.

Experiments 3–6 measured the gain-control factors that determine binocular dominance. In these experiments, a monocular masking stimulus was superimposed on the sinewave gratings whose phase was being judged. Experiment 3 investigated the question: When the spatial frequency for which binocular combination is being determined is f_0, how much do other spatial frequencies f_1 contribute to gain control? This was tested by superimposing a 2D bandpass noise on the sinewave grating in just one of the two eyes.

In experiment 4, a static vertical sinewave grating was used to mask the horizontal sinewaves whose position was being judged. The contrast and spatial frequency of the masking grating was varied from trial to trial. Spatial-frequency transfer functions were obtained.

In experiment 5, the binocular horizontal grating whose position was being judged was masked by a monocular moving vertical sinewave grating whose contrast and drift rate vary from trial to trial. Temporal-frequency transfer functions were obtained.

In experiment 6, the orientation of a static, sinewave masking grating was varied. Orientation tuning functions were obtained.

15.2   Methods

15.2.1   Apparatus

The purpose of the apparatus was to produce a binocular display in which each eye is presented with a horizontal sinewave grating, and the two eyes' images are optically superimposed. The two sinewave gratings are identical except for differences in phase and contrast. The reason for choosing sine waves is that the sum of two sine waves of the same wavelength is again a sine wave. Typically, for the parameters used in the experiments of this paper, the observer perceived a cyclopean sinewave grating. Sinewave gratings were horizontal to make the cyclopean image relatively independent of horizontal vergence angle. A high-contrast surrounding visual frame was used to assist the eyes in maintaining vergence. The task of the observer was to judge the position of the center of the dark stripe of the cyclopean sinewave gratings relative to two adjacent dark reference lines.

15.2.2 Display

The experiments were controlled by an 8600/250 Power Macintosh; stimuli were presented on a Nanao Technology monochrome monitor. The programs were written in Matlab, using the Psychophysics Toolbox extensions (Brainard, 1997; Pelli, 1997). A special circuit (Pelli and Zhang, 1991) was used to combine two eight-bit output channels of the video card to yield 6144 distinct gray-scale levels (12.6 bits). The luminance of the monitor with all pixels set to the minimum value was 0.38 cd/m^2; the luminance with all pixels set to the maximum value was 68.1 cd/m^2. The background level I_0 surrounding the sinewave gratings was set to 34.2 cd/m^2, and this was also used as the average luminance of the sine waves themselves. Displays were viewed in a mirror stereoscope and positioned optically 68 cm from the observer.

A psychophysical procedure was used to generate a linear look-up table. This look-up table was used, as required, in either of two ways: (1) to divide the entire dynamic range of the monitor into 256 evenly-spaced gray levels or (2) to select 256 evenly-spaced grey levels within a limited intensity range and thereby to obtain higher contrast resolution within that range (Lu and Sperling, 1999).

15.2.3 Stimuli

Horizontal gratings with sinusoidal luminance profiles were used as stimuli. To describe these stimuli we make the following definitions: I_0 is luminance of the background and the mean luminance of the sinewave gratings; m_L and m_R are the modulation contrasts of the left- and right-eye sinewave gratings, respectively; θ_L and θ_R are the corresponding phases. In experiments 3–6, a mask $\mathcal{M}(x, y)$ which consisted of either a bandpass noise or a sinewave grating was superimposed on the sinewave grating presented to one eye. The mask's modulation contrast is either n_L or n_R corresponding to adding the mask either to left or to right eye. The stimuli were windowed in a rectangular window both spatially and temporally. Equations (15.1) and (15.2) describe the stimuli to the left and right eyes respectively,

$$I_{L} = I_{0} - (m_{L}\cos(2\pi f_s x + \theta_{L}) + n_{L}\mathcal{M}(x,y))I_0 u(t,T)u(x+2\pi,4\pi)u(y+2\pi,4\pi) \tag{15.1}$$

$$I_{R} = I_{0} - (m_{R}\cos(2\pi f_s x + \theta_{R}) + n_{R}\mathcal{M}(x,y))I_0 u(t,T)u(x+2\pi,4\pi)u(y+2\pi,4\pi). \tag{15.2}$$

Stimuli appeared for a duration T defined as follows:

$$u(t, T) = \begin{cases} 1 & \text{if } 0 \le t \le T \\ 0 & \text{otherwise} \end{cases} . \tag{15.3}$$

In experiment 2, T varied from 50 ms to 1000 ms; in all other experiments, T was fixed at 1000 ms. In experiments 1 and 2, no mask was superimposed, i.e., $n_L = n_R = 0$. In all trials for all experiments, the spatial frequency of the gratings f_s was fixed at 0.68 cpd and there were exactly two cycles (4π) visible in each eye's sinewave grating. A reference line was shown on each side of the sinewave grating. A high-contrast, surrounding visual frame was presented from the start of the trial until the end of the stimulus presentation to assist observers in maintaining vergence (Figure 15.3).

15.2.4   Procedures: Sequence of events on a trial

Figure 15.3 shows the procedures used in experiment 1. The two left-hand columns show the stimuli presented to the left and the right eyes respectively. The right-hand column represents the cyclopean image perceived by an observer. Every trial began with two fixation crosses, each with two dots, presented to two eyes and arranged so that with correct vergence, a single cross with four symmetrically placed dots would be perceived (Figure 15.3a). Only after this cross with four symmetric dots was seen clearly, did the observer press a key to initiate the trial. The key press produced a screen with only the high-contrast frame (Figure 15.3b) for 500 ms followed by sinewave gratings presented to the two eyes for one second (Figure 15.3c). Stimulus presentation was followed by a blank screen of mean luminance until the observer responded.

The observer's task was to indicate the apparent location of the center of the dark stripe in the perceived cyclopean sinewave grating relative to a black horizontal reference line adjacent to its edge. If the reference line were judged above the dark cyclopean stripe, a key press indicating "above" was made; if the line were judged below, the "below" key press was made. After the response, the preparation for the next trial began with presentation of the cross-plus-dots fixation images.

In experiments 3–6, the procedures were exactly the same as that in experiment 1 except that a masking bandpass noise or a masking sinewave grating was randomly superimposed on one eye's sinewave grating.

15.2.5   Procedures: Adaptive concurrent staircases

An adaptive staircase procedure, with many concurrent staircases, was used in all experiments. Within a staircase, the position of the reference line was varied according to the response in the previous trial of that staircase. In each staircase, when the response was "Above," the reference line was moved down on the next trial of that staircase; when the response was "Below," the reference line was moved up in the next trial. For each condition, four staircases were interleaved randomly, corresponding to the four variations of each experimental condition: the higher-contrast sinewave grating presented either to the left or right eye with either the original display or a mirror reflection of the origial display around the horizontal midline. For an experiment with n

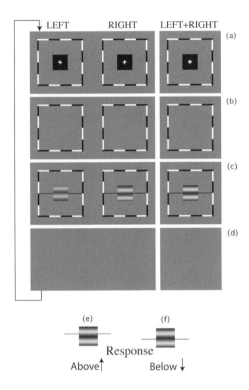

Figure 15.3. Procedure used in Experiments 1, 3, 4, 5, and 6. The column "LEFT" shows the stimuli presented to the left eye; the column "RIGHT" shows the stimuli presented to the right eye; the column "LEFT+RIGHT" illustrates the arithmetic sum of these stimuli. (a) A cross-hair with two dots was presented to each eye; when the eyes were correctly verged, a cyclopean cross with four dots was perceived. (b) Once vergence has been achieved, a key is pressed that changes the stimulus to a blank field (with only the surrounding frame) for 500 ms. (c) Horizontal sinewave gratings were presented to each eye for 1000 ms. Black horizontal reference lines were adjacent to the edges of the gratings. The cyclopean image was also a sinewave in which the observer judged the position of the reference line relative to the center of the central dark stripe of the grating. In experiment 3, a bandpass noise is added to one of the sinewave gratings in one eye; in experiments 4, 5 and 6, a masking sine wave was added to one eye's sinewave gratings. (d) A blank screen persisted until a response was made. (e) A cyclopean image for a response "reference line above dark stripe." (f) A cyclopean image for a response "reference line below dark stripe." After the response, the entire sequence repeated.

conditions, $4n$ staircases were run concurrently and interleaved randomly. Each staircase was run for a total of 50 trials.

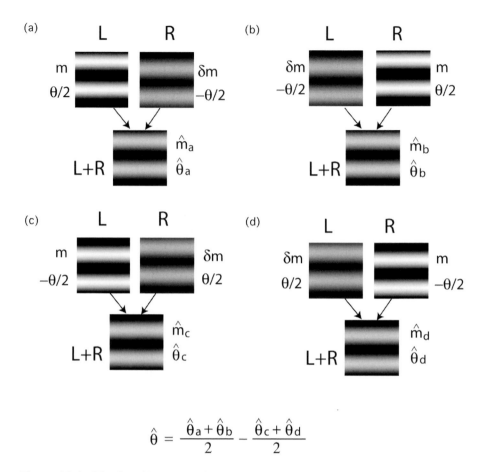

$$\hat{\theta} = \frac{\hat{\theta}_a + \hat{\theta}_b}{2} - \frac{\hat{\theta}_c + \hat{\theta}_d}{2}$$

Figure 15.4. The four binocular stimuli used to cancel position and eye biases and thereby to yield unbiased estimates of the perceived phase of cyclopean images produced by left-eye (L) and right-eye (R) gratings that differ in contrast by a factor of δ and in phase by θ. (a, L) High-contrast grating with modulation amplitude m in the left eye and with dark band $\theta/2$ above the midline. (a, R) A low-contrast grating with modulation δm, $0 \le \delta \le 1$, and with the dark band below the midline presented to the right eye. The cyclopean image perceived when L+R are presented has perceived contrast $\hat{m}_a$ and perceived phase $\hat{\theta}_a$. (b) High-contrast m in right eye, dark stripe $\theta/2$ (above midline). (c) High-contrast m in left eye, dark stripe $-\theta/2$ (below midline). (d) High-contrast m in right eye, dark stripe $-\theta/2$ (below midline). The estimated cyclopean phase shift $\hat{\theta}$ produced by left-eye and right-eye gratings that differed in contrast by δ and phase by θ is given by the formula at the bottom. Note that whenever $\delta = 1$, the expected value of $\hat{\theta} = 0$; whenever $\delta = 0$, the expected value of $\hat{\theta} = \theta$.

15.2.6 Procedures: Counterbalancing to control for eye and position biases

The basic stimuli used in all experiments are described by Eqs. (15.1) and (15.2) and Figure 15.3. A horizontal sinewave was presented to each eye. The contrast of the higher-contrast sinewave grating was m, the contrast of the lower-contrast sinewave grating was δm, where $0 \leq \delta \leq 1$. The phase difference between the left- and right-eye sinewave gratings was θ. For any given combination of m, δ, θ there were four alternative stimuli: The higher-contrast sinewave grating could be presented either to the left (Figures 15.4a and c) or to the right (Figures 15.4b and d) eye and the higher contrast can be assigned to either the upper (Figures 15.4a and b) or to the lower (Figures 15.4c and d) sinewave grating in the combination (causing the dark stripe to appear either above or below the midline).

For any condition (a combination of m, δ, θ) four independent staircases corresponding to the four configurations of Figure 15.4 were conducted. The four staircases for each condition were combined (see below) to give a single-valued dependent variable: the perceived phase shift between applying the higher contrast to the upper versus to the lower sine wave in the combination. This measure cancelled modest dominance biases in favor of one or the other eye, and perfectly cancelled up/down location biases in judging the position of the center of the cyclopean grating's dark band relative to the reference lines.

Figure 15.5 shows an example of how we measured the perceived phase shift for the following condition: $m = 10\%$, $\theta = 90°$, and $\delta = 0.5$ (i.e. the contrast of the higher-contrast sinewave grating was 10%, that of the lower-contrast sinewave grating was 5%). In viewing these stimuli, observers generally were unaware of having gratings of different contrast in each eye; they perceived only a cyclopean grating.

There were four alternative sine wave presentations of this combination of parameters, in each of which the dark band of one sine wave was $45°$ above the midline and the dark band of the other was $45°$ below the midline:

(a) The 10% grating was presented to the left eye and its dark band was the higher of the two sinewave components (Figure 15.4a), i.e. $m_L = 10\%$, $\theta_L = 45°$, $m_R = 5\%$ and $\theta_R = -45°$.

(b) The 10% grating was presented to the right eye and its dark band was the higher of the two sinewave components (Figure 15.4b), i.e. $m_L = 5\%$, $\theta_L = -45°$, $m_R = 10\%$ and $\theta_R = 45°$.

(c) The 10% grating was presented to the left eye and its dark band was the lower of the two sinewave components (Figure 15.4c), i.e. $m_L = 10\%$, $\theta_L = -45°$, $m_R = 5\%$ and $\theta_R = 45°$.

(d) The 10% grating was presented to the right eye and its dark band was the lower of the two sinewave components (Figure 15.4d), i.e. $m_L = 5\%$, $\theta_L = 45°$, $m_R = 10\%$ and $\theta_R = -45°$.

Let $\hat{\theta}_i$ be the perceived position of the dark stripe of the cyclopean sinewave in condition i ($i = a, b, c, d$). Then: $(\hat{\theta}_a + \hat{\theta}_c)/2$ and $(\hat{\theta}_b + \hat{\theta}_d)/2$ are measures of position bias; $\hat{\theta}_b - \hat{\theta}_a$ and $\hat{\theta}_d - \hat{\theta}_c$ are measures of eye bias; and $\hat{\theta}_a - \hat{\theta}_c$ and $\hat{\theta}_b - \hat{\theta}_d$ are left- and right-eye measures of a phase shift induced by unequal left- and right-eye grating contrasts. The left- and right-eye measures of phase shift can be combined into a single quantity, the perceived phase shift:

$$\hat{\theta} = \frac{\hat{\theta}_a + \hat{\theta}_b}{2} - \frac{\hat{\theta}_c + \hat{\theta}_d}{2}. \tag{15.4}$$

The perceived phase shift $\hat{\theta}$ has the useful property that, except for measurement error, when $\delta = 1$, $\hat{\theta} = 0$; when $\delta = 0$, $\hat{\theta} = \theta$. The perceived phase shift $\hat{\theta}$ is the dependent variable in all the experiments.

As shown in Figure 15.5, for a given condition of m, δ, and θ, each $\hat{\theta}_i$ ($i = $ a, b, c, d) was first measured by the corresponding psychometric function, and then the perceived phase shift $\hat{\theta}$ was calculated by Eq. (15.4).

15.2.7 Observers

Three observers were tested, the first author and two naïve observers, one of whom only participated in experiment 1. All had normal or corrected-to-normal vision.

15.3 Experiment 1. Binocular combination as determined by the interocular contrast ratio, the interocular grating phase difference, and overall contrast level

Experiment 1 measured the influence of the absolute contrast, relative contrast, and the relative phase of gratings in the left and right eyes on the cyclopean image.

15.3.1 Stimuli

The independent variables in the experiment were the contrast of the higher-contrast sinewave grating, $m = \max\{m_L, m_R\}$, the contrast of the lower-contrast sinewave grating which is expressed as a contrast ratio of lower/higher, $\delta = \min\{m_L, m_R\}/\max\{m_L, m_R\}$, and the phase difference, $\theta = \max\{\theta_L, \theta_R\} - \min\{\theta_L, \theta_R\}$, between the sinewave gratings presented to the left and right eyes. The duration of the stimulus T was fixed at 1000 ms.

15.3.2 Psychometric functions

The data are displayed as psychometric functions: the fraction of trials (converted to a probit) in which the reference line was judged to be above the middle of the dark band of the grating is plotted as a function of the vertical position of the reference line. Figure 15.5 illustrates four psychometric functions corresponding to four variations a, b, c and d (see also Figure 15.4) at a condition of $m = 10\%$, $\delta = 0.5$ and $\theta = 90$ for a single observer. In each plot, the abscissa is the position of the reference line in phase degrees relative to the center of the frame. The ordinate is the fraction of trials

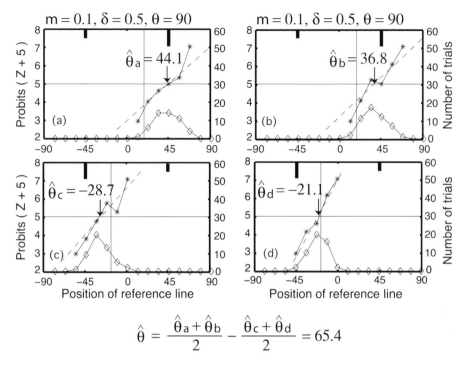

$$\hat{\theta} = \frac{\hat{\theta}_a + \hat{\theta}_b}{2} - \frac{\hat{\theta}_c + \hat{\theta}_d}{2} = 65.4$$

Figure 15.5. Psychometric functions and probit analyses. The data illustrated in panels (a), (b), (c), (d) correspond to the stimulus configurations (a), (b), (c), (d) of Figure 15.4. The left- and right-eye stimuli themselves are represented as bars at the top edge of the figure at $-45°$ and $+45°$, the length of the bar indicates the relative contrast. The abscissa is the position of the reference line measured in phase degrees of the sinewave grating; the ordinate is the fraction of trials on which the reference line was judged as being above the black stripe measured in probits (probits = Zscore + 5). Five probits corresponds to 50% probability. The bell-shaped curves at the bottom of the figure represent the number of trials actually conducted at the indicated position of the reference line; the right-hand ordinate indicates the number of trials. The dashed lines are maximum likelihood best fits (assuming Gaussian distributions) to the psychometric function data; their intersection with the horizontal 50% line represents the estimated cyclopean phase $\hat{\theta}_i$, i = a, b, c, d. The vertical lines represent predictions based on algebraic (linear) addition of the left- and right-eye stimuli and indicate a phase shift $\hat{\theta}_{linear}$ of $36°$ owing to unequal contrasts in the two eyes compared to the empirically observed phase shift of $\hat{\theta}$ of $65.4°$.

(converted to probits) on which the reference line was judged to be above the center of the dark band of the cyclopean grating. The ordinate is shown as probits (inverse normal density function, probits = Zscore + 5) so that if measurement errors were normally distributed, the data would fall on a straight line. Five probits corresponds to 50% probability.

Probits analysis (Finney, 1971) was used to fit the data. The slanted dashed line is the best-fitting straight line. The staircase procedure generated the most trials near 5 probits, and therefore these data have the most weight in the Maximum Likelihood Estimation of the best fit. The actual number of trials at each position of the reference line is illustrated at the bottom of each plot; the right-hand ordinate indicates the number of trials.

The apparent phase of the cyclopean grating is defined as the point at which the reference line is equally likely to be judged above and below the center of the dark band, i.e., the abscissa value at 5 probits, which we designate as $\hat{\theta}_i$ ($i = a, b, c, d$). The best-fitting straight line was determined by probit analysis. In the example of Figure 15.5a, the center of the dark band was judged to be higher above the center of the display, $\hat{\theta}_a = 44.1°$. The same analysis was applied to the data of conditions b, c and d (Figures 15.5b, c, and d, respectively), in which the apparent center of the dark band was judged to be at $\hat{\theta}_b = 36.8°$, $\hat{\theta}_c = -28.7°$, and $\hat{\theta}_d = -21.1°$, respectively.

Measurements $\hat{\theta}_a$, $\hat{\theta}_b$, $\hat{\theta}_c$, and $\hat{\theta}_d$ of the apparent phase shift tended to be biased slightly upwards. Whether this was due to a bias in the visual system, or due to the way pixels were designated in the display is immaterial because this bias is cancelled by considering only the difference given in Eq. (15.4), and never $\hat{\theta}_i$ ($i = a, b, c, d$) individually. The perceived phase shift $\hat{\theta}$ has two noteworthy properties: When there was no contrast difference between the left- and right-eye gratings, the displays of Figure 15.4a and Figure 15.4d are physically identical, as are the displays of Figure 15.4c and Figure 15.4b; therefore, the expected value of $\hat{\theta}$ is zero. When the lower-contrast grating has a contrast of zero, so that only the higher-contrast grating is visible, the expected value of $\hat{\theta}$ is simply the phase difference θ between the left- and right-eye gratings ($\theta = \theta_L - \theta_R = 90°$ in the example of Figure 15.5). The perceived phase shift $\hat{\theta}$ (Eq. (15.4)) measures how far a particular contrast ratio δ pushes the cyclopean perception $\hat{\theta}$ towards the maximum possible value θ (which is achieved when the left- and right-eye grating contrasts, respectively, are 1 and 0 ($\delta = 0$)).

The solid vertical lines in the plots of psychometric function (Figure 15.5) indicate the locations of the centers of the dark bands predicted by linear summation of the left- and right-eye images. The measured locations of the cyclopean gratings were more shifted toward the higher-contrast grating than predicted by simple linear addition of left- and right-eye inputs. This would occur if the linear prediction over-estimated the relative contribution of the lower-contrast grating to the cyclopean perception, i.e. if the effective $\hat{\delta}$ in this example were less than the the actual δ of 0.5.

15.3.3   Control conditions

We consider here the control conditions for experiment 1 in which the phase difference θ between the left- and right-eye sine waves was 90°. In the first set of control conditions, only one eye was presented with a sinewave grating, i.e. $\delta = 0$. This sinewave grating could be 45° above the midline in the left or right eye (conditions a and b, Figures 15.4a and 15.4b), or 45° below the midline (conditions c and d, Figures 15.4c and 15.4d). The perceived phase shift, $\hat{\theta}$ from Eq. (15.4), of cyclopean sinewave gratings should be the same as the actual phase difference θ of the input sinewave gratings, i.e. $\hat{\theta} = \theta = 90°$. Position bias can be evaluated in each control condition individually; it cancels in the difference.

In a second set of control conditions, the two eyes were presented with sinewave gratings of exactly the same contrast, i.e., $\delta = 1$. In this case, conditions a and d (as described above) were identical, as were conditions c and b. There would be a perceived difference between conditions a and b (left eye sinewave grating below or above midline) only if the left and right eyes did not have equal weight. For example, if the left eye was strongly dominant, then moving the dark band from above the midline to below the midline in the right eye (from a to b) would produce a big change in apparent position of the band. On the other hand, if the two eyes were equal in dominance, then there would be no perceived change. So, the subtraction $(b + c)$ minus $(a + d)$ gives an indication of the degree of difference in weights given to the left- and right-eye images.

Before formal data collection in an experiment session began, a preliminary session including two control conditions of $\delta = 0$ and $\delta = 1$ was carried out to evaluate position bias and ocular dominance. In fact, none of the three observers showed significant ocular dominance as tested with these sinewave gratings.

15.3.4 Results

Figure 15.6 shows the results of experiment 1. The data are the $\hat{\theta}$ values representing the perceived phase shift of cyclopean stimuli in which the dark band of the cyclopean sinewave grating (determined by the higher-contrast sine wave) was set above and below the midline position. The four different types of trials used to collect such a difference cancel linear components of position and eye bias. The contrast of the higher-contrast grating m took the following values, each of which is represented in an individual panel of Figure 15.6: (a) 5%, (b) 10%, (c) 20%, and (d) 40%. The phase difference θ took the values $45°$ (+), $90°$ (∗) and $135°$ (×), and the contrast ratio δ varied among 0.3, 0.5, 0.71, and 0.86 (abscissa). The ordinate is the perceived phase shift $\hat{\theta}$ produced by the asymmetry of the stimuli in the two eyes (see Eq. (15.4)). The dashed curves are predictions of the linear summation model. Linear summation gave a poor fit to the results except in the control conditions for which the predictions are trivial. In Figure 15.6, the solid lines are one-parameter fits to the data generated by the gain-control model described later in this article. Figures 15.7 and 15.8 show data for two additional observers.

All the data for all the observers lie above the linear prediction. This means that when the input contrasts to the two eyes are unequal, the higher-contrast grating has more weight (relative to the lower-contrast grating) in determining the cyclopean grating than predicted by linear summation of the inputs to the two eyes. In other words, the effective interocular contrast ratio $\hat{\delta}$, which can be calculated from the perceived phase shift $\hat{\theta}$, was smaller than the real contrast ratio. Figure 15.9 shows the effective interocular contrast ratio $\hat{\delta}$ as a function of the real contrast ratio δ in a log-log graph. The data are illustrated by lower-case letters that represent the experimental conditions. The dashed line is $\hat{\delta} = \delta$, the prediction of linear summation. The solid line with slope $1 + \gamma$ is $\hat{\delta} = \delta^{1+\gamma}$, the prediction of the gain-control model with best fitting γ from Figures 15.6, 15.7 and 15.8 for each observer. The greater spread of data for small δ is due to the fact that the variance of position judgements is relatively constant, independent of δ. Therefore the variance in $\log \hat{\delta}$ is proportional to $- \log(\delta)$.

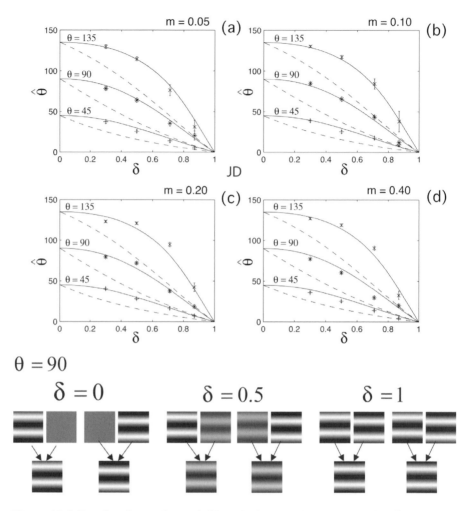

Figure 15.6. Results of experiment 1. How the interocular contrast ratio affects binocular combination: Perceived phase shift $\hat{\theta}$ as a function of the interocular contrast ratio for three phase differences of the interocular gratings and for four contrasts of the higher-contrast grating. Each panel shows the perceived phase shift $\hat{\theta}$ as a function of contrast ratio δ when the interocular grating phase difference θ is $45°$ (+), $90°$ (*), or $135°$ (×), and the greater contrast m was (a) 5%, (b) 10%, (c) 20%, or (d) 40%. The stimulus duration T was fixed at 1000 ms. The abscissa is the interocular contrast ratio δ; the ordinate is the measured cyclopean phase shift $\hat{\theta}$. The solid lines are best fits of the gain-control model (see below); the dashed lines are predictions of algebraic (linear) summation of the left- and right-eye stimuli. Inserts at the bottom show left- and right-eye stimuli together with the cyclopean (perceived) images for three contrast ratios δ with an interocular grating phase difference of $90°$. Observer JD.

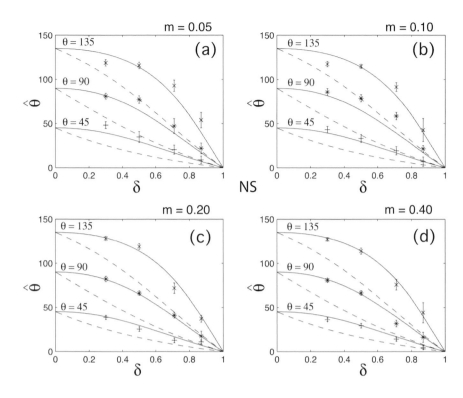

Figure 15.7. Results of experiment 1 for observer NS. See caption to Figure 15.6.

The data of experiment 1 are explained simply as the attenuation of the lower-contrast stimulus by a factor of δ^γ before binocular combination. This relationship is derived from the gain-control model. The following experiments investigate factors that determine the relative weights of the stimuli in the two eyes to enable estimation of other parameters of the gain-control model.

15.4 Experiment 2. Stimulus duration

15.4.1 High contrast energy vs. low contrast energy

The gain-control model of binocular combination described below has two properties that are relevant to experiment 1 and bear further investigation. As the contrast energy, $\mathcal{E}_L$ and $\mathcal{E}_R$, of input sinewave stimuli is reduced, the gain-control model asymptotically approaches simple linear summation. As the contrast energy $\mathcal{E}_{max}$ of the greater of two sinewave inputs is increased, the model's output becomes asymptotically independent of $\mathcal{E}_{max}$.

In experiment 1, the contrast energies $\mathcal{E}_{max}$ were quite high and, indeed, the shapes of the model predictions were virtually independent of the contrast of the higher-contrast sinewave grating. Experiment 2 was designed to investigate whether the gain-control

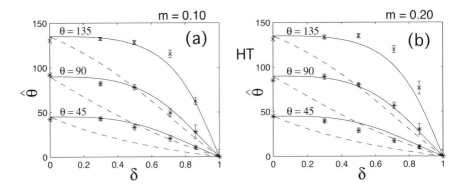

Figure 15.8. Results of experiment 1 for observer HT. See caption to Figure 15.6. The results for the control conditions $\delta = 0$, $\delta = 1$, are also shown here.

model remains valid when input gratings have low contrast energies, to investigate binocular combination over a range of contrast energies, and thereby to determine the time-constant of interocular gain control.

15.4.2 Stimuli

In experiment 1, the reference lines and the sinewave stimulus to be judged appeared simultaneously for 1000 ms. This simultaneity did not yield reliable data with very brief exposures. Figure 15.10 shows the slightly modified procedure used in experiment 2. Unlike experiment 1, the reference line was presented in advance of the input sinewave gratings. The reference line appeared 500 ms before the input sinewave grating was presented and remained on for 1500 ms. The duration of input sinewave gratings varied from 50 ms to 1000 ms. The stimuli used in experiment 2 are given by Eqs. (15.1) and (15.2) as in experiment 1 except that, where the stimulus duration T (Eq. (15.3)) in experiment 1 was fixed at 1000 ms, in experiment 2, T varied from 50 ms to 1000 ms.

Only one phase difference $\theta = 90°$ between the left- and right-eye sinewave gratings was used. Two contrasts of the higher-contrast grating were studied: 10% and 20%. The contrast ratio δ of the lower to the higher contrast sinewave grating took values of 0, 0.3, 0.5, 0.71, and 0.86. The following exposure durations were used: 50, 100, 200, 400, and 1000 ms. Each condition (m contrast of higher-contrast grating, δ contrast ratio, T exposure duration) was run in the four variations in Figure 15.4. All $2 \times 5 \times 5 \times 4 = 200$ conditions (10 000 trials) were run in a mixed-list design with interleaved up-down staircases. One experienced observer (HT) served as the observer.

15.4.3 Results

Figure 15.11 shows the results of experiment 2. Each panel shows a different combination of exposure duration and of contrast of the higher-contrast sine wave. In the control conditions, $\delta = 0$, the measured apparent phase difference was consistently very close to $90°$, indicating that the observer was able to make reliable judgments of

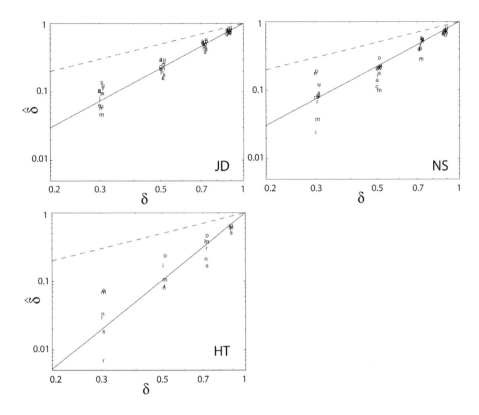

Figure 15.9. Experiment 1 analysis. How the interocular contrast ratio affects binocular combination: A log-log plot of the apparent interocular contrast ratio $\hat{\delta}$ as a function of the actual interocular contrast ratio δ. The apparent interocular contrast ratios $\hat{\delta}$ are calculated from the perceived phase shifts $\hat{\theta}$ of Figures 15.6, 15.7, and 15.8. The dashed lines are predicted by algebraic (linear) summation of left- and right-eye stimuli. The gain-control model predicts that, within measurement error, data for all interocular phase differences and for all contrasts of the higher-contrast grating collapse onto a single straight line with a slope equal to $1+\gamma$, where γ is the exponent of the rectifying power function in the gain-control path. For observers JD, NS, and HT, respectively, $\gamma = 1.18$, 1.17, and 2.27. The data points are represented by letters: a, $m = 0.05$ and $\theta = 45°$; c, $m = 0.05$ and $\theta = 90°$; e, $m = 0.05$ and $\theta = 135°$; i, $m = 0.10$ and $\theta = 45°$; m, $m = 0.10$ and $\theta = 90°$; n, $m = 0.10$ and $\theta = 135°$; o, $m = 0.20$ and $\theta = 45°$; r, $m = 0.20$ and $\theta = 90°$; s, $m = 0.20$ and $\theta = 135°$; u, $m = 0.40$ and $\theta = 45°$; v, $m = 0.40$ and $\theta = 90°$; x, $m = 0.40$ and $\theta = 135°$. The increase in log variability as δ decreases merely indicates that the variabilities of phase judgments tend to remain constant, independent of δ, and therefore for small δ log variability in $\hat{\delta}$ increases proportionally to $\log(1/\delta)$.

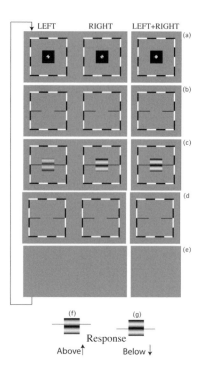

Figure 15.10. Procedure of experiment 2. How stimulus duration affects binocular combination. The procedure is similar to that of experiment 1 (see Figure 15.3). The differences are: (b) the reference lines appear 500 ms before the stimuli are presented; (c, d) the reference lines remain for 1500 ms; and the duration of the stimuli (c) varies from 50 ms to 1000 ms.

location. The dashed curves of Figure 15.11 are predictions of simple linear summation. The solid curves are the best fit of the gain-control model with one additional parameter, the time constant of interocular gain-control (563 ms).

For the short stimulus duration (50 ms) and lowest contrast (of the higher-contrast sinewave grating, 10%), the data are quite well described by linear summation of the inputs of the two eyes. However, as duration and contrast increased, the deviations from linear summation become greater. For the the highest contrast and duration, deviation from the linear model is extreme. Note also that in Figure 15.11, combinations with equal contrast energy produce similar data: e.g., $m = 0.1 \times T = 100$ and $m = 0.2 \times T = 50$, $m = 0.1 \times T = 200$ and $m = 0.2 \times T = 100$, and $m = 0.1 \times T = 400$ and $m = 0.2 \times T = 200$.

Figure 15.12 shows the results in a plot of the perceived phase shift $\hat{\theta}$ versus the stimulus duration T for a fixed contrast ratio of 0.5 for two observers. The data are the same as in Figure 15.11 when $\delta = 0.5$. The dashed line indicates the prediction of the linear model. The solid curve is derived from the same gain-control model as in Figure 15.11.

Figure 15.13 shows the effective interocular contrast ratio $\hat{\delta}$ as a function of the

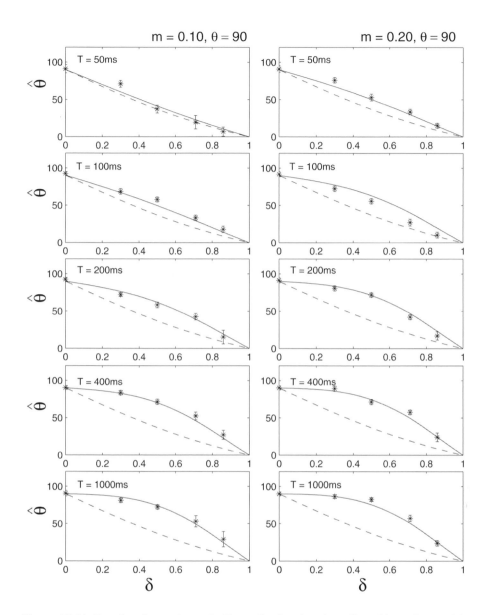

Figure 15.11. Results of experiment 2. How stimulus duration affects binocular combination. Perceived phase shift $\hat{\theta}$ as a function of interocular contrast ratio δ for stimulus durations from 50 ms to 1000 ms. Each row of panels shows a different duration T of the stimulus gratings. For the left column of panels, the contrast m of the higher-contrast grating is 0.10, for the right column, $m = 0.20$. The interocular grating phase difference θ was fixed at 90°. The dashed lines are the predictions based on algebraic (linear) summations of left- and right-eye stimuli; the solid lines are best fits of the gain-control model. Observer HT.

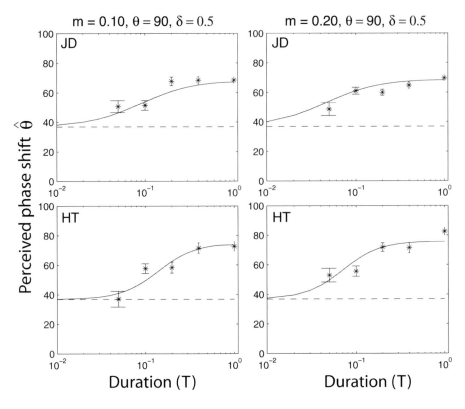

Figure 15.12. Summary of experiment 2. How stimulus duration affects binocular combination: Perceived phase shift $\hat{\theta}$ as a function of stimulus duration T for a fixed interocular contrast ratio $\delta = 0.5$. The interocular grating phase difference θ is 90°; the contrast m of the higher-contrast grating is 10% (left column) or 20% (right column). Top panels: Observer JD. Experimental data were obtained only for $\delta = 0.5$. Bottom panels: Observer HT. Data are taken from Figure 15.11 for $\delta = 0.5$. Dashed lines are predictions based on algebraic (linear) summations of the left- and right-eye stimuli; solid lines are best fits of the gain-control model.

actually presented contrast ratio δ in log-log coordinates. The solid curves are predictions from the best fitting gain-control model in Figure 15.11 transformed into this new coordinate system. All the data curves lie between the two asymptotes. The upper asymptote line is $\hat{\delta} = \delta$, the prediction from linear summation. The lower asymptote is $\hat{\delta} = \delta^{1+\gamma}$, the prediction from the same gain-control model with infinite contrast energy or, equivalently, $k = 0$. As the stimulus duration increased from 50 ms to 1000 ms and the contrast of higher-contrast sinewave grating increased from 10% to 20%, the stimulus contrast energy increased from the low values that approached the upper asymptote to high values of contrast energy that approached the lower asymptote. For all values of contrast energy, the data are confined to lie laminarly between these two asymptotes.

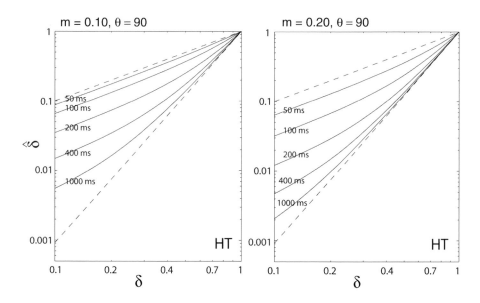

Figure 15.13. Experiment 2 analysis. How stimulus duration affects binocular combination. A log-log plot of the apparent interocular contrast ratio $\hat{\delta}$ as a function of the actual interocular contrast ratio δ for two contrasts of the higher-contrast stimulus and five different stimulus durations. The top dashed lines are derived from algebraic (linear) summations of the left- and right-eye images, i.e., $\hat{\delta} = \delta$. The solid lines are replotted from Figure 15.11 and represent the best fits of the gain-control model with the following parameters: a rectifying, power-law exponent $\gamma = 2.04$, a simple exponental temporal filter in the gain control path with time constant $\tau = 0.563$ s, and a gain-control threshold energy $k = 2.18 \times 10^{-4}$ s, e.g. 50 ms $\times$ contrast 0.436%. The bottom dashed lines are predictions of the gain-control model with a stimulus of infinite duration (or energy), or equivalently, when $k = 0$.

15.5 Experiment 3. Masking by spatial-frequency noise

15.5.1 Total contrast energy versus signal contrast energy

The gain-control model described by Eq. (15.9) predicts that the eye presented with a higher-contrast contrast energy stimulus will dominate binocular combination. In experiments 1 and 2, all contrast energies were perfectly correlated with the signal being judged. In experiments 3–6, one eye received an irrelevant stimulus, a "masking" stimulus, in addition to the stimulus being judged in order to determine the effect of the "mask" on ocular dominance. In all these experiments, the eyes were presented, as previously, with the 0.68° horizontal sinewave gratings in which the location of the cyclopean dark stripe was to be judged. The gratings were identical in contrast ($\delta = 1$) and differed only by a phase shift of $\theta = 90°$.

In experiment 3, the signal to one of the eyes also had added bandpass noise. If gain control was produced only by signal energy, the perceived phase shift would be

$0°$ for all levels of noise as $\delta = 1$. If the gain control were caused by the total contrast energy, the eye simultaneously presented with the added noise would dominate
in binocular combination because the eye receiving the added noise would have more
contrast energy.

15.5.2   Stimuli

In experiment 3, the two sinewave gratings being judged were both of contrast 0.1 and
differed in phase by $90°$. A bandpass noise, produced by filtering a two-dimensional
binary random noise $R(x, y)$ with a 2D isotropic bandpass filter (Rainville and Kingdom, 2002), was superimposed on the sinewave grating presented to one eye. In the
spatial frequency domain, the isotropic bandpass filters are defined as

$$Q(u, v, f_{s,N}) = \exp\left(-\frac{1}{2}\left(\frac{\ln(f/f_{s,N})}{\ln(\sigma)}\right)^2\right),   (15.5)$$

where u and v are the dimensions of a two-dimensional Cartesian spatial-frequency
coordinate system, f is defined as $\sqrt{u^2 + v^2}$, $f_{s,N}$ is the center spatial-frequency, and
σ determines the bandwidth of the filter. Six bandpass filters having different values of
center spatial-frequency were used in the experiment. Their center spatial-frequencies,
$f_{s,N}$, were separated by an octave, and are $\{0.34, 0.68, 1.36, 2.72, 5.44, 10.88 \text{ cpd}\}$.
The half-amplitude bandwidth of the various noise masks was a factor of 2.4 (1.26
octaves). A spatial bandpass filtered noise $\widetilde{\mathcal{M}}(x, y, f_{s,N})$ was obtained via a reverse
Fourier transform: $\widetilde{\mathcal{M}}(x, y, f_{s,N}) = Re(\mathcal{F}^{-1}\{Q(u, v, f_{s,N})\mathcal{F}(R(x, y))\})$. Normalizing a bandpass noise $\widetilde{\mathcal{M}}(x, y, f_{s,N})$ by its RMS contrast yielded a "standard" noise
$\mathcal{M}(x, y, f_{s,N})$ with RMS contrast 1.0, i.e.,

$$\mathcal{M}(x, y, f_{s,N}) = \frac{\widetilde{\mathcal{M}}(x, y, f_{s,N})}{\text{RMS}(\widetilde{\mathcal{M}}(x, y, f_{s,N}))}.   (15.6)$$

The stimuli in experiment 3 are given by Eqs. (15.1) and (15.2), where the mask
$\mathcal{M}$ is given by Eq. (15.6), $m_L = m_R$, $\theta_L - \theta_R = \pm 90°$, and one of n_L and n_R (the RMS
contrast of the bandpass masking noise in one eye) was set to be zero. The values of m
and n were constrained so that less than 5% of pixels fell outside the range of contrast
values that can be produced on the display screen.

Sample stimuli are shown in the top of Figure 15.14. Figure 15.14 (L) illustrates a
sinewave grating presented (for example) to the left eye and Figure 15.14 (R) illustrates
a similar grating presented to the right eye phase-shifted $90°$ and with added bandpass
noise. A sample of a signal plus noise in each frequency band is shown in the inset on
each plot.

The procedure for experiment 3 was the same as that for experiment 1. For each
combination of center spatial-frequencies, $f_{s,N}$, and noise-signal ratios $N/S = n/m$
there are four variations: dark stripe up/down × mask L/R. All $6 \times 4 \times 4 = 96$ conditions
were run in a mixed-list design with interleaved up-down staircases. Two experienced
observers served in the experiment.

15.5.3 Results

Figure 15.14 shows the results of experiment 3. The abscissa indicates the root-mean-square (RMS) contrast ratio of the noise to the signal (N/S), and the ordinate indicates perceived phase shift, $\hat{\theta}$. When $\hat{\theta} = 0$, both eyes have equal contributions to binocular combination. When $\hat{\theta} > 0$, it indicates that the eye with the added noise mask dominated the binocular combination. All of the data show that the eye which receives the added noise dominates binocular combination. The greater the noise energy, the greater the domination. Remarkably, the greatest domination occurred at a frequency (2.72 cpd) that is 4× the frequency being judged. At equal contrast ($N/S = 1$) there was almost complete domination, a phase shift of $80°$ out of a possible $90°$. Contrary to a Bayesian point of view which would suggest that a noisy stimulus should have less influence in binocular combination than a noiseless one, the noisy stimulus dominates up to and beyond the point where it has obliterated the stimulus being judged so that location judgments are no longer possible (e.g. Figure 15.14 b and c).

Figure 15.15 shows the data of a second observer. The spatial frequency modulation transfer function derived from these data is shown in the model section (below).

15.6 Experiment 4. Masking sinewave gratings of different spatial frequencies

15.6.1 Masking sinewave gratings in experiments 4, 5, and 6

In experiments 4, 5, and 6, as in experiment 3, the left- and right-eye sinewave gratings are of the same contrast and differ only in phase, $\theta = 90°$. A masking sinewave grating, given by

$$\mathcal{M}(x, y, f_{s,mask}, f_{t,mask}, \beta) = \sin(2\pi f_{s,mask}(x \cos \beta + y \sin \beta) \pm 2\pi f_{t,mask}t + \theta_{mask}),$$
$$(15.7)$$

was superimposed on one eye's sinewave grating.

15.6.2 Stimuli

In experiment 4, the stimuli are given by Eqs. (15.1) and (15.2) where $\mathcal{M}$ is given by Eq. (15.7), $m_L = m_R = 10\%$, $\theta_L - \theta_R = \pm 90°$, and one of n_L and n_R was set to be zero.

The mask was a static vertical sinewave grating; its spatial frequency $f_{s,mask}$ was chosen from among $\{0.34, 0.68, 1.36, 2.72, 5.44, 10.88\}$ cpd, $\beta = 90°$ (the angle between horizontal grating being judged and the the masking grating), and $f_{t,mask} = 0$. For each combination of the spatial frequency $f_{s,mask}$ and mask-to-signal contrast ratio M/S, there were four variations: dark stripe up/down × mask L/R. The procedure for experiment 4 was the same as that for experiment 1. All $6 \times 5 \times 4 = 120$ conditions were run in a mixed-list design with interleaved up-down staircases. Two experienced observers served in the experiment.

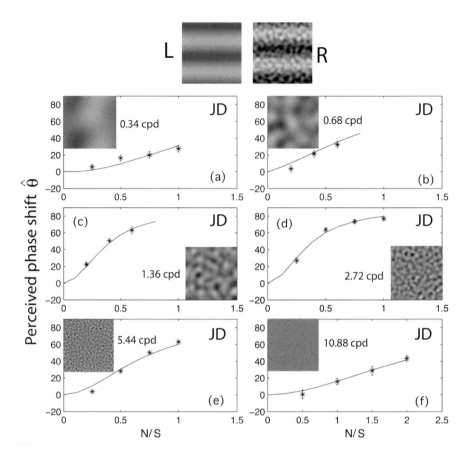

Figure 15.14. Experiment 3. How the spatial frequency and contrast of added 2D noise in one eye increase its binocular dominance. (L, R) A sample binocular stimulus to the left and right eyes. Panels (a)–(f) show the perceived phase shift $\hat{\theta}$ as a function of the ratio of RMS noise to RMS signal, N/S. The horizontal grating contrast (signal) S was 0.1 and was equal in both eyes (interocular contrast ratio $\delta = 1$). The interocular grating phase difference θ was $90°$. The central spatial frequency (in cycles per degree of visual angle, cpd) of the noise is indicated in each panel. The half-amplitude bandwidth of the various masking noise stimuli was a factor of 2.4 (1.26 octaves). The signal has a spatial frequency of 0.68 cpd. Data collection was continued until N/S was either too great to permit judgments of phase (e.g. panels (b), (c)) or until the limits of the apparatus were reached (other panels). The solid lines are the best fits derived from the gain-control model. Adding noise to one eye at 2.72 cpd with an RMS amplitude equal to that of the binocular signal being judged gave the masked eye virtually complete binocular domination, i.e. produced a phase shift of $80°$ of a maximum possible $90°$ (a $90°$ phase shift implies zero weight for the signal in the unmasked eye). Observer JD.

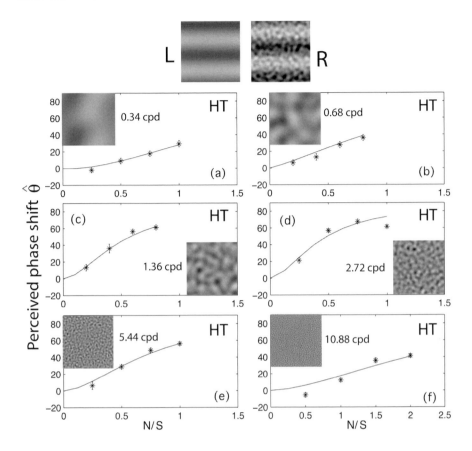

Figure 15.15. Experiment 3. How the spatial frequency and contrast of added 2D noise in one eye increases its binocular dominance. Observer HT. See caption to Figure 15.14.

15.6.3 Results

Figure 15.16 shows the results of experiment 4. The abscissa indicates the contrast ratio M/S of mask to signal, and the ordinate indicates the perceived phase shift, $\hat{\theta}$. As in experiment 3, the data show that the eye receiving the grating mask dominates the summation. As mask contrast increased, domination increased. The data for sinewave masking as a function of spatial frequency were quite similar to those obtained in experiment 3 for band-limited noise masking as a function of spatial frequency. Figure 15.17 shows the results of a second observer. The spatial frequency modulation transfer function will be considered in the model section.

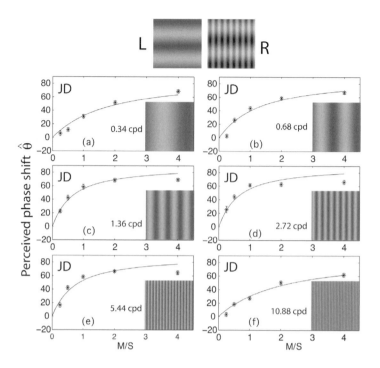

Figure 15.16. Results of experiment 4: How masking sinewave gratings of different spatial frequencies in one eye increase its dominance in binocular combination. (L, R) A sample binocular stimulus to the left and right eyes. Panels (a)–(f) show the perceived phase shift $\hat{\theta}$ as a function of the ratio M/S of the amplitude M of a vertical sinewave grating masking stimulus in one eye to the amplitude S of the binocular horizontal sinewave signal whose phase was being judged. The spatial frequency (in cycles per degree of visual angle, cpd) of the vertical masking grating was indicated in each panel. The horizontal signal grating contrast S was 0.1 and equal in both eyes (interocular contrast ratio $\delta = 1$). The interocular grating phase difference θ was 90°. The horizontal signal grating is 0.68 cpd. Data collection was continued until M/S was at the limits of the apparatus. The solid lines are the best fits derived from the gain-control model. A masking-to-signal ratio M/S ≥ 2 gave the masked eye overwhelming dominance in binocular combination. Observer JD.

15.7 Experiment 5. Temporal frequency masking

15.7.1 Stimuli

The procedure for experiment 5 was basically the same as that for experiment 4. The stimuli were the same as those in experiment 4, given by Eqs. (15.1) and (15.2) except that the added vertical mask was a drifting rather than a stationary sinewave grating. Mask parameters were $f_{s,mask} = 0.68$ cpd, the same spatial frequency as the signal, and $\beta = 90°$ (mask to signal angle, Eq. (15.7)).

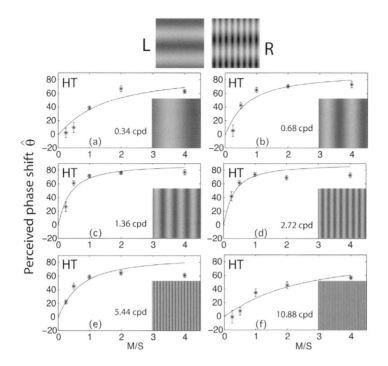

Figure 15.17. Results of experiment 4. How masking sinewave gratings of different spatial frequencies in one eye increase its dominance in binocular combination. Observer HT. See caption of Figure 15.16.

The independent variables were mask contrast, mask temporal frequency $f_{t,mask}$, four variations (dark stripe up/down × mask L/R), and mask movement direction (left, right). All $5×5×4×2 = 200$ conditions were run in a mixed-list design with interleaved up-down staircases (5 000 trials). Two experienced observers served in the experiment.

15.7.2 Results

Figure 15.18 shows the results of experiment 5. The abscissa indicates the contrast ratio of mask to signal (M/S), and the ordinate indicates the perceived phase shift, $\hat{\theta}$. Again, the data show that the eye receiving – in this case – a drifting masking grating dominated the binocular combination. As mask contrast increased, domination increases for all temporal frequencies. In Figure 15.18f, the data from 0 Hz and 30 Hz are plotted together to illustrate that these two masking functions differ mainly by a horizontal translation, i.e. there was proportionally less masking at 30 Hz than for a stationary grating – or for that matter any lower temporal frequency. This low-pass characteristic of the temporal frequency modulation transfer function will be further considered below in the model section. Figure 15.19 shows the data of a second observer.

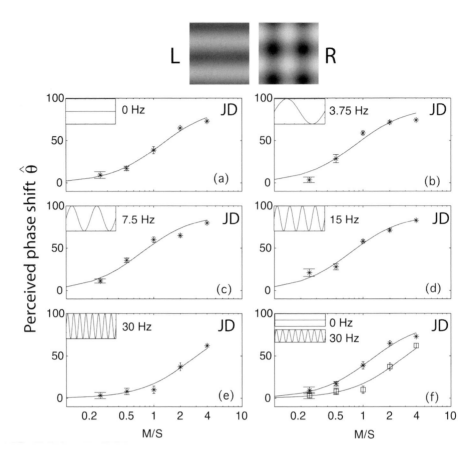

Figure 15.18. Results of experiment 5. How the temporal frequency and contrast of a dynamic masking grating in one eye increase its binocular dominance. (L, R) A sample left- and right-eye frame from a dynamic binocular stimulus. Panels (a)–(f) show the perceived phase shift $\hat{\theta}$ as a function of the ratio M/S of the amplitude M of a drifting vertical sinwave grating masking stimulus in one eye to the amplitude S of the binocular horizontal sinewave signal whose phase is being judged. The horizontal signal and vertical masking grating both have a spatial frequency of 0.68 cpd. The horizontal signal grating contrast S is 0.1 and equal in both eyes (interocular contrast ratio $\delta = 1$). The interocular grating phase difference θ is 90°. The vertical masking grating translates horizontally (randomly left or right from trial to trail) to produce temporal frequencies of 0–30 Hz as indicated in panels (a)–(f). For comparison, panel (f) shows the data for both 0 Hz masking (from panel a) and 30 Hz. Data collection is continued until M/S is at the limits of the apparatus. The solid lines are the best fits derived from the gain-control model. At all temporal frequencies 0–30 Hz, a masking-to-signal amplitude ratio of 4 gives the masked eye overwhelming dominance in binocular combination. Observer JD.

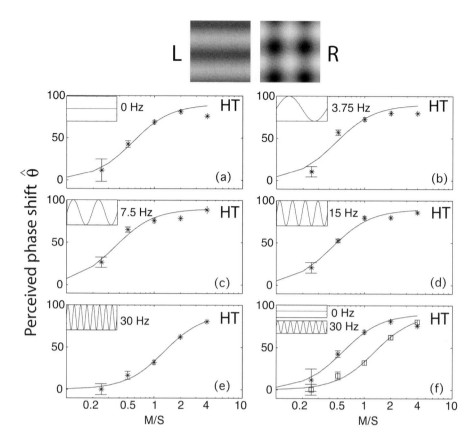

Figure 15.19. Results of experiment 5. How the temporal frequency and contrast of a dynamic masking grating in one eye increase its binocular dominance. Observer HT. See caption of Figure 15.18.

15.8 Experiment 6. Orientation masking

15.8.1 Stimuli

The procedure for experiment 6 was similar to that for experiment 4. The stimuli were the same as those in experiment 4, given by Eqs. (15.1) and (15.2), except that the orientation of the mask grating varied from trial to trial instead of being fixed at the vertical position. The parameters for the mask grating are described in Eq. (15.7): spatial frequency $f_{s,mask} = 5.44$ cpd (three octaves higher than that of the signal), temporal frequency $f_{t,mask} = 0$ (a static sinewave grating). The independent variables were mask contrast (5 levels) and mask orientation (9 levels). All $9 \times 5 \times 4 = 180$ conditions were run in a mixed-list design with interleaved up-down staircases. Two experienced observers served in the experiment.

15.8.2   Results

Figure 15.20 shows the results of Experiment 6. The abscissa indicates the contrast ratio of mask to signal (M/S) and the ordinate indicates the perceived phase shift, $\hat{\theta}$. Again, the data show that the eye receiving – in this case – an oriented, static masking grating dominates binocular combination. All orientations are effective in producing domination, but vertical and horizontal gratings seem to be somewhat better than diagonally oriented gratings. As mask contrast increases, domination increases for all orientations. That orientation angle affects masking indicates that the "receptive field" of the masking channels cannot be exclusively circularly symmetric which, in turn, implies that at least some portion of the gain control has a cortical origin. The orientation tuning function will be derived and discussed in the model section. Figure 15.21 shows the results of a second observer.

15.9   Model

There have been many experimental investigations and numerous theories proposed to describe binocular combination. A pervasive problem with these efforts has been that they typically operate on a principle that is less than a point-by-point binocular combination of images. Typically, the theories abstract a parameter from each eye's image (e.g., the maximum stimulus contrast or brightness, a contrast detection threshold, a signal-to-noise ratio, or the visual direction of a significant point) and combine the parameter values from each eye to predict the parameter value in the cyclopean image.

Previously (Ding and Sperling, 2006), we offered a gain-control theory that in principle could derive a cyclopean image from a point-by-point comparison of the monocular images, and which derived the desired cyclopean parameters from the cyclopean image itself (rather than simply from a combination of the monocular parameters). At present we have derived the parameters of the gain-control theory for just a single visual channel sensitive to horizontal sine waves around 0.68 cpd. It is not clear how these parameters will generalize to other channels nor how channels will combine. Nevertheless, this is a physiologically plausible approach to binocular processes in early vision. Here we represent the gain-control model, derive the model parameters from the experimental data, and show how the model can efficiently account for not less than 97% of the variance in the experimental data for all observers and experiments. We then extend the model's predictions, which here have been concerned entirely with the phase of binocularly combined gratings, to amplitude as well.

15.9.1   Linear summation

Suppose that binocular combination were a linear combination of the left- and right-eye images, i.e., $\hat{I}(x) = I_{\mathrm{L}}(x) + I_{\mathrm{R}}(x)$, where $I_{\mathrm{L}}(x)$ and $I_{\mathrm{R}}(x)$ are defined by Eqs. (15.1) and (15.2). The perceived phase shift $\hat{\theta}$ of $\hat{I}(x)$ (defined by Eq. (15.4)) is then given by

$$\hat{\theta} = 2\tan^{-1}\left(\frac{1-\delta}{1+\delta}\tan\left(\frac{\theta}{2}\right)\right). \qquad (15.8)$$

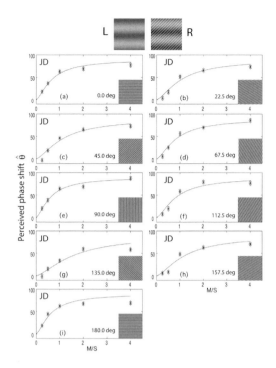

Figure 15.20. Results of experiment 6. How the orientation and contrast of a masking grating in one eye increase its binocular dominance. (L, R) A sample binocular stimulus to the left and right eyes. Panels (a)–(i) show the perceived phase shift $\hat{\theta}$ as a function of the ratio M/S of the amplitude M of a sinewave grating masking stimulus (in one eye) to the amplitude S of the binocular horizontal sinewave signal whose phase was being judged. The signal grating contrast S was 0.1 and was equal in both eyes (interocular contrast ratio $\delta = 1$). The interocular grating phase difference θ was 90°. The spatial frequency of the masking grating was 5.44 cpd, 3 octaves higher than that of the 0.68 cpd horizontal signal grating whose phase was being judged. The angle of the monocular masking grating (relative to the binocular signal grating) is indicated in each panel (a)–(i). Data collection was continued until M/S is at the limits of the apparatus. The solid lines are the best fits derived from the gain-control model. At all orientations, masking stimuli that have contrasts 2 times greater than the binocular stimulus being judged gave the masked eye almost total ocular dominance. Observer JD.

Equation 15.8 defines the dashed lines (linear predictions) in Figures 15.6, 15.7, 15.8, 15.11 and elsewhere. The linear summation model's prediction connects with the data only at the end points – the nominal control conditions – in which $\delta = 0$ and $\delta = 1$ (which do not require measurement). The linear prediction does not match any of the actual data except those obtained with near-threshold stimuli.

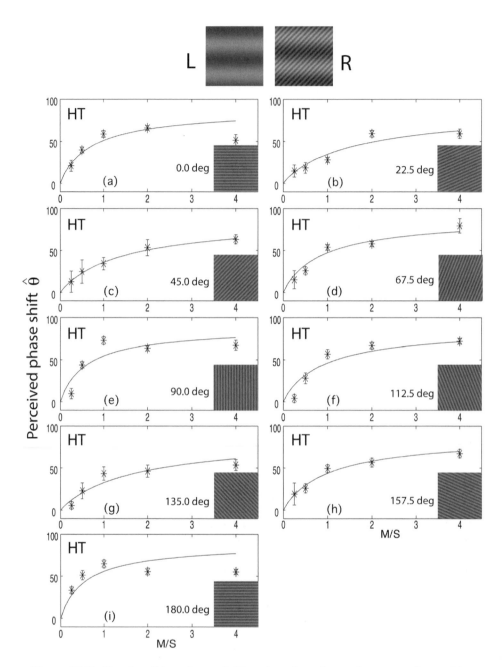

Figure 15.21. Results of experiment 6. How the orientation and contrast of a masking grating in one eye increase its binocular dominance. Observer HT. See caption of Figure 15.20.

15.9.2 Gain-control model

The problem with the linear model is that the eye with the higher-contrast stimulus has a greater advantage (or equivalently, the eye with the lower-contrast stimulus has a greater disadvantage, or both) than is predicted by algebraic addition of the stimuli. How does this come about? How does the brain attenuate the weaker stimulus prior to binocular combination? The gain-control model of Figure 15.22 (Ding and Sperling, 2006) is our attempt to answer this question. In every neighborhood, each eye exerts gain control on the other eye in proportion to the strength of its own input. The eye receiving the lower-contrast stimulus not only has a weaker stimulus but also receives the stronger gain-control signal from the other eye which has the higher-contrast stimulus.

Normalizing the gain control itself solves a lot of problems. We propose that an eye, say the left eye, not only gain-controls the right eye's output but also the right eye's attempt to control the left eye's output. These dual gain control mechanisms give the model the extraordinary property that, for equal stimuli to the two eyes which are sufficiently above threshold, closing one eye does not change the output of the model, emulating a profound property of natural vision. As shown in Figure 15.22a, the output $\hat{I}$ of the model is

$$\hat{I} = \frac{1 + \mathcal{E}_L}{1 + \mathcal{E}_L + \mathcal{E}_R} I_L + \frac{1 + \mathcal{E}_R}{1 + \mathcal{E}_L + \mathcal{E}_R} I_R, \tag{15.9}$$

where $\mathcal{E}_L$ and $\mathcal{E}_R$ are the total contrast energies of the images presented to the two eyes respectively. When $\mathcal{E}_L \gg 1$ and $\mathcal{E}_R \gg 1$, Eq. (15.9) becomes

$$\hat{I} \approx \frac{\mathcal{E}_L}{\mathcal{E}_L + \mathcal{E}_R} I_L + \frac{\mathcal{E}_R}{\mathcal{E}_L + \mathcal{E}_R} I_R, \tag{15.10}$$

from which the one-eye-equals-two-eyes property is immediately apparent.

15.9.3 Total visually weighted Contrast Energy (TCE)

The results from experiment 3 show that the gain-control mechanism depends not only on the stimulus contrast in the channel being judged, but on a wide range of channels, the most effective ones being $4\times$ higher in spatial frequency. The model assumes that a quantity, the "Total visually weighted Contrast Energy" (TCE) of a stimulus, is used for the gain-control mechanism. Experiment 2 showed that gain control depended on exposure duration or, more precisely, on total contrast energy. Spatial frequency (experiments 3,4), temporal frequency (experiment 5), and orientation of a masking stimulus (experiment 6) all affect binocular combination. We assume therefore that the gain-controlling contrast energy is a weighted sum over all spatial frequency channels. We have not investigated how the TCE depends on the spatial arrangement of the contributing channels.

Figure 15.22b illustrates the computation of Total visually-weighted Contrast Energy (TCE) for the left eye. Let I_L be the input image to the left eye and $I_{L,i}$ be the output of the temporal filter $h_{L,i}(t)$ within the ith spatial-frequency-and-orientation

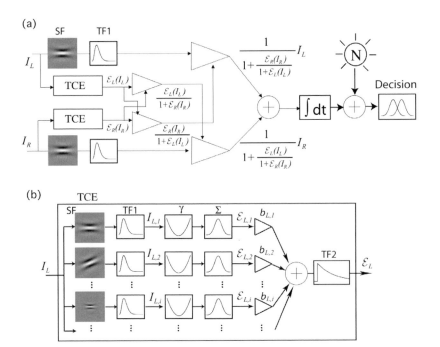

Figure 15.22. Gain-control model for binocular combination within a single binocular channel. (a) Block diagram of the model. The luminance stimuli to each eye, I_L and I_R, are considered as being split into two channels: a stimulus analysis channel which, in this case, is selective for 0.68 cpd horizontal sine waves, and a gain-control channel that computes the Total visually weighted Contrast Energy, TCE. The stimulus analysis channels from the two eyes add their outputs to produce the cyclopean image. Triangles indicate shunting gain-control "amplifiers" in which the input is divided by a gain-control signal to produce the output. Prior to the addition of the signal channels, the TCE in each eye exerts shunting gain control on the signal of the opposing eye (top and bottom triangles). Additionally, the TCE in each eye also exerts gain control on the other eye's gain-control signal (middle triangles). This model of binocular combination has the remarkable property that when only one eye has a stimulus and the other eye has a blank, the output is asymptotically the same as when both eyes have the same stimulus. To extend the model of binocular combination to apply to the present psychophysical experiments, three additional components are required. An integrator that integrates the total output of the model for the duration of a trial; random noise that is added to the integrated output; and a decision component that makes an optimal response based on the input it receives. (b) The computation of Total visually weighted Contrast Energy (TCE). The visual stimulus is processed separately in spatial-frequency-and-orientation channels, i.e. within each spatial frequency band, there are separate channels for each orientation. Channels overlap in spatial frequency, in orientation, and in space. In each gain-control channel, the signal is first temporally filtered by a lowpass filter (TF1) whose properties are defined by experiment 5, power-law rectified with exponent (γ), passed through a summing filter that sums over a wide spatial area ($\sum$), and assigned a weight $b_{L,i}$ that is specific for the particular pair of channels involved (signal, gain-control). TCE is the weighted sum of many such channels, only three of which are illustrated, and averaged over a relatively long period of time by a simple one stage RC filter TF2 whose time-constant is determined by experiment 2.

channel $g_{L,i}(x, y)$. Then

$$I_{L,i}(x, y, t) = \int g_{L,i}(x' - x, y' - y)h_{L,i}(t' - t)I_L(x', y', t')dx'dy'dt'. \quad (15.11)$$

The visually weighted contrast energy of the ith channel is given by

$$\mathcal{E}_{L,i}(I_L, x, y, t) = \int a_{L,i}(x' - x, y' - y)|I_{L,i}(x', y', t)|^\gamma dx'dy', \quad (15.12)$$

where $a_{L,i}(x, y)$ is a large-space constant spatial filter. The TCE, $\mathcal{E}_L(I_L)$ is the weighted sum over all spatial-frequency-and-orientation channels, i.e.

$$\mathcal{E}_L(I_L, x, y, t) = \sum_i b_{L,i}\mathcal{E}_{L,i}(I_L, x, y, t), \quad (15.13)$$

where $b_{L,i}$ is a gain-control weight that is specific to an output channel (e.g. the horizontal channel centered at 0.68 cpd).

15.9.4 How the gain-control model accounts for the data of experiment 1

The model deals with contrast energy $\mathcal{E}$ which, in experiment 1, is taken to be simply the contrast of the sinewave grating stimulus to each eye, m_L and m_R. We have $\mathcal{E}_L = b_S m_L^\gamma$ and $\mathcal{E}_R = b_S m_R^\gamma$, where b_S is the gain-control efficiency of the signal sinewave grating. In experiment 1, even the lowest-contrast stimuli are sufficiently strong that the total contrast energy $\mathcal{E}_L(I_L) \gg 1$. Therefore we can use Eq. (15.10) to fit the data of experiment 1. Given the estimated parameters, using Eq. (15.10) instead of Eq. (15.9) changes the predictions by less than 1%. Equation (15.10) is further simplified to yield:

$$\hat{I} \approx \frac{m_L^\gamma}{m_L^\gamma + m_R^\gamma}I_L + \frac{m_R^\gamma}{m_L^\gamma + m_R^\gamma}I_R. \quad (15.14)$$

The advantage of Eq. (15.14) over Eq. (15.9) is that together with Eqs. (15.1) and (15.2) it yields a simple expression for the perceived phase shift $\hat{\theta}$

$$\hat{\theta} \approx 2\tan^{-1}\left(\frac{1 - \delta^{\gamma+1}}{1 + \delta^{\gamma+1}}\tan\left(\frac{\theta}{2}\right)\right), \quad (15.15)$$

represented by the solid curves in Figures 15.6–15.8. Equations (15.15) and (15.8) yield the effective interocular contrast ratio as a power function of the actual interocular contrast ratio:

$$\hat{\delta} = \delta^{1+\gamma}, \quad (15.16)$$

which is plotted as solid lines in Figure 15.9 along with experimental data. In experiment 1, when $\mathcal{E}_L(I_L) \gg 1$ and $\mathcal{E}_R(I_R) \gg 1$, the gain control effectively attenuates the lower-contrast stimulus by a factor of δ^γ.

Using Eq. (15.14) (the close approximation for above-threshold stimuli to the full gain-control model) to fit the data, means only one free parameter γ needs to be estimated for each observer: $\gamma = 1.18$ for the observer JD whose data are shown in

Figure 15.6; $\gamma = 1.17$ for the observer NS in Figure 15.7; $\gamma = 2.27$ for the observer HT in Figure 15.8. Overall, this 1-estimated-parameter version of the gain-control model accounts for 99.4%, 99.0%, and 98.5%, respectively, of the variance of the data (48 conditions) for observers JD, HT, and NS.

15.9.5   How the gain-control model accounts for the data of experiment 2

The data of experiment 2 depend on the temporal filter $h(t)$

$$h(t) = \exp\left(\frac{-t}{\tau}\right), \tag{15.17}$$

in the model as shown in Figure 15.22b. For a pulse of duration T (Eq.(15.3)), the model output is given by

$$q(t) = \int_0^t u(t')h(t - t')dt'. \tag{15.18}$$

When inputs $I_L(x, y, t)$ and $I_R(x, y, t)$ are given by Eqs. (15.1) and (15.2), the contrast energies $\mathcal{E}_L(t)$ and $\mathcal{E}_R(t)$ are given by

$$\mathcal{E}_L(t) = b_S\left(m_L \int_0^t u(t')h(t - t')dt'\right)^\gamma = b_S m_L^\gamma q^\gamma(t), \tag{15.19}$$

$$\mathcal{E}_R(t) = b_S\left(m_R \int_0^t u(t')h(t - t')dt'\right)^\gamma = b_S m_R^\gamma q^\gamma(t). \tag{15.20}$$

From Eqs. (15.9), (15.19) and (15.20), a cyclopean stimulus $\hat{I}(x, y, t)$ is given by

$$\hat{I}(x, y, t) = \frac{k + m_L^\gamma q^\gamma(t)}{k + m_L^\gamma q^\gamma(t) + m_R^\gamma q^\gamma(t)} I_L(x, y, t) + \frac{k + m_R^\gamma q^\gamma(t)}{k + m_L^\gamma q^\gamma(t) + m_R^\gamma q^\gamma(t)} I_R(x, y, t), \tag{15.21}$$

where $k = 1/b_S$ is a gain-control threshold energy. Integrating $\hat{I}(x, y, t)$ over stimulus duration T yields $\hat{I}(x, y)$, i.e.

$$\hat{I}(x, y) = \int_0^T \hat{I}(x, y, t)dt, \tag{15.22}$$

a cyclopean sinewave grating whose phase is used to fit the data.

When the stimulus duration T is very brief, the output of temporal filter $h(t)$ is very small, and the total contrast energy TCE is too small to exert effective gain control in binocular combination; the behavior of the model approximates linear summation. As T increases, the contrast energy also increases, and the behavior of the model deviates from linear summation to become more and more nonlinear.

To fit the data of experiment 2, two new model parameters are needed in addition to the power-law rectification parameter γ from experiment 1: a threshold parameter

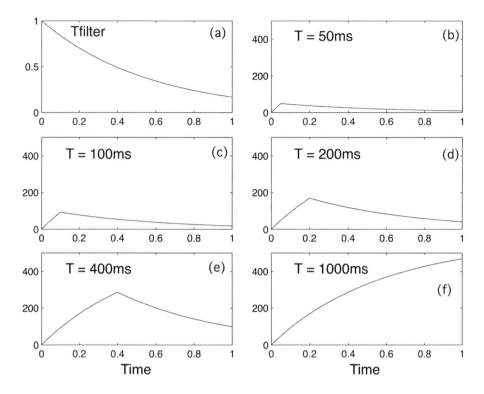

Figure 15.23. The temporal filter (TF) in the gain control circuit and the filter's response to square-wave stimuli of various durations. (a) Impulse response of the temporal filter. A time constant of 563 ms provides an optimal fit to the data of experiment 2. (b)–(f) Filter outputs when the input is a pulse of the indicated duration. In the model, the direct stimulus inputs are not subjected to frequency filtering – an adequate approximation for the current experiments – but the inputs are modified by gain control. In experiment 2, the input is zero when there is no stimulus; therefore gain control is effective only during the actual duration of the stimulus.

k, and the time-constant τ of the temporal filter. The best fitting parameters for data in Figure 15.11 are $\gamma = 2.04$, $k = 2.18 \times 10^{-4}$ s (e.g. 50 ms × 0.436%), and $\tau = 563$ ms. Figure 15.23a illustrates the simple exponential temporal filter, and Figures 15.23b-f illustrate its outputs as stimulus duration T varies from 50 ms to 1 000 ms. The percents of data variance accounted for by the model are 99.4% and 98.2%, respectively, for observers JD and HT.

15.9.6 How the gain-control model accounts for the data of experiment 3

In experiment 3, the contrasts of the sinewave grating stimuli to each eye were identical, i.e. $m_R = m_L = m$. Let the RMS contrast of a bandpass noise added to one eye, say the left eye, be n. The total contrast energy is $\mathcal{E}_L = b_S m^\gamma + b_N n^\gamma$ and $\mathcal{E}_R = b_S m^\gamma$. In experiment 3, the contrast energy $\mathcal{E}_L \gg 1$ and $\mathcal{E}_R \gg 1$, so for simplicity, we can use Eq. (15.10). Equation (15.10) becomes

$$\hat{I} = \frac{1 + b(f_{s,N})(N/S)^\gamma}{2 + b(f_{s,N})(N/S)^\gamma} I_L + \frac{1}{2 + b(f_{s,N})(N/S)^\gamma} I_R, \qquad (15.23)$$

where $N/S = n/m$ is a noise-to-signal RMS contrast ratio (here, m is defined as RMS contrast), and $b(f_{s,N}) = b_N/b_S$ is a relative contribution to gain control of the bandpass noise with central frequency of $f_{s,N}$. The free parameters for the model are γ_3 which is the average rectification power-law exponent for the signal and the various noise channels involved in experiment 3, and the $b(f_{s,N})$ that represent the domination efficiencies (relative to the 0.68 cpd horizontal sinewave grating being judged) of the various masking noise stimuli. The six solid curves in Figure 15.14 are the best fits using the gain-control model of Eq. (15.23). For observer JD, the best fitting parameters are $\gamma = 1.89$ and $b(f_{s,N}) = \{0.69, 1.0, 1.68, 3.61, 1.41, 0.42\}$; they yield the spatial frequency modulation transfer function (MTF) illustrated in the top of Figure 15.24. The bottom panel of Figure 15.24 shows the MTF for observer HT. For both observers, the gain-control efficiency of masking noise was at maximum when the noise frequency was at 2.72 cpd ($4\times$ the signal spatial frequency). The percents of data variance accounted for by the model are 99.3% and 98.4%, respectively, for observers JD and HT.

15.9.7   How the gain-control model accounts for the data of experiments 4–6

In experiments 4–6, when a mask sinewave grating was superimposed on, say, the left eye, the total contrast energy to each eye can be calculated similarly to experiment 3 as $\mathcal{E}_L = b_S m^\gamma + b_M n^\gamma$ and $\mathcal{E}_R = b_S m^\gamma$. Similarly, for the conditions of experiments 4, 5 and 6, the contrast energy $\mathcal{E}_L \gg 1$ and $\mathcal{E}_R \gg 1$. Again, Eq. (15.10) is sufficiently accurate and it simplifies to

$$\hat{I} = \frac{1 + b(f_{s,mask}, f_{t,mask})(M/S)^\gamma}{2 + b(f_{s,mask}, f_{t,mask})(M/S)^\gamma} I_L + \frac{1}{2 + b(f_{s,mask}, f_{t,mask})(M/S)^\gamma} I_R,$$
$$(15.24)$$

where $M/S = n/m$ is the mask-to-signal contrast ratio and $b(f_{s,mask}, f_{t,mask}) = b_M/b_S$ is the relative contribution to gain control of a masking sinewave grating.

In experiment 4, the spatial frequency of the masking sinewave grating $f_{s,mask}$ is an independent variable, and other parameters of the mask are constant. In Figure 15.16, the solid curves are the best fit of Eq. (15.24). The parameters are $\gamma_4 = 1.004$ and $b(f_{s,mask}) = \{0.81, 1.13, 2.20, 2.27, 1.97, 0.74\}$. The $b(f_{s,mask})$ are plotted against $f_{s,mask}$ to yield the spatial frequency MTF for observer JD, in Figure 15.25 upper right. Figure 15.25 lower right shows spatial frequency MTF for observer HT. For both observers, the maximum gain-control efficiency was at $f_{s,mask} = 2.72$ cpd, the same as that for the bandpass noise in experiment 3. The percents of data variance accounted for by the model are 98.6% and 97.7%, respectively, for the observers JD and HT.

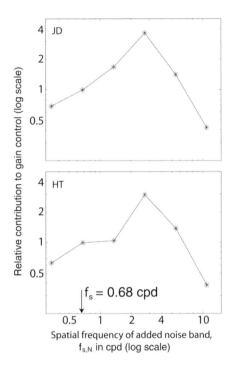

Figure 15.24. How noise of different spatial frequencies increases the weight in binocular combination of the eye to which it is added. Noise in one eye (like all other stimuli) exerts gain control on the opposing eye. The ordinate shows the contribution to gain control, relative to the stimulus grating being judged (0.68 cpd), of the added noise as derived from the gain-control model. The abscissa indicates the central frequency of the added noise. Based on data of experiment 3 for two observers. For both observers, maximum gain-control efficiency occurred at 2.72 cpd (4× the signal frequency).

In the left column of Figure 15.25 the perceived phase shift $\hat{\theta}$ is plotted against $f_{s,mask}$ at different contrast levels. For both observers, at low contrast levels, the curves have peaks at $f_{s,mask} = 2.72$ cpd. However, at high contrast levels, the curves are flat; the contrast efficiencies are similar for all spatial frequencies.

In experiment 5 the temporal frequency of the masking sinewave grating $f_{t,mask}$ is an independent variable, and the other mask parameters are constant. In Figure 15.18, the solid curves are the best fits using Eq. (15.24). The best fitting parameters are $\gamma_5 = 1.43$ and $b(f_{t,mask}) = \{1.06, 1.54, 1.72, 1.74, 0.49\}$, which are plotted against $f_{t,mask}$ to yield the temporal frequency MTF for observer JD in Figure 15.26 upper right. Figure 15.26 lower right shows temporal frequency MTF for observer HT. For both observers, the corner frequency was about 15 Hz. In the left column of Figure 15.26, the perceived phase shift $\hat{\theta}$ is plotted against $f_{t,mask}$ at different contrast levels; at low contrast levels, the corner frequency is at 15 Hz, but at high contrast levels, the MTF becomes quite flat. The percents of data variance accounted for by the model are 99.2% and 99.3%, respectively, for observers JD and HT.

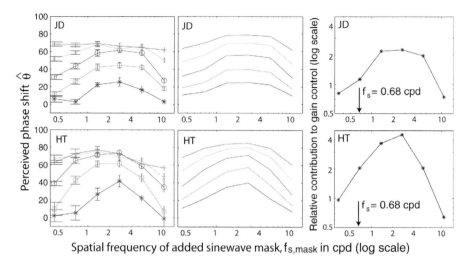

Figure 15.25. The transformation of a single gain-control efficiency function for spatial frequency masking into multiple modulation transfer functions that depend on stimulus contrast. (Left column) Spatial frequency modulation transfer functions. Perceived phase shift $\hat{\theta}$ as a function of the spatial frequency of a masking sine wave grating added in one eye, shown for mask contrast amplitudes of 2.5% (∗), 5% (□), 10% (○), 20% (×), and 40% (+). (Right column) Gain-control efficiency of a masking grating in one eye as a function of its spatial frequency. These efficiencies (weighting parameters in the gain-control model) are used to fit the model to the data of experiment 4, i.e. to generate the predicted perceived phase shifts $\hat{\theta}$ in the center column, which are the gain-control model's best fits to the data panels on the left. Observers JD, HT.

For experiment 6, the orientation β of the masking sinewave grating, is an independent variable, and other parameters of the mask are fixed. In Figure 15.27, the solid curves in the center panels are the best fits derived from Eq. (15.24). The best fitting parameters are $\gamma_6 = 1.42$ and $b(\beta) = \{1.92, 1.21, 1.13, 1.52, 2.11, 1.54, 0.81, 1.06, 2.07\}$; these are plotted against orientation β in Figure 15.27 upper right to yield the orientation tuning function for observer JD. Figure 15.27 (lower right) shows the orientation tuning function for observer HT. For both observers, the vertical and horizontal gratings contributed more to the total contrast energy than the gratings in ±45° orientations. In the left column of Figure 15.27, the perceived phase shift $\hat{\theta}$ is plotted against β at different contrast levels. The percents of data variance accounted for by the model are 98.6% and 96.9%, respectively, for observers JD and HT.

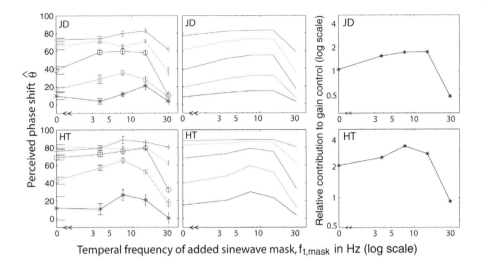

Figure 15.26. The transformation of a single gain-control efficiency function for temporal frequency masking into multiple modulation transfer functions that depend on stimulus contrast. (Left column) Temporal frequency modulation transfer functions. Perceived phase shift $\hat{\theta}$ as a function of the temporal frequency of a masking sine wave grating added to one eye, shown for mask contrast levels of 2.5% ($*$), 5% ($\square$), 10% ($\circ$), 20% ($\times$), and 40% ($+$). (Right column) Gain-control efficiency of a masking grating in one eye as a function of its temporal frequency. These efficiencies (weighting parameters in the gain-control model) are used to fit the model to the data of experiment 5, i.e. to generate the predicted perceived phase shifts $\hat{\theta}$ in the center column, which are the gain-control model's best fits to data panels on the left. Observers JD, HT.

15.10   Discussion

15.10.1   Binocular iso-contrast contours

The present experiments have not dealt with amplitude, only with phase, i.e. the perceived location of the dark stripe of a cyclopean grating. Here we investigate the gain-control model's predictions for the perceived contrast of cyclopean gratings, specifically, iso-contrast contours.

Consider sinewave gratings, identical except for contrast, that are presented to the left and right eyes, i.e., $I_L = m_L \sin x$ and $I_R = m_R \sin x$. According to the model, $\mathcal{E}_L(I_L) = bm_L^\gamma$ and $\mathcal{E}_R(I_R) = bm_R^\gamma$. To simplify the expressions, replace k with $1/b$. This yields an expression for the perceived cyclopean contrast $\hat{m}$

$$\hat{m} = \frac{k + m_L^\gamma}{k + m_L^\gamma + m_R^\gamma} m_L + \frac{k + m_R^\gamma}{k + m_L^\gamma + m_R^\gamma} m_R. \tag{15.25}$$

At very low contrast-energy levels, $m_L^\gamma \ll k$ and $m_R^\gamma \ll k$, the equal contrast contours

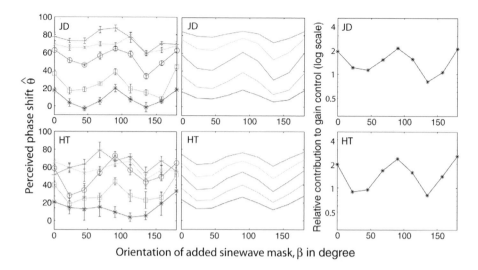

Figure 15.27. The transformation of a single gain-control efficiency function for orientation masking into multiple modulation transfer functions that depend on stimulus contrast. (Left column) Orientation modulation transfer functions: Perceived phase shift $\hat{\theta}$ as a function of the angle relative to the horizontal stimulus being judged of a masking sine wave grating added to one eye, shown for contrasts of 2.5% (*), 5% ($\square$), 10% ($\circ$), 20% ($\times$), and 40% ($+$). Zero on the abscissa indicates parallel stimulus and masking gratings. (Right column) Gain-control efficiency of a masking grating in one eye as a function of its orientation relative to the stimulus being judged. These orientation efficiencies (weighting parameters in the gain-control model) are used to fit the model to the data of experiment 6, i.e. to generate the predicted perceived phase shifts $\hat{\theta}$ in the center column, which are the gain-control model's best fits to data panels on the left. Observers JD, HT.

on a graph of m_R versus m_L are almost linear, i.e.

$$\hat{m} \approx m_L + m_R. \tag{15.26}$$

At high contrast-energy levels, $m_L^\gamma \gg k$ and $m_R^\gamma \gg k$, we have,

$$\hat{m} \approx \frac{m_L^\gamma}{m_L^\gamma + m_R^\gamma} m_L + \frac{m_R^\gamma}{m_L^\gamma + m_R^\gamma} m_R, \tag{15.27}$$

which is contrast-weighted summation.

Legge and Rubin (1981) studied binocular combination in a supra-threshold contrast matching task that involved left- and right-eye sinewave gratings with different contrasts combined into a cyclopean grating.

Figure 15.28a shows examples of binocular iso-contrast contours extracted from Legge and Rubin (1981). To smooth their data, all points shown in Figure 15.28a, except the points at the ends of contours, are averaged with their two nearest neighbors. The two resulting contours represent Legge and Rubin's highest and lowest iso-perceived-contrast contours. The dashed line is a prediction of linear summation.

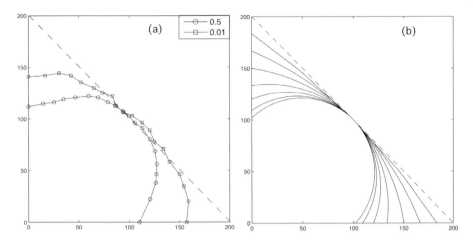

Figure 15.28. Binocular perceived iso-contrast contours. Combinations of left- and right-eye grating contrasts that produce equal cyclopean perceived contrasts. (a) Replot of two binocular iso-contrast contours from Legge and Rubin (1981, Figure 4B, p. 55). Except the data points at the ends of the plot, each plotted point is an average of the original point at that location with its two neighbors. (b) Binocular iso-contrast contours generated by the gain-control model. Sinewave gratings presented to two eyes are identical except for their contrasts. The abscissa is the contrast of the left-eye grating; the ordinate is the contrast of the right-eye grating. The curves are binocular iso-contrast contours. The model parameters are assumed to be $k = 0.02$ s and $\gamma = 1$. The dashed lines are the predictions from linear summation of the contrasts in the two eyes. The solid lines are normalized predictions from the gain-control model at contrast levels of 0.002, 0.005, 0.01, 0.02, 0.04, 0.1, and 0.5 corresponding from top to bottom. Both the model and the data at high (but not at low) contrast exhibit Fechner's paradox; i.e. replacing a zero-contrast stimulus in one eye with a low-contrast stimulus (thereby increasing the total contrast energy presented to the observer) reduces apparent cyclopean contrast and requires an increase in the contrast of the high-contrast grating to maintain perceived iso-contrast.

Figure 15.28b shows the full gamut of iso-perceived-contrast contours derived from a simulation of the gain-control model for various contrast levels from very low contrast (0.002) to very high contrast (0.50) with model parameters $k = 0.02$ and $\gamma = 1$. Generally, the features of the data and of the model correspond very well. At a low contrast level (0.01), the data contour approaches the limiting straight line expected from linear summation at extremely low contrast energies. At a high stimulus contrast level (0.50), the data contour is highly nonlinear and it looks quite similar to the 0.50 contour of the model.

Both the data and the model demonstrate Fechner's paradox in the high-contrast iso-contrast contours but not in low-contrast contours. Fechner observed that when the contrast of the grating in one eye is zero, increasing the contrast in that grating initially decreases the (perceived) cyclopean contrast even though overall contrast energy has increased. In the model, Fechner's paradox occurs because the gain control from the low-contrast eye has a greater divisive effect in reducing the output of the high-contrast eye than an additive effect in contributing to the summed output, especially as its output is being attenuated by intense gain control from the competing eye which is receiving a high-contrast grating.

15.10.2   Binocular power summation

Legge (1984b) proposed a binocular quadratic summation to explain his data derived from binocular combination experiments. Similarly, Anderson and Movshon (1989) reported that, in a binocular detection task for vertical sinewave gratings, the iso-effectiveness contour for binocular summation could be well described by a power-summation equation of the form

$$\hat{m}^\sigma = m_R^\sigma + m_L^\sigma, \tag{15.28}$$

with an exponent σ near 2. Binocular power summation implies that the contrast signal in each eye is subjected to a power-law transformation prior to binocular summation. For example, one implication for experiment 1 would be that the effective interocular contrast ratio would be $\hat{\delta} = \delta^\sigma$. If we take $\sigma = 1 + \gamma$, it turns out that both the power summation model and the gain-control model give the same effective interocular contrast ratio. This apparently happy coincidence of two theories is superficial. A power-law transform applies only to weak stimuli. For high-contrast stimuli addition of the two eyes' power-law-transformed stimuli would grossly violate the one-eye-equals-both-eyes constraint for equal stimuli to both eyes.

   The data of experiment 2 (exposure duration) offer very clear limits on the exponent of a power law that could operate on monocular signals before they were added in binocular combination. We consider here the graphs of $\hat{\theta}$ versus δ (e.g. Figure 15.11) and a log-log graph of $\hat{\delta}$ versus δ (e.g. Figure 15.13). Data from threshold-level stimuli were not obtained here but experiment 2 provides data concerning the binocular summation of fairly low contrast-energy stimuli in the condition: exposure duration 50 ms, grating contrast 0.10. In Figure 15.29, these data from experiment 2 are displayed on the two graphical forms described above. The solid line is the best fit from the gain-control model. The dashed lines are predictions from a power-summation model (Eq. (15.28)) with power-law exponent $\sigma = \{1, 1.2, 1.4, 1.7, 2, 2.5, 3\}$ corresponding to the dashed lines from bottom to top in Figure 15.29a and from top to bottom in Figure 15.29b. With the possible exception of a point for $\delta = 0.2$ (where log variability is greatest), the data are consistent with a power-law exponent of 1.0, and clearly rule out exponents greater than 1.20. The conclusion is that monocular inputs, at least from grating stimuli, combine linearly, or nearly so, prior to binocular combination. Apparent similarity (when it occurs) to a power-law transformation prior to binocular combination derives from quite different processes.

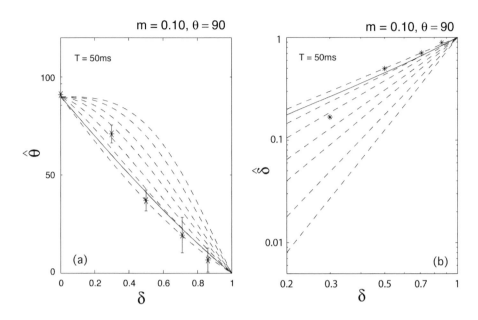

Figure 15.29. Is the monocular signal transformed nonlinearly by a power law prior to binocular combination? Comparison of the gain-control model with a power-law transformation. Power-law transformations are most effective at near-threshold contrasts, so we consider the subset of data from experiment 2, Figure 15.11, in which the contrast of the higher-contrast grating is 0.1, the contrast of the lower-contrast grating is 0.1δ and the exposure duration is 50 ms (the lowest energy stimuli tested). The solid curve is the prediction of the gain-control model (linear transduction, no input power-law transformation). The dashed lines are predictions from a power-law transduction model with power-law exponents $\sigma = 1, 1.2, 1.4, 1.7, 2, 2.5, 3$ corresponding to the dashed lines from bottom to top. (b) A log-log plot of the apparent interocular contrast ratio $\hat{\delta}$ as a function of the actual interocular contrast ratio δ. The solid curve is a prediction of the gain-control model; the dashed lines are predictions based on a power-law transformation prior to binocular combination with power-law exponents $\sigma = 1, 1.2, 1.4, 1.7, 2, 2.5, 3$ corresponding to the dashed lines from top to bottom. Conclusion: Prior to binocular combination, the input contrast is represented linearly or very nearly linearly.

15.11 Summary and conclusions

Six experiments were performed. In experiment 1, static sinewave gratings of different modulation contrasts and in different phases were presented to the left and right eyes. Stimuli were viewed for 1 s. The data consist of 48 combinations of contrasts of the left- and right-eye stimuli and of their relative phases. From the judged phase of the cyclopean grating relative to a reference marker, we inferred the ratio of the contributions of the two eyes to the cyclopean image. In all cases, the stimulus with greater contrast had more weight in binocular combination than predicted by simple linear summation.

A one-parameter gain-control model accounted for 98% of the variance of the data. The gain-control model predicts that when the contrast energy is much smaller than a particular constant in the gain-control equation, binocular combination will be perfectly described by linear summation. The deviations from perfect summation (nonlinearity) become increasingly important as the contrast energy of the stimulus increases. The model also correctly predicts that for idential stimuli to both eyes at moderate and high contrasts, the perceived cyclopean image will be the same whether viewed with one or both eyes.

Experiment 2 investagated the effect of varying grating contrast and exposure duration as multiplicative contributers to contrast energy. The stimuli and procedure were similar to experiment 1 except that the duration was varied in the range from 50 ms to 1000 ms to create low-energy stimuli (50 ms, contrast 0.1) ranging to very strong stimuli (1000 ms, contrast 0.2). The results show that for low-contrast-energy stimuli binocular combination is well described by algebraic summation of the two physical images – no gain control is observed. As stimulus duration and/or contrast is increased, algebraic summation of left- and right-eye images increasingly fails to account for perception. This increasing deviation of observed binocular combination from linear summation is well modeled by a gain-control pathway that has an exponential decay filter with a time constant of 563 ms.

Experiment 3 investigated the question: When the spatial frequency for which binocular combination is being determined is f_0, how much do other spatial frequencies f_1 contribute to gain control? Each eye was presented with a sinewave grating, the interocular phase difference was 90°, and bandpass spatial noise was added to the grating in one eye. The eye with the added noise dominated binocular combination. Noise in a 4× higher frequency band than the signal being judged was the most effective stimulus for producing dominance. Adding noise is inconsistent with a Bayesian model that would give less weight to noisy signals, but it is totally consistent with a gain-control model in which Total visually weighted Contrast Energy (TCE) determines the interocular gain control.

Experiments 4–6 were designed to measure the contribution of various frequency components to TCE and thereby to ocular dominance. The paradigms were the same as in experiment 3 in that 90°. out-of-phase grating stimuli were presented to both eyes and a masking grating was added to only one eye's stimulus. The contrasts of the masking sinewave gratings were varied. Experiment 4 also varied the spatial frequency of a sinewave masking grating that was perpendicular to the grating whose phase was being judged and it produced similar results to experiment 3 in which bandpass noise was added. Experiment 5 varied the temporal frequency to reveal a low-pass characteristic with a corner frequency of about 15 Hz. Experiment 6 varied orientation. Spatial, temporal, and orientation modulation transfer functions were derived to describe the TCE gain-control parameters and thereby to characterize the increase in dominance provided by the various masking stimuli. The gain-control model accurately described the change in dominance as the ratio of the two eyes' contrasts varied and as the overall contrast energy level varied, accounting for at least 97% of the data variance for all observers in all experiments. In experiment 6, added orientation gratings were most effective at inceasing ocular dominance when their orientation was vertical or horizontal versus diagonal, implicating at least a partial cortical origin for interocular gain control.

References and further reading

Anderson, P. A. and Movshon, J. A. (1989). Binocular combination of contrast signals. *Vis. Res.*, **29**, 1115–1132.

Bearse Jr., M. A. and Freeman, R. D. (1994). Binocular summation in orientation discrimination depends on stimulus contrast and duration *Vis. Res.*, **34**, 19–29.

Blake, R. (2003). In L. M. Chalupa and J. Warner, eds., *The Visual Neurosciences*. Cambridge, MA: MIT Press.

Bolanowski Jr., S. J. (1987). Contourless stimuli produce binocular brightness summation. *Vis. Res.*, **27**, 1943–1951.

Brainard, D. H. (1997). The Psychophysics Toolbox, *Spat. Vis.*, **10**, 433–436.

De Weert, C. M. M. and Levelt, W. J. M. (1974) Binocular brightness combinations: Additive and nonadditive aspects. *Percept. Psychophys.*, **15**, 551–562.

Ding, J. and Sperling, G. (2006). A gain-control theory of binocular combination. *Proc. Natl. Acad. Sci. USA*, **103**, 1141–1146.

Finney, D. J. (1971), *Probit Analysis*, third edition. Cambridge: Cambridge University Press.

Legge, G. E. (1979). Spatial frequency masking in human vision: binocular interactions. *J. Opt. Soc. Am. A*, **69**, 838–847.

Legge, G. E. (1984a). Binocular contrast summation–I. Detection and discrimination *Vis. Res.*, **24**, 373–383.

Legge, G. E. (1984b). Binocular contrast summation–II. Quadratic summation *Vis. Res.*, **24**, 373–383.

Legge, G. E. and Rubin, G. S. (1981). Binocular interactions in suprathreshold contrast perception. *Percept. Psychophys.*, **30**, 49–61.

Levelt, W. J. M. (1965a). *On Binocular Rivalry*. Institute for Perception RVO-TNO, Soesterberg, The Netherlands.

Levelt, W. J. M. (1965b). Binocular brightness averaging and contour information. *British J. Psych.*, **56**, 1–13.

Lu, Z. L. and Sperling, G. (1999). Second-order reversed phi. *Percept. Psychophys.*, **61**, 1075–1088.

Mansfield, J. S. and Legge, G. E. (1996). The binocular computation of visual direction. *Vis. Res.*, **36**, 27–41.

Pelli, D. G. (1997). The VideoToolbox software for visual psychophysics: Transforming numbers into movies. *Spat. Vis.*, **10**, 437–442.

Pelli, D. G. and Zhang, L. (1991). Accurate control of contrast on microcomputer displays. *Vis. Res.*, **31**, 1337–1350.

Rainville, S. J. M. and Kingdom, F. A. A. (2002) Scale invariance is driven by stimulus density. *Vis. Res.*, **42**, 351–367.

Author index

Subject index

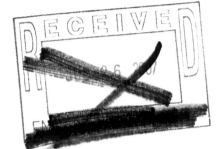